Success in Academic Surgery

Series Editors

Lillian Kao, McGovern School, The University of Texas Health Science Centre
Houston, TX, USA

Herbert Chen, Department of Surgery, University of Alabama at Birmingham
Birmingham, AL, USA

All of the intended volume editors are highly successful academic surgeons with expertise in the respective fields of basic science, clinical trials, health services research, and surgical education research. They are all also leaders within the Association for Academic Surgery (AAS). The previous AAS book, Success in Academic Surgery: Part I provided an overview with regards to the different types of surgical research, beginning one's academic career, and balancing work and life commitments. The aims and scopes of this series of books will be to provide specifics with regards to becoming successful academic surgeons with focuses on the different types of research and academic careers (basic science, clinical trials, health services research, and surgical education). These books will provide information beyond that in the introductory book and even beyond that provided in the Fall and International Courses. The target audience would be medical students, surgical residents, and young surgical faculty. We would promote bulk sales at the Association for Academic Surgery (AAS) Fall Courses (www.aasurg.org) which take place prior to the American College of Surgeons meeting in October, as well as the AAS International Courses which take place year-round in Australasia, Colombia, West Africa, and France. Courses are also planned for India, Italy, and Germany and potentially in the United Kingdom and Saudi Arabia. As the AAS expands the course into other parts of the world, there is a greater need for an accompanying series of textbooks. The AAS has already received requests for translation of the book into Italian. These books would be closely linked with the course content and be sold as part of the registration. In 2011, there were 270 participants in the Fall Courses. In addition, we would anticipate several hundred participants combined per year at all of the international courses.

Andrea Gillis • Cary B. Aarons
Editors

A How To Guide For Medical Students

Second Edition 2024

Springer

Editors
Andrea Gillis
Department of Surgery
University of Alabama at Birmingham
Birmingham, AL, USA

Cary B. Aarons
Division of Colon and Rectal Surgery
Columbia University Irving Medical Center
New York, NY, USA

ISSN 2194-7481 ISSN 2194-749X (electronic)
Success in Academic Surgery
ISBN 978-3-031-66010-8 ISBN 978-3-031-66011-5 (eBook)
https://doi.org/10.1007/978-3-031-66011-5

This Springer imprint is published by the registered company Springer Nature Switzerland AG
The registered company address is: Gewerbestrasse 11, 6330 Cham, Switzerland

Contents

Contributors

Tania K. Arora Division of Surgical Oncology, Department of Surgery, Birmingham, AL, USA

Alison S. Baskin, MD Department of Surgery, University of California, San Francisco, CA, USA

Julia L. Beilis Cleveland Clinic Cole Eye Institute, Cleveland, OH, USA

Simryn Covarrubias Center for Mindfulness in Surgery, University of California San Francisco, San Francisco, CA, USA

Lauren Curwick University of Alabama at Birmingham, Birmingham, AL, USA

Jonathan Dort Department of Surgery, Inova Health System, Inova Fairfax Medical Campus, Falls Church, VA, USA

Lesly A. Dossett University of Michigan, Ann Arbor, MI, USA

Vikas Dudeja Division of Surgical Oncology, Department of Surgery, Birmingham, AL, USA

Chukwuma Eruchalu Department of Surgery, University of Michigan, Ann Arbor, MI, USA

Department of Surgery, Massachusetts General Hospital, Boston, MA, USA

Robert George Division of Plastic and Reconstructive Surgery, University of Wisconsin, Madison, WI, USA

Amir A. Ghaferi Froedtert and the Medical College of Wisconsin, Milwaukee, WI, USA

Suzanne Gillern, MD Tripler Army Medical Center, Honolulu, HI, USA

Islam Hasasna West Virginia School of Osteopathic Medicine, Lewisburg, WV, USA

J. W. Awori Hayanga Division of Thoracic Surgery, Department of Cardiovascular and Thoracic Surgery, Morgantown, WV, USA

Emon K. Javadi Center for Mindfulness in Surgery, University of California San Francisco, San Francisco, CA, USA

St. George's University School of Medicine, Saint George, Grenada

Kennedy Jensen Department of Surgery, Salt Lake City, UT, USA

William D. Jordan Jr Division of Vascular Surgery and Endovascular Therapy, University of Alabama-Birmingham, Birmingham, AL, USA

Kristen Laaman Department of Surgery, Bassett Healthcare Network, Cooperstown, NY, USA

Jennifer LaFemina Department of Surgery, University of Massachusetts Chan Medical School, Worcester, MA, USA

Carter C. Lebares Center for Mindfulness in Surgery, University of California San Francisco, San Francisco, CA, USA

Department of Surgery, University of California San Francisco, San Francisco, CA, USA

James A. Lee Department of Surgery, Columbia University Medical Center, New York, NY, USA

Major Kenneth I. V. Lee Department of Surgery, Perelman School of Medicine at the University of Pennsylvania, Philadelphia, PA, USA

Brenessa Lindeman University of Alabama at Birmingham, Birmingham, AL, USA

Sophie E. Mayeux Department of Surgery, Columbia University Irving Medical Center, New York, NY, USA

Imani E McElroy, MD, MPH Department of Surgery, Massachusetts General Hospital, Boston, MA, USA

Sophia K. McKinley, MD, MEd Department of Surgery, Massachusetts General Hospital, Boston, MA, USA

Catherine McManus Department of Surgery, Columbia University Irving Medical Center, New York, NY, USA

Steven Molina Center for Mindfulness in Surgery, University of California San Francisco, San Francisco, CA, USA

UCR School of Medicine, University of California Riverside, Riverside, CA, USA

Gabrielle Moore Department of Surgery, Medical College of Georgia, Augusta, GA, USA

Rebecca Moreci Department of Surgery, Louisiana State University, New Orleans, LA, USA

Ofelia Negrete Vasquez Department of Surgery, University of Texas Southwestern Medical Center, Dallas, TX, USA

Ariel Nehemiah Department of Surgery, Perelman School of Medicine, University of Pennsylvania, Philadelphia, PA, USA

Jesse Passman Department of Surgery, Perelman School of Medicine at the University of Pennsylvania, Philadelphia, PA, USA

Benjamin J. Pearce Division of Vascular Surgery and Endovascular Therapy, University of Alabama-Birmingham, Birmingham, AL, USA

Roy Phitayakorn, MD, MHPE Massachusetts General Hospital, Boston, MA, USA

Samuel Poore Division of Plastic and Reconstructive Surgery, University of Wisconsin, Madison, WI, USA

Hayley Reddington Department of Surgery, University of Massachusetts Chan Medical School, Worcester, MA, USA

Courtney Rentas Department of Surgery, University of Michigan, Ann Arbor, MI, USA

Department of Surgery, Massachusetts General Hospital, Boston, MA, USA

Paul Rothenberg West Virginia University, Morgantown, WV, USA

WVU Heart and Vascular Institute, Morgantown, WV, USA

Deanna L. Palenzuela Rothman, MD Department of Surgery, Massachusetts General Hospital, Boston, MA, USA

Massachusetts General Hospital, Boston, MA, USA

Joon K. Shim Department of Surgery, Bassett Healthcare Network, Cooperstown, NY, USA

Julie Ann Sosa, MD, MA Department of Surgery, University of California, San Francisco, CA, USA

Crystal D. Taylor University of Michigan, Ann Arbor, MI, USA

Noah Tocci Department of Surgery, Cleveland, OH, USA

Paul E. Wise Department of Surgery, Washington University School of Medicine in St. Louis, St. Louis, MO, USA

Jennifer Yu Abdominal Transplant Surgery, Washington University School of Medicine in St. Louis, St. Louis, MO, USA

Jessica Zagory Louisiana State University Health New Orleans, Children's Hospital New Orleans, New Orleans, LA, USA

Part I
Exploring Surgical Specialties and Practice Settings

Chapter 1
Assessing your Interests, Skills, and Values

Amir A. Ghaferi

Abstract Leadership, communication, and resilience are three traits that are the marker of a successful surgical resident and future surgical leader. The following will help you assess your preparedness in these essential domains and help you determine where you need to focus your attention in the coming years. We are all lifelong learners, not only of the technical aspects of surgery, but also of professional development and self-improvement.

1.1 The Goal: Understanding your Personal Strengths and Opportunities as you Embark on a Career in Surgery

Students who choose to pursue a career in surgery have self selected as future leaders. Surgery is inherently a contact sport with surgeons, nurses, scrub technicians, and patients occupying the same octagon. Fortunately, they are all fighting the same opponent—surgical disease. This is a team of professionals who do not choose each other, but rather they are often thrown together during a critically important episode of care. It is important that they are immediately cohesive, confident, and focused. Most importantly, no one ever conquers a surgical disease without a surgeon who is an effective leader, a master communicator, and resilient in the face of adversity.

Leadership, communication, and resilience are three traits that are the marker of a wildly successful surgical resident and future surgical leader. The following will help you assess your preparedness in these essential domains and help you determine where you need to focus your attention in the coming years. We are all lifelong learners, not only of the technical aspects of surgery, but also of the professional development and self-improvement.

A. A. Ghaferi (✉)
Froedtert and the Medical College of Wisconsin, Milwaukee, WI, USA
e-mail: aghaferi@mcw.edu

A. Gillis, C. B. Aarons (eds.), *A How To Guide For Medical Students*, Success in Academic Surgery, https://doi.org/10.1007/978-3-031-66011-5_1

1.2 Leadership Development

What are the core values every leader possesses? The following are neither all encompassing nor developed by consensus—respect, integrity, authenticity, service, humility, and wisdom. As a surgery resident, you will be called upon to be a follower and a leader at various times during your training. It is incumbent upon you to seek experiences during medical school to help foster these traits and/or develop them *de novo*. Leadership is not an inherent characteristic, rather it requires deliberate awareness of oneself and continually seeking to improve.

Surgical residents are recognized leaders in the hospital. There are stories of surgical residents being the "go-to" physician in the hospital whenever there was a crisis. The respect garnered by surgical chief residents was an important responsibility that they carried with them daily. However, there are also anecdotes of surgical chief residents being ineffective due largely to their leadership style. Leadership, practiced at its best, is the art and science of calling to the hearts and minds of others. It is engaging others in an enterprise of sound strategic focus, where they can experience a sense of ownership, of making a difference, of being valued and adding value. These attributes are important to the cohesiveness needed in the healthcare setting to care for the sickest and most complex patients.

As a result, surgery program directors are aware of the need for selecting medical students who have demonstrated the ability to lead others by example, by inspiring, and by learning. The question remains how to acquire the necessary experiences and skills to become an effective leader. While some leaders are born, the majority of people must seek development opportunities or are a product of the circumstances they find themselves in.

First, one should identify a mentor or individual whose leadership style resonates with him or her. Ideally this individual holds defined leadership roles, such as an administrative chief resident, leader of a clinical program, division chief, or director of a research program. Simply observing them in their habitat can be profoundly educational and inspirational. One should pay attention to the short-term goals set by the leader and how the team is motivated to achieve excellence and success. Beyond the short term, observe how the leader outlines a vision for the group. A vision gives everyone engaged something to shoot for and a larger context within which to plan and set strategy. It provides everyone with an essential sense of direction and purpose, whether it is which part of the task to own, or more profoundly, who and what the team is striving to become.

Second, discover an organization that resonates with your personal values and beliefs, such as a fraternity or sorority, charity group, religious organization, or educational mission. Fully engage in the group by organizing an event, keynote lecture, symposium, group meeting, workshop, or outreach activity. The key is to be wholeheartedly invested in the success and growth of the group. Substance over quantity is key here. Being a member in multiple organizations as a follower demonstrates the ability to attend meetings and eat a free lunch. Being a leader requires courage and dedication. The seven acts of courage laid out by Robert Staub in *The Heart of Leadership* include:

1. The courage to dream and put forth that dream.
2. The courage to see current reality.
3. The courage to confront.
4. The courage to be confronted.
5. The courage to learn and grow.
6. The courage to be vulnerable
7. The courage to act.

Finally, be flexible in your leadership style and seek continuous feedback on how to improve. This may take the form of actively seeking feedback from peers, superiors, and juniors. Remember, seeking a pat on the back is not the goal here. It is important to create an environment where honest feedback is given without fear of offending you, creating an awkward work environment, or worry about reprimand. Often the best way of doing this is using anonymous feedback tools such as "360 evaluations" or online survey tools such as Qualtrics. This is becoming a widespread and accepted practice in medicine, especially surgery. There are many valuable resources such as books and online tools that also provide instruments for assessing your leadership style, your individual blind spots in leadership, and methods for improving daily.

1.3 Communication Skills

The ability to communicate with peers, consultants, and patients is of utmost importance to a career in surgery. We are often faced with difficult, complex patients with multidisciplinary pathology. Surgeons are expected to be the clinical champion for many patients by synthesizing input from multiple providers, the patients themselves, and family members. The ability to effectively communicate important facts and views is an invaluable attribute of a successful surgeon.

This begins during residency where an intern is viewed as a reporter of information. This is encapsulated in the notes that they write as communication to other providers and verbal communication to patients, families, and superiors. Toward the end of internship, surgical house officers are expected to begin synthesizing information into relevant pieces that explain the clinical story of the patient in a clear and concise manner. The learning curve is steep and there is always room for improvement. During the ensuing years, residents are expected create a more cohesive interpretation of objective and subjective data elicited from the patient, providers, physical examinations, and laboratory and radiologic studies.

Building and honing these skills is not a simple task. Much like leadership, this is a lifelong endeavor that requires hard work and a willingness to adapt, grow, and accept feedback. The following are some strategies on how to begin working on communication skills during medical school.

First, writing is one of the most important skills that all professionals should maintain and cultivate during their careers. The most obvious times that surgeons need to be effective writers are through operative notes, clinic notes, and letters to consulting physicians. In academic surgery, one of the most recognizable currencies is peer reviewed manuscripts. Each of these forms of writing require the ability to communicate plainly and succinctly without missing important details.

Medical students have the opportunity to write clinic and progress notes. This may be viewed as grunt work, and it is if there is no feedback loop. The act of writing notes is important and the more practice the better one becomes. However, it is important to seek meaningful feedback from other students, junior and senior residents, and faculty. The most powerful feedback comes during these formative years of training. Entering residency with sharpened writing skills can prove to be a valuable asset.

Another opportunity to practice writing is through manuscripts. While the research opportunities will vary across medical schools, there are many chances to write case reports, viewpoints, and review articles. Manuscript preparation is very much like patient care. It requires identifying a problem or question, gathering data, analyzing and interpreting facts, drawing conclusions from that information, and finally communicating it through writing.

Another important method of sharing research brings to light the second form of communication that is vital to a successful surgical resident/surgeon—speaking. Increasingly, local and national meetings are encouraging the participation of medical students in their programs. These meetings provide an exceptional occasion for students to gain exposure to high level research discussions, present their work and gain insight from others about their research, and to meet new people from medical schools and surgical residencies around the country. Depending on the environment of various medical schools, it may be easier or more difficult to access these types of events. However, seeking the input or mentorship of people outside your home institution is also encouraged.

1.4 Resilience

Resilience is a hot topic and buzz word in both business and medicine today. Surgery by essence is a field that requires the ability to constantly bounce back from difficult situations. Surgical training is a time that tests an individual's ability to tolerate grueling work hours, intense physical and emotional stress, and maximum absorption and comprehension of vast amounts of medical and surgical knowledge. There is no doubt that every surgical resident has at some point felt the elation and despair of patient care.

There are three key principles or characteristics of resilient people that Diane Coutu puts forth in a poignant Harvard Business Review article entitled *How Resilience Works*—face down reality, search for meaning, and continually improvise. Resilient people possessed three defining characteristics. They coolly accept the harsh realities facing them. They find meaning in terrible times. And they have an uncanny ability to improvise, making do with whatever is at hand.

A common belief about resilience is that it stems from an optimistic nature. That is true but only as long as such optimism does not distort one's sense of reality. In extremely adverse situations, rose-colored thinking can actually spell disaster. Instead of slipping into denial to cope with hardship, one should take a silver "I'm a down-to-earth" view of the reality of one's situation. One will prepare themself to act in ways that enables one to endure—training oneself to survive before the fact. So, face down reality.

When hard times strike, a resident should resist any impulse to view oneself as a victim and to cry, "Why me?" Rather, they should devise constructs about their suffering to create meaning for oneself and others. One can build bridges from the present-day ordeal to a fuller, better future. Those bridges will make the present manageable, by removing the sense that the present is overwhelming. So, search for meaning.

When disaster hits, one should be inventive—even if that means letting one's inner child out in a world that is dominated by gravity and urgency. Individuals should make the most of what they have, putting resources to unfamiliar uses and imagining possibilities others do not see. So, continually improvise.

1.5 Summary

Surgical residency is a privilege and honor. Patients welcome surgeons into the most vulnerable moments and aspects of their lives. With this honor there comes significant responsibility to respect and value the day to day interactions needed to provide quality surgical care. The core of becoming a successful surgeon starts within oneself. The need to foster an environment conducive to effective teamwork, communication, and leadership is paramount to the performance of surgical teams. Continual self reflection and improvement is key to making this work. It is never too early to start.

Suggested Readings

1. Staub R. Heart of leadership. Executive Excellence Publishing; 2000.
2. Coutu DL. How resilience works. Harvard Bus Rev. 2002;80(5):46–56.
3. Cameron KS, et al. Competing values leadership. Cheltenham: Edward Elgar Publishing; 2014.
4. Kouzes J, Posner B. The leadership challenge: how to make extraordinary things happen. Atlanta: Better World Books; 2012.

Chapter 2
Choosing a Surgery Training Environment: Military Programs

Suzanne Gillern

Abstract Making the decision to commit to military surgical training has a significant implication for the rest of one's surgical career. A military surgical career provides the unique opportunity to utilize one's surgical skills while serving the nation. However, this commitment comes with potential limitations on ability to make decisions about one's individual career path. One should give thoughtful consideration of the pros and cons before committing to military surgical training.

2.1 Choosing a Military General Surgery Career

The motivation for starting a military surgical career is often based in pride for serving one's country and the opportunity to practice surgical skills in austere environments serving soldiers, sailors, airmen, and marines willing to sacrifice their lives in the line of duty for the United States.

When one makes the choice to become a military general surgeon, they are taking on two jobs: *General Surgeon* and *Military Officer*. There are additional responsibilities for a military officer, including mandatory physical fitness standards, weapons qualification, as well as leadership training. While the number one priority of a military general surgeon is to be a safe, compassionate, and competent surgeon, when joining the military, one is also dedicating themselves to the values and principles of military service as an officer and making a strong commitment to leadership. This commitment cannot be forgotten and should be considered when choosing to train in the military.

S. Gillern (✉)
Tripler Army Medical Center, Honolulu, HI, USA

A. Gillis, C. B. Aarons (eds.), *A How To Guide For Medical Students*, Success in Academic Surgery, https://doi.org/10.1007/978-3-031-66011-5_2

2.2 Benefits of Choosing a Military General Surgery Career

One of the most significant advantages of training in a military residency program is decreased financial stress during training. Students are entering residency with zero or minimal debt due to their military scholarship. In addition, the base salary for a PGY1, who is commissioned as an Active Duty Captain (Army and Air Force) or Lieutenant (Navy) is approximately $60,000–$80,000. In addition to one's base pay, a resident will get additional compensation referred to as Basic Allowance for Subsidence (BAS) and Basic Allowance for Housing (BAH) that is based on the location of the resident's program. This amount can range from an additional $21,500–$48,000 per year depending on location and if a resident has dependents. Therefore, more expensive locations will get a higher amount of money to offset the expensive cost of living. In addition, medical care is provided without any additional charge and family members are covered as well.

In addition to better financial well-being during residency, having the military career provides a sense of security throughout residency and one's surgical career. If a resident needs to take an extended leave of absence due to medical or family issues, they are still compensated. Military residencies offer significant paid time off for both maternity and paternity leave. Compared to civilian residencies, the only consideration when determining time off when having a family as a resident is how much time to miss from residency training and is not financially driven.

Distinct to a military career are opportunities to travel and encounter professionals and patients from all over the world. This opportunity can lead to learning about different cultures and practices and serves to further cultivate a well-balanced General Surgeon. It is possible to be stationed at remote geographic locations and support smaller medical facilities that can provide both unique personal and professional experiences.

Deployments are to be expected at the completion of surgical training. In no situation will a resident be pulled from resident training to be deployed. Deployments can be considered both a pro and a con to a military surgical career. On the positive note, they provide a sense of pride and a unique opportunity to practice surgical skills in a variety of different environments. These environments include but are not limited to field hospitals, air craft carriers, or far forward austere environments supporting active combat operations, and in particular, Special Operations Forces. The professional challenge as well as the ability to use one's surgical skills to serve those in need can result in significant professional and personal gratification.

2.3 Negative Implications of Military General Surgery Training

Although General Surgery military training programs provide equivalent training to civilian programs, it is one's surgical practice after graduation in the military system that is often a challenge. The operative case volume is often significantly decreased compared to civilian surgical practice. The variety and severity of cases will depend on the duty location, if there are specialists co-located, presence of an Intensive Care Unit, and the number of other surgeons present. Depending on where one is assigned, there are often Off Duty Employment (ODE) opportunities to both make additional money and gain increased operative experience by working in civilian facilities. While the pay during residency is far above the national average, compensation for General Surgeons and General Surgery Sub-specialists in the military is not competitive with most civilian positions. The military offers opportunities for getting additional significant monetary bonuses but this requires incurring additional time in the military.

After graduation, the surgeon does not necessarily get to choose where they will be stationed. That could mean being stationed far from family or in locations not personally desirable. Depending on one's military branch, there is also the expectation that a surgeon may need to move every 2–3 years. This lack of control over one's future can be frustrating at times.

Another important aspect of post-surgical training which is important to consider is the desire to complete a fellowship. While most General Surgery specialties are still needed in the military hospitals, there are some specialties in which only a few specialists are required. A resident or staff surgeon can only apply to a fellowship if their specific branch of the military needs a specialist in that specific area at that specific time. For example, if the Army is not in need of any surgical oncologist, and an Army General Surgery Resident wishes to pursue a fellowship in surgical oncology, the resident will need to wait until the Army gives them permission to apply. Therefore, one may have to wait several years or never be allowed to apply for a fellowship in the specialty of their choice. If a surgeon is granted permission by the military to apply for fellowship, they can then apply for civilian fellowships. The surgeon will incur a 1-for-1 year of obligation for each year of fellowship that is completed.

As previously mentioned, deployments are to be expected after completion of residency training. The frequency of deployments will depend on the current world and US military operational environment. Deployments can be extremely fulfilling or very frustrating depending on military operative tempo of one's deployment location. Deployments will be a disruption to one's surgical practice, which can be a source of dissatisfaction, especially if one is not performing many or any operations on deployment. In addition, deployment may serve as a stressor due to prolonged time away from family and significant others.

2.4 Military Surgical Career Opportunities

The Military provides unique career opportunities to the General Surgeon. Inherent to being a general surgeon in the military, one is also taking on the role of an officer and, therefore, a leader. This may involve running a team in a high-pressured deployment setting or taking on leadership roles in one's medical facility. Some military surgeons may choose to seek out additional military leadership courses available in all military branches and pursue elite positions in the military, such as Hospital Commanders, Consultants to the Surgeon General, Surgeon General or other high ranking positions that can provide the opportunity to effect change in medical processes throughout the military and across the nation.

Also unique to the military surgeon is the opportunity to take on more operational roles. Positions such as Forward Surgical Team or Fleet Surgical Team (FST) Commanders are readily available to general surgeons. These jobs allow a surgeon to both incorporate medical training, leadership, and military strategy in preparing to care for service members in forward settings. In addition, military surgeons may choose to pursue a career in working closely with special operation units which involves additional non-medical military training.

An academic career is also possible within the military surgical community. There is a large opportunity for research funding and avenues to pursue research both military oriented as well as clinically relevant. In addition, the presence of residency training programs, rotating Uniformed Services University (USU) medical students, and physician assistant training programs, allows exposure to teaching and involvement in advanced surgical education.

2.5 Who Can Apply to Military Training Programs

Only medical students who are a participant of a Health Professions Scholarship Program (HPSP) or attending Uniformed Services University (USU) are able to apply to a Military Training program. Uniformed Services University is an accredited medical school located in Bethesda, Maryland. Before entering school, students will select their desired service, predominantly the Army, Navy, and Air Force. At USU, a student is on active duty status and receives the salary of a First Lieutenant or Ensign. All books, study materials and required travel are paid for. Attending USU requires the student to pay back 7 years of military service after residency is complete. Refer to the USU webpage (www.usuhs.edu) for further information.

HPSP scholarships are offered for the Army, Navy and Airforce. Tuition is covered by the government and students receive a monthly living stipend. Reimbursement is also provided for required books, equipment and supplies. There is often times a monetary signing bonus offered. While on an HPSP scholarship, students are on Individual Ready Reserve (IRR). For both USU and HPSP students, medical training is the priority and there is no risk of being pulled from school for deployments or other military trainings. HPSP scholarships require an obligation for a 1-to-1 commitment to military service based on the number of years of a scholarship the student receives. Of note, many military surgical programs are 6 years. There is no payback required for intern year, but if one attends a civilian or military residency program that is 6 or more years, they will need to pay back 5 years, even if they received a 4 year or less scholarship. For more information refer to the HPSP website (medicineandthemilitary.com).

2.6 Application Process to a Military General Surgery Program

There are major differences in the application process for military residency programs compared to civilian residency programs. There is a separate on-line application system, Medical Operation Database System (MODS). MODS can only be accessed on computers with a military network or when using a Common Access Card (CAC). All letters of recommendation and other supplemental information will need to be emailed to the student's respective service GME office.

The process for residency application starts earlier in the military system. The initial intent to apply is required by the end of August, any supplemental documentation is required by mid-October and the military residency and fellowship match results are released early/mid December. See Table 2.1 for an overview of the timeline. Besides the military residency programs in each specialty, there are the several military/civilian partnerships available, but the specific civilian programs available and number of available positions vary from year to year and with each military branch of service. Military/civilian partnerships are an opportunity to train in a civilian program while still getting paid the salary of active duty resident and being on active duty status. Interviews for these positions occur in late summer and early fall. These programs are part of the military match and therefore occurs with the MODS system with results released in December. The military match determines if a student is deferred to the civilian match. A student may rank all of the military programs available in their service (see Table 2.2), military-civilian partnerships and the desire to be deferred to the civilian match. All military applicants from both

Table 2.1 Military residency training Application timeline

July 1: MODs application opens
End of August: Submission of application
Mid October: Submission of all supporting documentation
Mid October: Applicant submits final rankings
Mid December: Match results released

Table 2.2 Military residency training locations

Program	Location	Military branch
Walter Reed National Military Medical Center	Bethesda, Maryland	Army & Navy
Eisenhower Army Medical Center	Augusta, Georgia	Army
Womack Army Medical Center	Fayetteville, North Carolina	Army
San Antonio Uniformed Services Health Education Consortium	San Antonio, Texas	Army & Air Force
William Beaumont Army Medical Center	El Paso, Texas	Army
Madigan Army Medical Center	Tacoma, Washington	Army
Tripler Army Medical Center	Honolulu, Hawaii	Army
Naval Medical Center San Diego	San Diego, California	Navy
Naval Medical Center Portsmouth	Portsmouth, Virginia	Navy
Wright Patterson Air Force Base/Wright-State University	Dayton, Ohio	Air Force
Nellis Air Force Base/UNLV	Las Vegas, Nevada	Air Force
Travis Air Force Base/UC Davis	Davis, California	Air Force
Keesler Air Force Base	Biloxi, Mississippi	Air Force

HPSP and USU should complete an ERAS application in addition to the MODs application. Students will not know until mid-December if they have been deferred for a civilian residency and therefore need to already have submitted the ERAS application.

The process for interviewing for military programs is also different. Students are encouraged to visit potential military programs and complete four-week interview rotations. Depending on one's branch of service, the military will fund one or two of these rotations, referred to as Active Duty Training (ADT) rotations. These rotations allow the student to get a good understanding of the program by first hand experiencing the academics, witnessing the operative experience, the graded level of responsibility awarded to residents, as well as the overall culture of the program. The program also gets a more comprehensive understanding of the candidate and idea of how they would function in the program. Non-ADT rotations are not funded and therefore travel and housing will need to be provided by the applicant. Ideally, an applicant performs three interview rotations, but at the very least, two rotations. If a student is unable to visit a program, they should reach out in July to set up a virtual interview with the remaining programs. The appropriate time to start reaching out to military programs to set up interviewing rotations is December through March of the third year of Medical School.

2.7 Overview of Military General Surgery Training

There is minimal difference in the actual surgical training between a military general surgery residency and a civilian residency. Most military surgical residencies are a 6-year program with a required research year. Most general surgery residents will be allowed to proceed directly through their medical training without interruption, however a small percentage of Navy general surgery interns will need to complete a tour as a General Medical Officer (GMO) before proceeding and completing surgical training.

Military hospitals care for active duty members, dependents (spouses and children), as well as retired military members and veterans. Therefore, all age groups with a variety of pathology is encountered in training. Most military programs have multiple civilian rotations incorporated into the curriculum, allowing the residents experience in both civilian and military settings. For the most part, military residents will not be training alongside fellows as there are only two military fellowships, Vascular Surgery at Walter Reed National Military Medical Center and Trauma/Critical Care at San Antonio Uniformed Services Health Education Consortium. Military Programs have a higher than average pass rate for Board Certification and typically average around the 50th percentile for cases performed by graduating residents.

2.8 Conclusion

In conclusion, a military surgical career can be filled with opportunities for adventure and gratifying professional experiences not available to civilian counterparts. However, a military surgical career can limit opportunities that would otherwise be obtainable. Careful consideration should occur, of both the benefits and limitations, before pursuing a military surgical career.

Chapter 3
Choosing a Surgery Training Environment: Independent Programs

Jonathan Dort

Abstract A surgical training program is defined as independent when it is connected to an academic medical center but not governed by a university based medical school. Approximately one third of the surgical training programs in the US fit into this category. Additionally, compared to their university-affiliated peers, these graduates have been shown to have increased confidence to practice independently, as well as enjoying improved program support and equivalent success with fellowship matches and practice opportunities. Herein, we describe the landscape of independent residency training programs in the United States.

A surgical training program is defined as independent when it is connected to an academic medical center but not governed by a university-based medical school. Approximately one third of the surgical training programs in the US fit into this category. While they are not geographically connected to medical schools, many of these programs will have an affiliation with a medical school that allows those students to rotate through the different surgical services. One misconception about independent programs is that they are either less academic or not academic at all and therefore do not carry the same potential for fellowship placement, employment opportunity, or research capabilities. This is not true, as studies have shown that graduates of these programs have equivalent success with fellowship matches and practice opportunities. Additionally, these graduates have been shown to have increased confidence to practice independently, as well as enjoying improved program support [1–4]. Independent programs lack only the physical presence of a four-year university, but many are otherwise fully resourced academic medical centers in every other way.

While sharing this common definition, independent programs can vary widely in their resident complement, geography, urban or rural setting, and focus of training. It is important when researching programs to determine which ones match your desired class size, history of placing graduates in practice in the community or into

J. Dort (✉)
Department of Surgery, Inova Health System, Inova Fairfax Medical Campus, Falls Church, VA, USA
e-mail: Jonathan.Dort@inova.org

A. Gillis, C. B. Aarons (eds.), *A How To Guide For Medical Students*, Success in Academic Surgery, https://doi.org/10.1007/978-3-031-66011-5_3

fellowships, requirement or allowance of research years, and strengths of the clinical services. This type of information can be found on program websites, social media accounts, or communication with residents and leadership within a program. Additional information to ascertain about programs include the presence of an affiliated medical school that provides opportunities for teaching and mentoring, the presence of advance practice providers that can assist with patient care without interfering with educational opportunities, and the amount and types of fellowships in the center. Fellows can offer great mentorship and enhance the educational experience of all the learners; however, it is important to gain assurance that they do not adversely affect the operative and patient care experience of the residents.

There are no specific circumstances or career pathways that cannot be achieved through an independent program. However, applicants looking for mandatory research years with entrenched basic science research opportunities within the home program are more likely to find those in university-based programs. While many independent programs offer strong opportunities in clinical outcomes, patient safety and quality, and educational research, their focus tends to be more in the clinical space and are generally not as likely to offer matured pathways to funded bench research. Many independent programs do allow for research years after the PGY 2 or PGY 3 clinical years, so applicants looking for this capability should investigate what specific programs are currently allowing and what their plans are for the future.

Contributing to the increased confidence of the graduates of independent programs are the traditional strengths of these programs, which include high operative volumes and case numbers, paucity of fellowship programs that can adversely affect the resident operative experience, and close mentorship relationships with faculty. Because medical students are most exposed to university-based surgeons, a bias against independent programs can exist because of a lack of familiarity with their resources and structure. This underscores the necessity for medical students to utilize the mechanisms available to research these programs so that they are in a position to make the best choices in applying for the programs that will offer the optimal environment to ensure the realization of their desired career paths.

References

1. Friedell ML, VanderMeer TJ, Cheatham ML, et al. Perceptions of graduating surgery chief residents: are they confident in their training? J Am Coll Surg. 2014;218:695–703.
2. Sullivan MC, Sue G, Bucholz E, et al. Effect of program type on the training experiences of 248 university, community, and US military-based general surgery residencies. J Am Coll Surg. 2012;214:53–60.
3. Adra SW, Trickey AW, Crosby ME, Kurtzman SH, Friedell ML, Reines HD. General surgery vs fellowship: the role of the Independent Academic Medical Center. J Surg Educ. 2012;69:740–5.
4. Jarman BT, Joshi ART, Trickey AW, Dort JM, Kallies KJ, Sidwell RA. Factors and influences that determine the choices of surgery residency applicants. J Surg Educ. 2015;72(6):e163–71.

Chapter 4
Choosing a Surgery Training Environment: Rural Surgery Programs

Kristen Laaman and Joon K. Shim

Abstract Rural surgery is the closest experience to practicing as a general surgeon in the twenty-first century, permitting a surgeon to pursue a broad scope of practice. It is recognized that 20% of the US population live in rural areas, but only 10% of physicians practice in these areas. In this section, we want to help medical students navigate the current system by discussing the topic of rural surgery, its rewards and challenges, career goals, rural surgery residency programs and tracks, support and mentorship and the rewarding career of a rural surgeon.

4.1 Rural Surgery

A career in rural surgery can be a stimulating and rewarding one. Rural surgeons have the opportunity to find creative solutions for patient care in lower-resource settings, utilize a broad scope of surgical skills in a diverse operative caseload, and contribute to making a difference within their community. Compared to their urban counterparts, rural surgeons perform more procedures each year and complete a broader variety of operations [1]. A rural surgeon may be the only surgeon practicing in a hospital that serves multiple counties. He or she may be the primary endoscopist for an area, performing cancer-screening colonoscopies and life-saving EGDs to treat upper GI bleeds. They may also be trained and required to perform c-sections and hysterectomies, plastic surgery, and urologic procedures such as vasectomies or hyrdrocelectomies and frequently also perform more specialized general surgery operations, such as parathyroidectomies, video-assisted throacoscopic surgery, and carotid endarterectomies [2]. Often rural hospitals are lower-resourced environments, and general surgeons may need to perform stabilizing surgeries such as for trauma patients prior to transfer. While it is true that rural surgeons need to be broad-based general surgeons, there are many opportunities and

K. Laaman · J. K. Shim (✉)
Department of Surgery, Bassett Healthcare Network, Cooperstown, NY, USA
e-mail: kristen.laaman@bassett.org; joon.shim@bassett.org

A. Gillis, C. B. Aarons (eds.), *A How To Guide For Medical Students*, Success in Academic Surgery, https://doi.org/10.1007/978-3-031-66011-5_4

needs in rural communities for these surgeons to also be sub-specialized—for colorectal and hepatobiliary surgeons taking care of cancer patients in the community, minimally invasive surgeons offering bariatric surgery, and trauma surgeons contributing to protocols and training such as for farming equipment usage or all-terrain vehicle (ATV) safety. From our experience working in smaller communities, general surgeons have the unique opportunity to often care for multiple members of a family, forming meaningful physician-patient relationships. In addition, rural surgeons can serve as mentors and guides for students in rural areas, an underrepresented group in health professions.

Rural surgery has become a much-discussed topic in academic surgery over recent years due to an anticipated rural surgeon shortage, with surgeon supply to rural areas dropping by nearly 30% in the past 20 years [3]. Lack of a general surgeon contributes to the closure of many critical access hospitals and limits access to care amongst rural populations [4]. About 20% of the US population is rural, but only 12.8% of US surgeons work in these areas [3]. In a study looking at surgery positions in two US states, rural surgery jobs made up almost 50% of the available general surgery positions [5]. Choosing to practice surgery in rural America is an excellent choice for a surgeon passionate about mitigating healthcare disparities and caring for underserved populations.

4.2 Rural Surgery Career Considerations

It is important to start thinking about what a career would look like for a medical student considering general surgery. A career in rural surgery is not for everyone, but for those who choose to practice in rural surgery, it can have lifelong rewards. There is a symbolic relationship between the small community and the surgeon where a surgeon may operate on the child, parent and grandparents. It's not unusual for a surgeon to walk into a local supermarket and see patients greeting them and thanking them.

The scope of practice is broader in spectrum, and a rural surgeon can wear many hats, performing a wide range of procedures beyond the scope of general surgery in urban settings. This can include appendectomies, cholecystectomies, hernia repairs, fracture repairs, joint replacements, cystoscopies, vasectomies, cesarean sections, hysterectomies, and tonsillectomies. In addition, unlike larger hospitals, rural settings often lack immediate access to specialist surgeons. This requires rural surgeons to be adaptable, resourceful, and comfortable managing a wider range of conditions independently.

There are rewards and challenges of being a rural surgeon. A rural surgeon can enjoy a high degree of autonomy in their decision-making. He or she can see direct results of their work on the lives of their patients given the longitudinal aspect. And while demanding, rural life can offer a slower pace than urban centers, potentially allowing for better work-life balance. It also should be stated that access to professional development opportunities and collaboration with specialists can be limited but if a rural surgeon is proactive, one can stay updated and connected.

As a medical student considering rural surgery as a career, one must consider the following questions: (1) Do you thrive in a close-knit community and enjoy building relationships? (2) Are you comfortable with a broad range of surgical procedures and independent decision-making? (3) Are you adaptable and resourceful in challenging situations? (4) Can you handle a demanding workload and unpredictable schedules? (5) Are you motivated by making a direct impact on the lives of your surgical patients? In a way, rural surgery seems to highlight all the ideals that should lead someone to follow a surgical career: diversity of cases, provision of services to those in need, and commitment of surgical services to local communities to improve people's lives [6].

4.3 Choosing a Program

Different options and types of programs exist for an applicant interested in pursuing surgery in a rural location. As the importance of rural surgery has become more highlighted over recent years, many residency programs have stepped up to develop tracks to foster rural surgical training, while select other programs have been committed to training rural general surgeons for decades. When choosing programs to apply to or rank, it is important to determine what your goals and priorities are in a program and to be well-informed about the strengths and weaknesses of each rural training program. The Advisory Council on Rural Surgery (ACRS) of the American College of Surgeons has identified four components considered essential for rural surgical training. These include rotations in a rural setting, broad exposure to surgical specialties, endoscopy experience, and lack of competing specialty learners [7]. When considering where to train, recognize that the goal of all general surgery residencies should be to produce competent general surgeons who are comfortable performing "bread-and-butter" general surgery cases. However, with the trend toward most trainees seeking fellowships after residency, residents often begin to already "subspecialize" during training [8]. In addition, with duty hour restrictions, more residents are finding fellowship necessary to become comfortable with general cases. Beyond this, what truly sets the requirements of rural training apart are the many other cases that a surgeon in a rural area may be required to perform. Some of these are within the realm of general surgery training, such as a VATS, arteriovenous fistula, or advanced endoscopic case, and others are in other surgical specialties like gynecology or urology. In the following section, we have categorized the programs with rural training components [2, 7, 9–12]. Of note, not all of these programs include the four components identified by the ACRS, but this will give you a starting place in your research of rural residency programs. Something else to consider is where graduates go after training. If a residency program has a list of their alumni, take a look at the percentage who go to fellowship versus practice.

4.3.1 Rural Program

Only a few programs exist in this category. The advantage of these programs is that one is truly immersed in a rural area and the challenges and rewards that this brings. Trainees in these programs have ample opportunity in endoscopy skills and other surgical specialties, with some programs having required rotations in ob-gyn or others and also offering elective time to further focus on gaining comfort in these "non-general" surgery cases. These programs also have a strong history of producing a high percentage of surgeons who practice in rural areas after graduation. The disadvantage of these programs is that trainees may not get as much exposure to more complex surgical oncology cases or other cases that are only performed at highly specialized centers. In addition, there is not often the option of completing a research year(s) during training.

Program	Location	Things of note
Bassett Healthcare Network	Cooperstown, NY	4 categoricals Rural location and additional rotations at critical access hospitals Gyn, Plastics, ENT, and urology experience
Gundersen Health System	La Crosse, WI	3 categoricals Optional 2 months in rural location, but strong subspecialty training, endoscopy experience, history of producing rural surgeons
Marshall Community Health Consortium Program	Huntington, WV	3 categoricals 50% of experience in rural location, 50% in Huntington
Marshfield Clinic	Marshfield, WI	3 categoricals Gyn, urology, and ENT experience

4.3.2 Rural Surgery "Tracks"

Many programs in this category require an applicant to apply specifically to the "rural track" with one or two positions available each year, and this is a separate National Resident Matching Program (NRMP) code. The programs typically consist of various surgical rotations at the main location and then a dedicated year in postgraduate year 3 (PGY3) or postgraduate year 4 (PGY4) of rural training at a partner hospital. During this year, residents may experience more of an apprenticeship model of training with one or more rural surgeons. Some programs do have more than just one year of rural training with dedicated months in rural locations scattered throughout the rest of the 5 years. The benefits of such programs are that trainees have hybrid training, receiving much of their training at a large university hospital and in larger programs than those that exist in rural locations. Some of these programs also do give the opportunity for the rural-track residents to do research years, though this varies. For disadvantages, during the time that a resident is not in a rural location, they may be competing with fellowship or other surgical specialty trainees for cases. Some may also find it isolating to leave their colleagues for a year of training. In addition, during the dedicated rural portion, some programs may be more focused on the "bread-and-butter" cases. These programs tend to be more newly developed and do not always have as strong of a record in producing rural surgeons, though residents trained in these programs are more likely to go straight into general practice, which indicates strong general surgical training [13]. Some of these programs, such as Gundersen, do have a long history of dedication and strong track record of training rural surgeons.

Program	Location	Rural track	Things of note
East Tennessee State University	Johnson City, TN	Optional year between PGY3 and PGY4 to do ortho, ENT, uro, gyn	Large rural catchment area Optional international elective
Maine Medical Center	Portland, ME	Not specified	Optional international elective
Mayo Clinic College of Medicine and Science	Rochester, MN	6–12 months	1/year, gynecology, orthopedic surgery, urology, otolaryngology, and plastic surgery. Began 2015, all have gone into general practice
Medical College of Wisconsin	Milwaukee, WI	10 months total, PGY 1–5	Optional international elective
Oregon Health and Science University	Portland, OR	12 months during PGY4 6 months PGY3 or PGY4 at additional location	General, vascular, endoscopy, urology, OB/GYN and orthopedics cases
Texas Tech University	Lubbock, TX	Not specified, but throughout all years	Time dedicated to endoscopy, IR, obstetrics & gynecology, ENT, and urology
University of Minnesota	Twin Cities, Minnesota	24 months, PGY4 and 5	Final 2 years completed at rural site
University of North Dakota	Grand Forks, ND	3 months in rural surgery, 6 months of subspecialty electives PGY 2–4	Almost 40% of all graduates practicing rurally
University of Utah	Salt Lake City, UT	Optional year instead of research in subspecialty training, 2 months during normal training	Gyn and ortho experiences
University of Wisconsin	Madison, WI	12 months total PGY2–5, 5 months of elective time in subspecialties	Mentorship program for rural track
UC Davis Health	Sacramento, CA	3 months during PGY4 rural with subspecialties, global elective	Rural and global surgery track Option for MPH during research years
Western Michigan University	Kalamazoo, MI	20 months of rural and subspecialty training throughout PGY2–5	Focus on medically underserved areas

4.3.3 Rural Surgery Rotation

These programs have optional or required rural surgery rotations during training. These rotations vary in length, and some programs have optional/required rotations spread across multiple years in training resulting in up to 9 months of dedicated rural training by the end of residency. Some of these programs do also offer rotations or electives in other surgical specialties such as urology or ENT. The advantage of these programs is a resident does not need to match into a single position like for a rural track, and, depending on the program, can somewhat shape their rural experience. You will find a wide variation in the commitment to and focus on rural surgery in these programs, so take your time researching them and developing questions for your interview to help you determine which programs will best meet your training goals and feel like a fit for you.

Program	Location	Rural surgery months
Atrium Health	Charlotte, NC	3 months optional PGY3–5
Emory University	Atlanta, GA	Unspecified, PGY3–5
East Carolina University	Greenville, NC	1 month PGY$
Southern Illinois University	Springfield, IL	Optional 1–4 months
St. Luke's Hospital	Bethlehem, PA	1 month PGY2, additional 2 months of electives
University of South Dakota School of Medicine	Sioux Falls, SD	3.5 months, PGY2 and 3, required
University of Tennessee	Knovxville, TN	2 months PGY4 Urology rotation
Carillion Clinic	Roanoke, VA	6 months total, PGY2, 3, 5
Indiana University	Indianapolis, IN	2 months, PGY3
Mountain Area Health Education Center	Asheville, NC	Rotations throughout residency in subspecialties and rural locations
Ochsner Clinic Foundation	New Orleans, LA	9 months total, PGY1–5
Prisma Health	Columbia, SC	2 months, PGY 3, 4 Urology and plastics rotations
Southern Illinois University	Springfield, IL	Optional rotation PGY3 and PGY4
University of Arizona	Tucson, AZ	2 months PGY2
University of Colorado	Denver, CO	1 month optional elective
University of Iowa	Iowa City, IA	2 months, PGY3
University of Kentucky	Lexington, KY	2 months, PGY2
University of Louisville	Louisville, KY	3 months total, PGY2–4
University of Mississippi	Jackson, MS	5 months total, PGY3, PGY4
University of Nebraska	Omaha, NE	1 month PGY3
University of Oklahoma	Tulsa, OK	6 months, PGY2–4 at VA
University of Tennessee, Chattanooga	Chattanooga, TN	2 months, PGY3

Program	Location	Rural surgery months
Western Michigan University	Kalamazoo, MI	Optional 3 months, PGY3–5
West Virginia University	Morgantown, WV	1 month, PGY3

4.3.4 *Rural Location*

There are a few additional programs with training primarily in a rural location. We have kept these separate from the "rural programs" because these programs do not necessarily have any focus in rural surgical training beyond the location of the hospital, and the percentage of graduates who end up practicing rurally varies. The advantage of these programs is a trainee does get full exposure to caring for a rural population while sometimes also having the opportunity to do dedicated research time. However, trainees at these locations may not gain experience in other surgical specialties and may compete with fellows for some general surgery cases.

Program	Location
Conemaugh Memorial Medical Center	Johnstown, PA
Dartmouth Hitchcock Medical Center	Lebanon, NH
Geisinger Health System Program	Danville, PA
Guthrie Clinic	Sayre, PA
University of Vermont Medical Center	Burlington, VT

4.4 Rural Surgery Mentorship

Having a rural surgery role model while in medical school can improve exposure to rural surgery and consequently increase a career and commitment to rural surgery. Providing opportunities in mentorship can increase awareness of the life of rural surgeons and increase medical students' interests. One of the ways to address mentorship could be social media and advertising. More websites can be created to provide lists and contacts for practicing rural surgeons who are willing to allow medical students to rotate with them.

One study reviewed primary areas for rural exposure before selecting practice location by having volunteers complete a survey [14]. Out of the 416 respondent in this survey, 75% of the respondents with prior rural experience selected rural surgery practice stating lifestyle, broad scope of practice, and family were the top three reasons for their decision. With regards to rural exposure before selecting rural surgery, more seems to gravitate towards this career due to having grown up in rural areas or having exposure during residency training. It was less likely due to medical school clerkship and exposure during undergraduate or earlier because of the lack of opportunities. More and more studies show that having rural training experiences in medical school seem to be associated with an increased likelihood of pursuing a rural practice, by building a clinical or personal interest [15].

A unified database of available mentors and rural/academic exposure opportunities can help medical students. This can also promote the highlights of rural life and family support with outreach programs. Other benefits such as loan repayments and scholarships can also help recruit rural surgeons. With the existing residency programs as listed earlier, a medical student can contact program directors to see if they can do an away rotation in these rural environments. And if this is not possible, they can still correspond with those program directors and faculty members in those institutions to navigate potential future opportunities in rural surgery. And for those medical students considering rural or community surgery careers, procedural training, case volume, and the number of fellows at residency programs should be considered during the application and residency interview process.

Some studies have looked at longitudinal integrated clerkships as efforts to increase special interest in rural medicine and surgery [16]. Skube et al. examined outcomes of those becoming surgeons after completing a rural focused longitudinal integrated clerkship. It is one of the first studies to demonstrate a high rate of rural practice in general surgeons with medical school education in a longitudinal integrated clerkship.

Medical students need exposure to rural surgery early as a potential option for their future career. It starts with defining students' needs such as those with specific expertise, perspectives and supportive faculty. With regards to network, professional connections can facilitate recruitment of medical students into rural surgery. The maintenance of a complete and updated list that identifies training programs and mentors can help in these efforts [17]. Online communities, professional social media, and surgical mentorship platforms can connect medical students seeking mentors. It will be prudent for medical students interested in rural surgery to personalize their approach with their potential mentor, that is to research their potential mentor and highlight their shared interests and explain their specific needs. The medical student can ask for an informational virtual interview to learn more about each other and gauge potential fit outlining expectations for each other's time and boundaries.

4.5 Rewarding Career in Rural Surgery

A surgeon's experience is personal. It starts with knowing what the medical student wants in their career while knowing that it may pivot as they further their career and interest levels may change with time. That being said, it is important that the student seeks out as much information as possible so they can make informed decisions. A lifelong commitment to rural surgery signifies a deep dedication to serving underserved communities in remote areas through the practice of surgery. It can delve into a core set of values and motivations that drive a surgeon throughout their professional journey. A lifelong commitment prioritizes the well-being of rural communities with investment in improving healthcare access and outcomes of rural residents. A rural surgeon will be adaptable and resourceful as rural settings often present unique challenges with limited resources and specialists. This commitment fosters the ability to adapt to diverse situations, at times improvising solutions and utilizing effectively available resources.

A rural surgeon is a mentor and leader. Sharing knowledge and skills with other healthcare professionals and students in rural areas fosters future generations of dedicated rural surgeons. A medical student considering a career in rural surgery should also recognize that not all rural areas are the same. Each rural community has its own resources, geographic barriers, staff, financial, and local challenges. Rural surgeons enjoy the close-knit community and life-long relationships with their patients and families. The doctor-patient relationship is made even stronger as rural surgeons provide a variety of life-saving and elective services to multiple generations of the same family.

References

1. Heneghan SJ, Bordley J, Dietz PA, Gold MS, Jenkins PL, Zuckerman RJ. Comparison of urban and rural general surgeons: motivations for practice location, practice patterns, and education requirements. J Am Coll Surg. 2005;201:732–6.
2. Stiles R, Reyes J, Helmer SD, Vincent KB. What procedures are rural general surgeons performing and are they prepared to perform specialty procedures in practice? Am Surg. 2019;85:587–94.
3. Larson EH, Andrilla CHA, Kearny J, Garberson LA, Patterson DG. The distribution of the general surgery workforce in rural and urban America in 2019. Policy Brief. WWAMI Rural Health Research Center, University of Washington; 2021.
4. Walker JP. Status of the rural surgical workforce. Surg Clin N Am. 2020;100:869–77.
5. Decker MR, Bronson NW, Greenberg CC, Dolan JP, Kent KC, Hunter JG. The general surgery job market: analysis of current demand for general surgeons and their specialized skills. J Am Coll Surg. 2013;217:1133–9.
6. Moris D, Karachaliou GS, Pawlick TM, Nwomeh B. Attrition in general surgery residency: can global and rural surgery shift paradigm? J Surg Res. 2017;224:166–8.
7. Rossi I, Rossi M, Mclaughlin E, Minor D, Smithson L, Borgstrom D, Sarap M, Deveney K. Rural surgical training in the United States: delineating essential components within existing programs. Am Surg. 2020;86:1485–91.
8. Woeste MR, Salyer CE, Hammaker AC, Dodwad S-J, Foote DC, Nahmias JT, Callahan ZM, Quillin RC, Cortez AR. Do general surgery residents begin specializing before fellowship? A multi-institutional study from the US Rope Consortium. J Am Coll Surg. 2022;235:799–808.
9. Freida Residency Program Database: Medical fellowship database: AMA. In: FREIDA. https://freida.ama-assn.org/search/list?spec=43326. Accessed 25 Dec 2023.
10. Rural surgery program. In: ACS. https://www.facs.org/for-medical-professionals/education/programs/so-you-want-to-be-a-surgeon/section-iii-surgical-specialties/rural-surgery-program/. Accessed 25 Dec 2023.
11. Mercier PJ, Skube SJ, Leonard SL, McElroy AN, Goettl TG, Najarian MM, Termuhlen PM, Chipman JG. Creating a rural surgery track and a review of rural surgery training programs. J Surg Educ. 2019;76:459–68.
12. Rural Health Information Hub. https://www.ruralhealthinfo.org/. Accessed 25 Dec 2023.

13. Halline CG, Mokhashi N, De Bie FR, Greenwood-Ericksen MB, Zonfrillo MR. An examination of general surgery residency programs with a rural track. J Surg Educ. 2022;79:315–21.
14. Frohne N, Sarap M, Alseidi A, Buckingham L, Parikh PP. Why interested surgeon are not choosing rural surgery: what can we do now? J Surg Res. 2021;263:358–64.
15. Deal SB, Cook MR, Hughes D, Sarap M, Hughes TG, Brasel K, Alseidi AA. Training for a career in rural and nonmetropolitian surgery—a practical need assessment. J Surg Educ. 2018;75:e229–33.
16. Skube SJ, Thorndal N, Bougler JG, Clark K, Coverdill JE, Termuhlen PM, Chipman JG, Acton RD. Outcomes and influences of rural-focused integrated clerkship programs in general surgery. Am J Surg. 2020;219:355–8.
17. Rossi IR, Wiegmann AL, Schou P, Borgstrom DC, Rossi MB. Reap what you sow: which rural surgery training programs currently exist and do medical students know of their existence? J Surg Educ. 2017;75:697–701.

Chapter 5
Choosing a Surgery Training Environment: University-Based Programs

Jesse Passman and Major Kenneth Lee IV

Abstract There is no strict definition of an "academic" surgical program and this is a designation not solely limited to university-based programs. Affiliation with a university is the most typical consideration. Using that criterion alone, an applicant will encounter a large number of programs that vary in size, length, caseloads, and research opportunities. Applicants seeking a university-based program may have particular interests and goals satisfied by some but not all of these programs. Here we will attempt to broadly characterize the attributes of university programs and the applicant group to which these programs may appeal.

5.1 The Clinical Experience

Major university-based academic programs are typically associated with tertiary or quaternary care centers rather than smaller, independent medical centers. Surgeons at these programs are expected to perform highly specialized procedures safely and with outcomes exceeding those of smaller centers [1]. Newer approaches and techniques become entrenched more quickly— institutions with greater resources have greater access to newer methodologies, and surgeons are expected to offer these approaches. The technical experience of the trainee can change significantly over a 5–10 year period. Open surgical procedures, minimally invasive approaches, and even specialized approaches tailored to individual anatomic considerations may all be present in abundance. There is typically a large faculty. The same specialized procedure may be done by several different surgeons with slightly different approaches. This affords a vast and diverse technical training.

Beyond the technical experience, the clinical experience can be quite different in this environment. Trainees not only study but also manage complex surgical

J. Passman · M. K. Lee IV (✉)
Department of Surgery, Perelman School of Medicine at the University of Pennsylvania, Philadelphia, PA, USA
e-mail: Major.Lee@pennmedicine.upenn.edu

A. Gillis, C. B. Aarons (eds.), *A How To Guide For Medical Students*, Success in Academic Surgery, https://doi.org/10.1007/978-3-031-66011-5_5

conditions not seen outside of tertiary care centers. Physicians at these centers manage patients with multiple comorbidities affording a level of medical expertise that is unsurpassed. Because difficult procedures are performed on highly comorbid patients, trainees develop an ability to recognize and manage complications independently. ICU experiences can be particularly formative, as cutting-edge practices are adopted early and evidence-based practice can be expected. The outpatient experience is also robust. Many patients are managed in multidisciplinary fashion with several providers. Communication and collaboration are inherent. Trainees witness this routinely and can also participate with some frequency. Involvement in these endeavors teaches the trainee surgical practice at the highest level.

As a resident, there are advantages and disadvantages to this construct. Trainees can become accustomed to the majority of approaches and techniques. Most trainees from university-based programs pursue fellowship, and they enter those fellowships having some familiarity with virtually everything. In short, training at major university-based, academic centers ideally engenders competence with core procedures but also provides a foundation for specialty training. The tradeoff is typically in autonomy. Surgical training conceptually progresses to independent performance of core procedures. However, it is unrealistic to expect a trainee to independently perform unique procedures that are foreign to most fully-trained surgeons. The pressures to complete these procedures quickly and safely can relegate the trainee to an observer rather than a doer. In the worst case, trainees feel ill-equipped to operate independently and graduate without the ability to perform even core procedures autonomously. This has been a noteworthy concern as surgical training has evolved [2, 3]. Smaller programs that perform fewer, less complex, core procedures may allow the trainee more progress toward independent practice even if the diversity of the experience is relatively limited. Smaller faculty also engender personal familiarity and investment—an individual trainee can gain comfort in repetition with the same teacher. Lastly, major university-based specialty centers often harbor significant numbers of fellows and/or integrated residents. This can create conflict and limit case numbers, though it can be mitigated by surgical volume [4].

5.2 Didactics

All programs are required to have protected didactic time for trainees. These curricula are typically based on readily available entities such as the Surgical Council on Resident Education (SCORE) curriculum, textbooks, and/or question banks available to any resident. The major underpinnings of curricula thus tend to be similar.

University-based programs typically have large faculty, many of whom are experts in their field. Didactic sessions may therefore be more in-depth and up-to-date since providers are aware of new developments. Further, the multidisciplinary nature of patient management at these entities exposes trainees to well-attended tumor boards and other conferences where nuanced management decisions are made collectively. This can certainly help to prepare the resident for fellowship or the transition to clinical practice. However, university-based, academic programs have not been clearly shown to increase board pass rates [5, 6].

Virtually all surgical programs also have well-entrenched simulation curricula. These are often better developed at larger programs simply due to resources and access. Most of these endeavors require disposable accessories, dry/wet lab access, and even available robotic platforms for practice. These are often better advertised and more available at larger programs whether academic or community-based.

5.3 The Research Experience

University-based, academic training programs universally offer the option of dedicated, protected, and typically funded research/professional development time. Some programs mandate two such years while others present 1–2 years as optional. The ability to fully commit to non-clinical development offers several advantages.

First, there is concern that current graduates typically have little interest in academic projects and cannot develop questions/studies that can advance the field [3]. This can be mitigated by early exposure to research. Residents may not even realize their interest or aptitude for research if they have never had the opportunity. University programs that mandate this can convert undifferentiated residents to surgeon-scientists.

Second, dedicated research time is associated with increased academic productivity [7]. Residents with barren CV's are typically poor candidates for the most competitive fellowships. Non-clinical accomplishments are essentially required. While a five-year community program is not a complete obstacle to research productivity, the rigors of clinical training may place those trainees at a disadvantage relative to others who have two years to fully commit to research.

Third, attendance and presentation at national meetings is an unparalleled networking opportunity for a resident. Constructing presentations and manuscripts that are subject to outsider critique is an invaluable experience. Successful trainees can become known entities before applying to fellowship. These connections and skillsets are less relevant for a budding community general surgeon, but their value to a candidate seeking a fellowship and academic appointment is significant.

Fourth, dedicated research time builds mentor-mentee relationships between residents and faculty that are not as well-developed in the clinical venue. These relationships can persist well beyond training and can even be formative in the early career of a junior faculty member.

For these and other reasons, dedicated research time has been shown to increase faculty appointments and early-career grant funding [8]. This suggests that university-based, academic training programs best promote the development of academic surgeons and future surgical leaders. While community programs can build paradigms to promote research productivity, there is no substitute for protected research time in residency. The impact of the university program in this regard is well supported by data.

5.4 Summary: Understanding your Personal Goals

An applicant must integrate a wide variety of considerations in identifying their ideal program. These include the competitiveness of their application, preferred geography, family considerations, preferred specialty, career goals, and other aspects. The residency selection process is a match, and many applicants apply to a large number of university and community-based programs since the ultimate outcome can be unpredictable. A few questions are worth asking as one moves forward:

1. What type of surgeon do I want to be? Specialty or general?
2. What type of career do I want? Do I want a significant commitment besides surgery (research, teaching, program building, etc.)? Would I want to have a regional/national presence and impact?
3. What is my preferred geography? Rural or urban? Where is my family support and how important is that?
4. What is my preferred learning style? Integrating strategies from many mentors or working with a very limited number of people consistently?

University-based programs offer a number of advantages, but there is data suggesting that choosing a program based solely on name/reputation is associated with increased attrition [9]. There are many paths to being a successful surgeon. Determining what qualities will promote an applicant's individual success is the first step in choosing a program.

References

1. Ramadan OI, Rosenbaum PR, Reiter JG, Jain S, Hill AS, Hashemi S, et al. Impact of hospital affiliation with a flagship hospital system on surgical outcomes. Ann Surg. 2024;279(4):631–9.
2. Napolitano LM, Savarise M, Paramo JC, Soot LC, Todd SR, Gregory J, et al. Are general surgery residents ready to practice? A survey of the American College of Surgeons Board of Governors and Young Fellows Association. J Am Coll Surg. 2014;218(5):1063–72.e31.
3. Mattar SG, Alseidi AA, Jones DB, Jeyarajah DR, Swanstrom LL, Aye RW, et al. General surgery residency inadequately prepares trainees for fellowship: results of a survey of fellowship program directors. Ann Surg. 2013;258(3):440–9.
4. Driedger MR, Groeschl R, Yohanathan L, Starlinger P, Grotz TE, Smoot RL, et al. Finding the balance: general surgery resident versus fellow training and exposure in hepatobiliary and pancreatic surgery. J Surg Educ. 2021;78(3):875–84.
5. Jones AT, Biester TW, Lewis FR Jr, Malangoni MA. Review courses for the American Board of Surgery certifying examination do not provide an advantage. Surgery. 2015;158(4):890–6; discussion 6–8.
6. Caldwell KE, Clanahan JM, Klingensmith ME, Wise PE, Awad MM, Dickinson KJ. National ABSITE preparation practices: a survey of general surgery residency program directors. J Surg Educ. 2024;81(1):56–63.
7. Papasavas P, Filippa D, Reilly P, Chandawarkar R, Kirton O. Effect of a mandatory research requirement on categorical resident academic productivity in a university-based general surgery residency. J Surg Educ. 2013;70(6):715–9.

8. Andriole DA, Klingensmith ME, Fields RC, Jeffe DB. Is dedicated research time during surgery residency associated with surgeons' future career paths?: a national study. Ann Surg. 2020;271(3):590–7.
9. Abelson JS, Sosa JA, Symer MM, Mao J, Michelassi F, Bell R, et al. Association of expectations of training with attrition in general surgery residents. JAMA Surg. 2018;153(8):712–7.

Chapter 6
Overview of the Surgical Subspecialties: Plastic and Reconstructive Surgery

Robert George and Samuel Poore

Abstract Plastic surgery, derived from the Greek word *plastikos* meaning moldable, has evolved significantly since its first mention in 1838. The field's rich history spans from ancient reconstructive techniques to modern advancements in aesthetic and reconstructive surgery. This evolution reflects the specialty's innovative spirit, demonstrated by early pioneers and continuing into contemporary practices. Modern plastic surgery encompasses a wide range of procedures affecting nearly all parts of the human body. It uniquely integrates aesthetic and reconstructive surgery. The specialty's dual nature often blurs the lines between aesthetic and reconstructive aims, emphasizing the comprehensive approach plastic surgeons take to patient care. The journey to becoming a plastic surgeon involves extensive training, either through the traditional independent model following a residency in a related field or the integrated model starting directly after medical school. While it is a competitive field to match into, the field attracts individuals with a passion for problem-solving, creativity, and lifelong learning. Plastic and reconstructive surgery represents a dynamic and fulfilling specialty characterized by constant innovation and a deep commitment to improving patients' lives.

6.1 Introduction and History

What is plastic surgery? This is a more difficult question to answer than one might initially suspect. To the less acquainted, plastic surgery evokes images of rhinoplasties (nose jobs), breast augmentations, or facelifts. However, plastic surgery is a broad field which encompasses a vast range of procedures affecting almost every part of human anatomy. The name "plastic surgery" was first introduced in 1838 by Eduard Zeis [1]. The etymology of "plastic" stems from the Greek word *plastikos*, meaning moldable [2].

R. George · S. Poore (✉)
Division of Plastic and Reconstructive Surgery, University of Wisconsin, Madison, WI, USA
e-mail: rgeorge6@wisc.edu; poore@surgery.wisc.edu

A. Gillis, C. B. Aarons (eds.), *A How To Guide For Medical Students*, Success in Academic Surgery, https://doi.org/10.1007/978-3-031-66011-5_6

While the term "plastic surgery" arrived in the 1800s, procedures that relate to those under the modern umbrella of plastic surgery have existed for thousands of years. A physician named Sushruta from what is now India described a technique to reconstruct the nose using a flap of tissue from the forehead around 600 BCE [3]. We still use this surgery for nasal reconstruction today. Approaching more modern times, Sir Harold Gillies advanced many aspects of plastic surgery via gender affirming surgery and reconstruction of facial trauma sustained by soldiers in World War I [4]. Interestingly, Dr. Joseph Murray, a plastic surgeon who served in the US Army, performed the first successful kidney transplant in 1954, showcasing the field's innovative spirit [5].

6.2 Breadth of Plastic Surgery

The rich history of plastic surgery has led to what is now a diverse specialty, with operations that focus on bone, nerves, blood vessels, lymphatic channels, and soft-tissue. The two arms of plastic surgery, aesthetic and reconstructive surgery, also highlight the complexity of the field. Aesthetic, also known as cosmetic, surgery is when a plastic surgeon enhances, or augments features that a patient already possesses. In contrast, reconstructive surgery consists of a procedure to restore anatomy that was damaged by conditions including trauma, cancer, or birth defects [6, 7]. In reality, the line between aesthetic and reconstructive surgery is not always a definitive one, and the optimal treatment of a patient often consists of a combined aesthetic and reconstructive approach. Furthermore, both cosmetic and reconstructive surgery can have tremendous value to a patient's psyche and sense of self [8, 9].

Within the realm of aesthetic surgery, procedures are geared towards improving the features of a patient or rejuvenation to combat the effects of aging. Augmentation procedures include breast augmentation, abdominoplasty (tummy tuck), gluteal augmentation, liposuction to contour the body, or injection of materials ranging from the patient's own fat to fillers in order to sculpt the body. Rejuvenation procedures include facelifting, breast lift, or an arm lift. Certainly, a surgery can have the dual goals of augmentation and rejuvenation.

The realm of reconstructive surgery is vast, often containing secondary goals consisting of aesthetic aims. In general, the goals of reconstructive surgery are to restore anatomy and a patient's sense of self, reduce pain, decrease risk of infection, and improve function. For someone who enjoys problem solving and creativity, reconstructive surgery can provide a satisfying career with continual learning. Furthermore, reconstructive surgeons have the privilege of collaborating with other specialties to improve the lives of patients. For example, plastic and orthopedic surgeons often work closely with patients presenting with lower extremity trauma. The orthopedist will fixate the fractures and the plastic surgeon will determine how to provide soft-tissue coverage over the hardware. This regularly requires free tissue transfer, meaning surgically removing tissue with an associated blood supply and reconnecting the arteries and veins elsewhere in the body. Free tissue transfer exists under the subspecialty of microsurgery with utilization of a microscope in the operating room, and is one of the many reasons why those who love the intricacy of anatomy often enjoy the study of plastic surgery. Different areas of collaboration with other surgeons include assisting neurosurgeons with covering the brain and/or skull with healthy tissue or covering the heart/sternum for cardiac surgeons. Other examples of reconstructive surgery are breast reconstruction for patients with breast cancer. The opportunity to help a patient feel more like themselves as they recover from both the physical and emotional aspects of breast cancer is truly a privilege for plastic surgeons. Other interesting areas of reconstruction include reattaching fingers after they are traumatically removed, restoring someone's ability to smile after facial nerve paralysis, and delicately repairing cleft lip and palates.

6.3 Path to Becoming a Plastic Surgeon

Because of the breadth and variety afforded by the field of plastic surgery, a significant amount of training is necessary to pursue it. There are two routes for aspiring plastic surgeons. The older path is the independent model, and the newer approach is the integrated model. An independent program consists of three additional years of plastic surgery training after completion of a residency in general surgery, otolaryngology, neurosurgery, urology, orthopedics, or oral-maxillofacial surgery [10]. The newer integrated residency was created in 1995 and consists of 6 years of training without a prerequisite of different residency [11]. Overtime, the integrated model has become more and more common while the number of independent training positions has gradually decreased [10, 12].

Medical students interested in plastic surgery should not be dissuaded if interested in the field, but should be aware that it is one of the most competitive specialties to match into [13, 14]. The match rate of U.S. MD seniors in 2022 was 62.7% [15]. This is mentioned not to intimidate future candidates, but to help them reflect on how they can strategize and plan to strengthen their applications. With Step 1 shifting to pass/fail, research is one avenue that applicants may consider to distinguish themselves [16]. For example, the mean number of abstracts, presentations, and publications of matched applicants was 28.4 vs 13.8 for unmatched applicants. In order to bolster their research skills and productivity, more and more medical students are participating in dedicated research years [16]. A secondary benefit of a dedicated research year is that it can increase exposure with faculty and assist in obtaining a high quality letter of recommendation, which is regarded as one of the most important components of applicant selection [17]. Admission into the Alpha Omega Alpha honor society can also benefit applicants, with 38% of matched US MD seniors possessing this status vs 20% of unmatched applicants [15]. Furthermore, away rotations are emphasized as a way to improve match success, obtain letters of recommendation, and allow both programs and applicants to know if there is a good fit between students and institution [18]. Networking at regional and national conferences is another way students can build relationships with programs, leading to an increased likelihood of mentorship and opportunities.

Beyond residency, there are several avenues for graduates to pursue. After completing a residency in plastic surgery, surgeons have the option of going into practice as an attending surgeon. In addition, graduates may undergo a fellowship to receive advanced training and specialization. Most fellowships are one year in duration. Common fellowships trainees to do after residency are hand and peripheral nerve surgery, microsurgery, craniofacial surgery, aesthetic surgery, gender affirmation surgery, body contouring, or burn surgery. The multitude of fellowship options truly reflects the diversity of plastic and reconstructive surgery. Another appealing aspect of the specialty is that plastic surgeons, if they desire, have the ability to perform operations pertaining to different subdisciplines of plastic surgery and are not limited in scope. Table 6.1 demonstrates the branches of plastic surgery with examples of each subdiscipline.

6.4 Conclusion

Plastic surgery can be a very rewarding field in a philosophical sense. Rather than taking things from patients, plastic surgeons are often giving something to patients, whether it is helping them appear outwardly in a manner that aligns with how they feel emotionally, removing pain and improving function via peripheral nerve surgery, enhancing dexterity with tendon transfers, or granting someone the freedom to move through society without unwanted attention after correction of a deformity.

Table 6.1 Plastic surgery subdisciplines

Subdiscipline	Examples
Craniofacial surgery	Facial trauma Craniosynostosis Facial reanimation
Microsurgery	Breast reconstruction Lymphatic reconstruction Lower extremity reconstruction
Pediatric plastic surgery	Pollicization Cleft lip/palate Otoplasty
Aesthetic surgery	Breast augmentation Rhinoplasty Body contouring
Hand surgery	Digital replantation Peripheral nerve transfers Distal radius fracture fixation
Gender surgery	Penile inversion vaginoplasty Phalloplasty Gender affirming mastectomy

Moreover, plastic surgery is a fulfilling field that allows for lifelong learning and excitement in the form of constantly striving to improve one's craft. The inherent problem solving and attention to detail that are associated with the specialty provide daily cognitive stimulation and opportunities for creativity. Furthermore, while a surgeon spends a significant amount of time in the operating room, plastic surgeons have the opportunity to enjoy profound relationships with their patients both before and after a procedure. Patients entrust plastic surgeons to operate on them while they are under anesthesia with results that often affect their lives in very tangible and personal ways. This contributes to a patient-doctor relationship that is very rewarding and provides meaning during a plastic surgeon's career.

References

1. Macionis V. History of plastic surgery: art, philosophy, and rhinoplasty. J Plast Reconstr Aesthet Surg. 2018;71(7):1086–92. https://doi.org/10.1016/j.bjps.2018.03.001.
2. Bouhadana G, Aljerian A, Thibaudeau S. The reconstruction of plastic surgery: a historical perspective on the etymology of plastic and reconstructive surgery. Plast Surg. 2023;31(4):366–70. https://doi.org/10.1177/22925503211064377.
3. Bath K, Aggarwal S, Sharma V. Sushruta: father of plastic surgery in Benares. J Med Biogr. 2019;27(1):2–3. https://doi.org/10.1177/0967772016643463.
4. Solish MJ, Roller JM, Zhong T. Sir Harold Gillies: the modern father of plastic surgery. Plast Reconstr Surg. 2023;152(1):203e–4e. https://doi.org/10.1097/PRS.0000000000010279.
5. Deivasigamani S, Phillips B, Yeo CJ, et al. Joseph Murray: pioneering plastic surgeon and father of the first organ transplant. Am Surg. 2023;89(4):871–4. https://doi.org/10.1177/00031348211048843.
6. Wei X, Gu B, Li Q. Defining plastic, reconstructive, aesthetic, and cosmetic surgeries: what can get lost and found in translation. Ann Plast Surg. 2019;83(6):609. https://doi.org/10.1097/SAP.0000000000002068.
7. Tansley P, Hodgkinson D, Brown T. Comments on "Defining Plastic, Reconstructive, Aesthetic, and Cosmetic Surgeries: What Can Get Lost and Found in Translation.". Ann Plast Surg. 2021;86(4):487. https://doi.org/10.1097/SAP.0000000000002498.
8. Margraf J, Meyer AH, Lavallee KL. Well-being from the knife? Psychological effects of aesthetic surgery. Clin Psychol Sci. 2013;1(3):239–52. https://doi.org/10.1177/2167702612471660.
9. Chen W, Lv X, Xu X, et al. Meta-analysis for psychological impact of breast reconstruction in patients with breast cancer. Breast Cancer. 2018;25(4):464–9. https://doi.org/10.1007/s12282-018-0846-8.
10. Erpenbeck SP, Bustos SS, Smith BT, et al. Independent or integrated plastic surgery residency pathways: trends in representation in academic plastic surgery in the United States. Ann Plast Surg. 2021;87(4):467–71. https://doi.org/10.1097/SAP.0000000000002926.
11. Asserson DB, Sarac BA, Janis JE. A 5-year analysis of the integrated plastic surgery residency match: the most competitive specialty? J Surg Res. 2022;277:303–9. https://doi.org/10.1016/j.jss.2022.04.023.
12. Amro C, McGraw JR, Broach R, et al. 40. An update on the independent plastic surgery match: recent trends and predictors of successful match (2019–2022). Plast Reconstr Surg Glob Open. 2023;11(2S):24. https://doi.org/10.1097/01.GOX.0000921708.65389.f7.
13. Morzycki A, Bezuhly M, Williams JG. How competitive is plastic surgery? An analysis of the Canadian and American residency match. Plast Surg (Oakv). 2018;26(1):46–51. https://doi.org/10.1177/2292550317749507.

14. Sarac BA, Janis JE. Matching into plastic surgery: insights into the data. Plast Reconstr Surg Glob Open. 2022;10(5):e4323. https://doi.org/10.1097/GOX.0000000000004323.
15. Anonymous. National Resident Matching Program, Charting outcomes in the match: senior students of U.S. medical schools, 2022. National Resident Matching Program, Washington, DC 2022. n.d.
16. Applebaum SA, Stoehr JR, Bacos JT, et al. Do dedicated research years during medical school predict academic productivity during residency? Plast Reconstr Surg Glob Open. 2021;9(10):e3849. https://doi.org/10.1097/GOX.0000000000003849.
17. Schultz KP, Shih L, Davis MJ, et al. Integrated plastic surgery applicant review: important factors and selection criteria. Plast Reconstr Surg Glob Open. 2020;8(7):e2892. https://doi.org/10.1097/GOX.0000000000002892.
18. Drolet BC, Brower JP, Lifchez SD, et al. Away rotations and matching in integrated plastic surgery residency: applicant and program director perspectives. Plast Reconstr Surg. 2016;137(4):1337–43. https://doi.org/10.1097/PRS.0000000000002029.

Chapter 7
Overview of the Surgical Subspecialties: Vascular Surgery

Benjamin J. Pearce and William D. Jordan Jr

Abstract Vascular surgery is an exciting and rewarding subspeciality of surgical discipline which has seen tremendous growth and is well positioned as a viable career path for the foreseeable future. In the most foundational explanation, Vascular surgery is the evaluation and management of disease involving the arterial and venous structures which are non-cardiac and extracranial. Unlike other medical specialties that treat vascular disorders, Vascular surgeons are able to offer patients the optimal management whether it be non-operative therapy, minimally invasive endovascular procedures or traditional open surgical correction. No other specialty is trained and board certified in all three domains. To accommodate the entry into endovascular procedures and to position the specialty for the future, Vascular surgery has broaden the training paradigm to encompass both a post surgery fellowship and a direct match into residency from medical school. Both paradigms produce surgeons of the highest calibre and allow prospective surgeons to select the path optimal for themselves.

7.1 Introduction

The field of Vascular surgery has seen tremendous change in the twenty-first century. This has been manifest in the training paradigms required to be board certified in Vascular surgery, an increase the options for surgical intervention including an exponential growth in minimally invasive procedures, and diverse site of service practices that allow surgeons to better balance work/life needs. Historically, Vascular surgery required completion of a full General surgery residency(5 years) followed by a 2 year fellowship in Vascular surgery. While that is still a viable training paradigm, students can now match directly into Vascular surgery Integrated Residencies

B. J. Pearce (✉) · W. D. Jordan Jr
Division of Vascular Surgery and Endovascular Therapy, University of Alabama-Birmingham, Birmingham, AL, USA
e-mail: bjpearce@uabmc.edu

A. Gillis, C. B. Aarons (eds.), *A How To Guide For Medical Students*, Success in Academic Surgery, https://doi.org/10.1007/978-3-031-66011-5_7

at over 94 programs in the United States. This has resulted in both a condensed time dedicated to training as well as an increase in the exposure of trainees to Vascular specific cases during residency.

The catalyst for this intensive and alternate training pathway has been the adoption by Vascular surgery of innovative, minimally invasive techniques using fluoroscopic and ultrasound guidance. This new field was heralded by the introduction of endovascular stent graft repairs (EVAR) for abdominal aortic aneurysm (AAA) pathology in 1999. These devices allowed surgeons to repair AAA remotely through femoral artery cutdown procedures and transform a surgery that traditionally required a surgical mortality of 5% [1] and an attendant hospital stay of 7–10 days into a near outpatient procedure. Over the ensuing two decades, significant engineering improvements have allowed these procedures to be performed completely percutaneously and encompass more complex anatomy, incorporating renal and visceral vessels into the repair. Further, this experience with image guidance and various catheter skills has enabled Vascular surgeons to branch out into other vessel pathology with minimal techniques such as angioplasty and stenting of peripheral vessels, percutaneous thrombectomy of occluded arteries and veins, and stenting of carotid arteries to prevent stroke.

Coincident with the rise of endovascular technique, many Vascular procedures have been shifted to the outpatient setting. At time of this chapter, it is estimated that ~60% of Vascular surgery procedures in the US are performed in outpatient Angiographic or Venous office settings [2]. By moving these procedures into the physician office, many Vascular surgeons have been able to improve their financial situation by controlling the costs of care more closely and improve work/life balance as they have significantly improved operative efficiency [3].

Historically, Vascular surgery has been an exciting specialty due to the life and death nature of many Vascular procedures, the breadth of operations offered and varied anatomic locations all vascular surgeons operate in, and the longitudinal care provided to patients. A hallmark tenet of Vascular surgery is the surveillance of intervention and maintenance of patency in the treated vessels. As such, most Vascular surgeons have long standing patients with whom they develop meaningful relationships.

At the core of most vascular disease is the hallmark triad of atherosclerosis—diabetes, hypertension and smoking. Given the current diabetes epidemic, the future need of Vascular surgery expertise is predicted to be at the top of surgical specialties [4]. Many specialties are competing for these patients, especially cardiology and interventional radiology. However, those specialties can only offer minimally invasive therapy to patients, whereas Vascular surgeons are the only professionals who can offer medical, endovascular and surgical therapy to patients with vascular conditions. These factors are promising for the job satisfaction and stability in the future.

7.2 Scope of Practice

Vascular surgery is rooted in the traditional open surgical techniques of endarterectomy, thrombectomy and bypass refined throughout the second half of the twentieth century. Several landmark randomized, prospective control trials were performed that defined the benefit of both therapeutic and preventative Vascular operations (see Suggested Reading). These studies have been repeated with newer technology, often helping to define the procedure of choice for a given clinical scenario. This allows Vascular surgeons to provide the best treatment plan for each individual patient.

The intent of this chapter is not to teach the gamut of Vascular surgery conditions and treatment options. However, given the impact of vascular conditions on so many medical specialities, a basic understanding of the major conditions/procedures performed in routine Vascular care and the underlying evidence that guides decision making is critical for all medical professionals.

7.2.1 General Vascular Exam

Almost every specialty in medicine will have some degree of cross over with Vascular surgery. A fundamental understanding of rudimentary evaluation of a patient for ischemia is crucial to trauma care, emergency medicine, primary care, neurosurgery, orthopedics, general surgery, and wound care. Multiple patient visits are related to back or extremity pain, of which, underlying vascular insufficiency or aneurysm must be within the differential. Further, the major complication of almost all surgical, cardiology or radiology interventions is difficult to control hemorrhage from vascular structures. As such, any surgical specialty from urology to gynecology should understand how to do an evaluation of arterial and venous structures for safe conduct of surgical intervention.

The hallmark of the evaluation of a patient presenting with ischemia is a dedicated pulse exam. While the validity and reliability of the pedal pulse palpation has been shown to be quite poor [5], learning a focused exam can be a critical step to ordering proper work up studies and expediting patient evaluation. A good pulse exam should include evaluation of the trophic appearance of the limb including turgor of the skin, color, capillary refill and distribution of nutrient hair growth on the lower limb and foot/hand. Once a general inspection is done, pedal pulse should be palpated with the patient supine or semi-recumbent on an exam table with the medical professional seated at the foot of the bed. The dorsalis pedis (DP) pulse should be felt with the pads of the first three fingers just lateral to the extensor hallucis longis tendon using the corresponding hand of the extremity being studied. For example, when palpating the patient's left DP, the examiner should use their left hand. The examiner should then switch to the opposition hand and use the pads of the first 3 digits to feel the posterior tibial (PT) artery underneath the medial malleolus of the ankle. Applying medium pressure at most with the pads of the fingers prevents complete compression of the vessel which can lead to spurious results. The examiner should quantify the pulse as either 2+, 1+ or absent, or as easily palpable, palpaple or absent.

Absence of a palpable pulse does not mean that the patient's limb is ischemic. In fact, radiographic and cadaveric studies have demonstrated an incidence of congenitally absent distal anterior tibial artery/dorsalis pedis artery in 6–8% of people [6]. Further, many patients with chronic PAD may have absent pulses, but excellent collateral flow to the pedal circulation and have robust doppler signals despite nonpalpable pulse. The absence of a palpable pulse should prompt the examiner to obtain a hand held continuous wave doppler to assess for arterial flow. True arterialized flow will be either monophasic, biphasic or triphasic and can be distinguished from venous flow as it should not vary with respiratory cycle or manual compression of the forefoot.

Using the handheld Doppler and a manual blood pressure cuff, anyone can perform a bedside ankle-brachial index (ABI). By taking bilateral brachial blood pressures and comparing it to the best of the DP and PT at each ankle, a ratio of Ankle:Brachial pressure is created. This is an excellent screening tool for ischemia both chronic and acute (Vascular etiology or traumatic). A normal quality Doppler signal and ABI $<1.4 > 0.9$ should exclude any acute vascular pathology from consideration in a patient presenting with limb complaints/trauma. A more formal evaluation with a dedicated ABI and Pulse Volume Recording (PVR) can be performed by a Vascular laboratory technician to aid in diagnosis if needed.

7.2.2 *Peripheral Arterial Disease (PAD)*

The logarithmic rise in the incidence of Diabetes in the general population has resulted in a dramatic increase in the incidence of lower extremity peripheral vascular disease. Historically, Vascular surgeons treated patients with the classic triad of hyperlipidemia, smoking and hypertension. Now, many patients, even those in the 3/4th decade of life are presenting with mixed neuropathic and ischemic ulcerations due to diabetic complication [7]. In fact, every 1% increase in glycosalated hemoglobin (HbA1c) over 7% carries a 26% increased risk of major lower extremity amputation compared to well controlled diabetic patients [8].

The classic framework for the evaluation of ischemia in patient's with lower extremity vascular disease is a continuum:

Asymptomatic → Claudication → Ischemic Rest Pain → Tissue Loss

This basic understanding is a good foundation for medical students evaluating patients with leg complaints in the Vascular, primary care, neurosurgery, rehabilitation medicine, or orthopedic clinic. It should be noted that patients with diabetic related wounds may not fit the classic continuum as wounds in diabetics can be present due to abnormal sensation (neuropathy) and no vascular occlusion, or the normal presenting pain syndromes with ambulation or at rest may be blunted by abnormal sensation [7]. As such, any leg complaints in a diabetic patient should prompt non-invasive vascular testing.

Based on the duration of a patient's PAD and their level of physical activity, many sedentary patients can have abnormal circulation but remain asymptomatic. The next phase of PAD usually manifests as claudication (from the Latin "to limp") which is pain in a lower extremity muscle during exertion which alleviates at rest. This is analogous to the more commonly understood "exertional angina". In claudication, the muscle group immediately perfused by the occluded segment will be well supplied in a sedentary state by collateral flow, but then have a perfusion mismatch when in use resulting in build of anaerobic metabolites that cause pain. A good history and physical exam can delineate the level of occlusion. For example, patients with buttock and thigh claudication and absent femoral pulsations will have aortic/iliac level occlusion. Conversely, classic calf claudication is caused by an intact inflow to the profunda femoris artery but superficial femoral (SFA) or popliteal artery occlusion. Discrimination of the level of occlusion and relative severity of the claudication can be obtained with Lower Extremity Arterial studies (LEA) combined with PVR using the same machine as an ABI (Fig. 7.1). Some patients with chronic occlusion and robust collaterals may have a normal ABI at rest but a decrease with ambulation. Use of ABI testing with treadmill walking test can help to differentiate between PAD related leg complaints and other disease such as radiculopathy.

Once the ABI drops <0.4, the patient is at risk for Critical Limb Threatening Ischemia (CLTI) which can be manifest as pain in the foot at rest and/or ischemic wounds to the lower extremity. Untreated, CLTI carries a >50% risk of limb loss and 25% 2 year overall mortality secondary to wound complications. Further, those who succumb to amputation have an overall mortality of 30% after 2 years [9].

The treatment of PAD in the modern interventional milieu is too complex for a medical student level review. However, the basic tenets of the approach to treatment of the atherosclerotic patient is warranted. All patients with PAD will benefit from lifestyle modifications targeted at smoking cessation, avoidance of all tobacco products, increased physical activity, cholesterol lowering diet, maintenance of optimum weight, control of hypertension and euglycemia. The majority of patients with proven atherosclerotic burden will benefit from administration of a statin medication, even in the setting of normal lipid numbers, due to the pleotropic effects of statins on plaque inflammation. Anti-platelet, anti-thrombotic management is recommended in some form for most patients with symptomatic disease and all who receive an intervention.

While other vascular conditions may require prophylactic intervention, it should be well understood that asymptomatic patients with PAD do not benefit from any intervention. The first line of therapy for patients with claudication is also non-operative. After appropriate life style modification and pharmacotherapy as outline above, randomized controlled trials have proven that a supervised exercise regimen (SET) combined with smoking cessation has superior limb salvage compared to intervention [10]. Endovascular or surgical intervention for claudication should

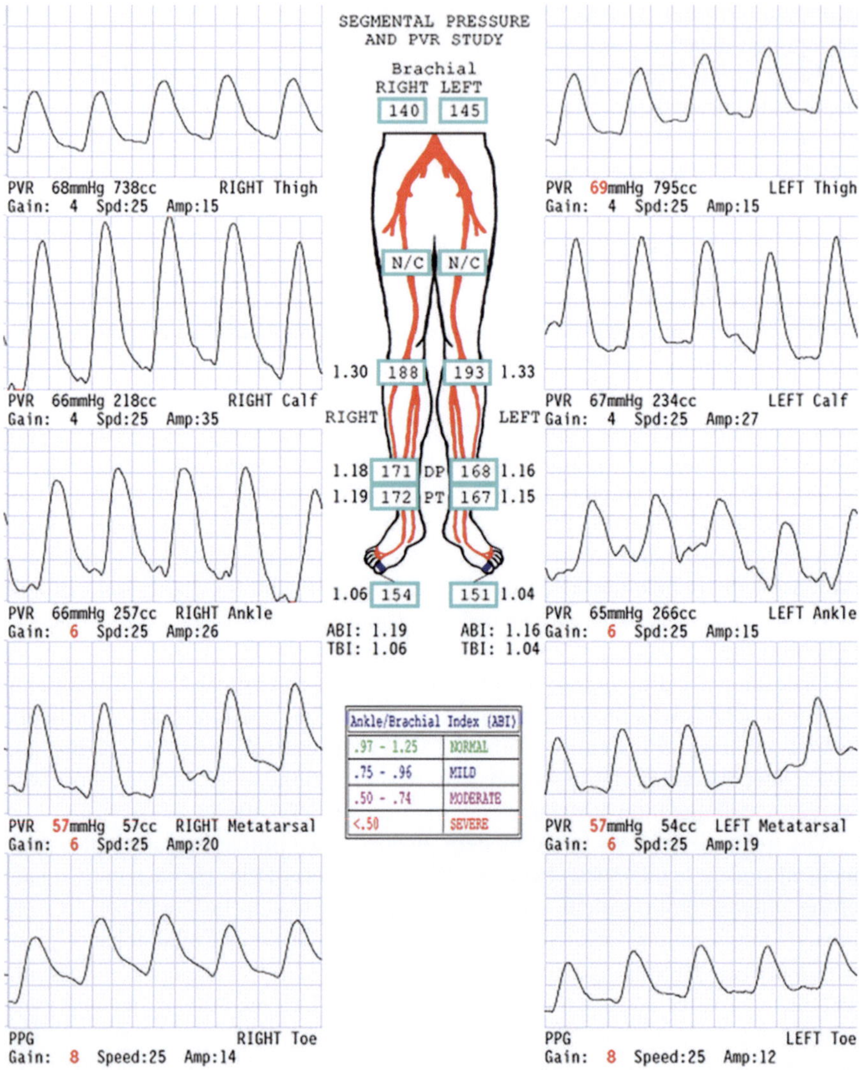

Fig. 7.1 Lower Extremity Arterial Study (LEA). Example of normal LEA with segmental pressures and list of Ankle Brachial Index (ABI) and Toe Brachial Index (TBI) as well as Pulse Volume Recording (PVR) waveforms for quantitative anlaysis of peripheral arterial disease (PAD). UAB Patient

only be offered to patients who have had at least a 3 month trial of lifestyle modification and exercise regimen.

The nuances of appropriate surgical and endovascular intervention are too great to delineate here. For the purposes of a medical student level rotation, the classic tenets of vascular surgery remain. Whether using endovascular technique or surgical therapy, one must be able to connect a healthy artery above the occlusion to a healthy artery below using an appropriate conduit or device. The suggested readings can be used for more in depth understanding of the various techniques used to achieve limb salvage.

7.2.3 *Aortic Aneurysm*

Aneurysmal degeneration of the aorta can occur at any level and is a complex cellular interaction with multiple underlying mechanisms that can influence surgical decision making. True aneurysms involve all 3 layers of the arterial wall, as opposed to pseudo-aneurysm which are typically a focal defect in the arterial wall with attending tamponade from adjacent structures. The overwhelming majority of aortic aneurysms are degenerative in nature and share the same underlying risks as classic PAD—atheroma, smoking and hypertension. Diabetes, while not prohibitive, has actually been demonstrated to be protective against aneurysm disease in population study [11]. Other underlying mechanism included connective tissue disorders (such as Marfan's disease, Loey's Dietz syndrome, or Vascular Ehlors Danlo) or congenital anomalies. Further, traumatic or infectious aneurysm often are lumped into aneurysm disease categories although these are typically pseudo-aneurysms.

The basic understanding of aortic aneurysm at the medical student level should focus on abdominal aortic aneurysm (AAA) which is the most frequently repaired aortic aneurysm in the US. Unlike PAD, Vascular surgeons often treat AAA prophylactically to prevent rupture. Indications for repair typically are related to the diameter of the largest centerline measurement of the AAA as this is a surrogate for the wall stress. The original studies recommending repair were based on physical exam measurements, however modern recommendation are based upon axial computed tomography or ultrasound imaging modalities. The UK (United Kingdom) Small aneurysm trial [12] and the concurrent VA (Veterans Administration) Aneurysm Detection and Management Trial [13] did an excellent job of defining the safe size measurements and surveillance intervals to decrease mortality in patients with asymptomatic AAA (See Fig. 7.2). In general, AAA in men can be safely observed in a routine ultrasound imaging surveillance schedule until the aneurysm is >5.5 cm in maximum diameter with the corresponding size threshold in women to be 5.0 cm. In both sexes, a rapid rate of growth >5 mm in 6 months or >9 mm in one year is also an indication for repair.

Some patients with impending rupture will present with an intact but symptomatic AAA. These patients will begin having significant abdominal and back pain which is unrelenting. The pain is often exacerbated with hypertension and will actually improve with blood pressure control—a tip to help differentiate abdominal pain syndromes in patients with AAA and possible other pathology. Tenderness over the palpable aneurysm further confirms the diagnose of symptomatic aneurysm and repair should be conducted within 24 h of onset of symptoms.

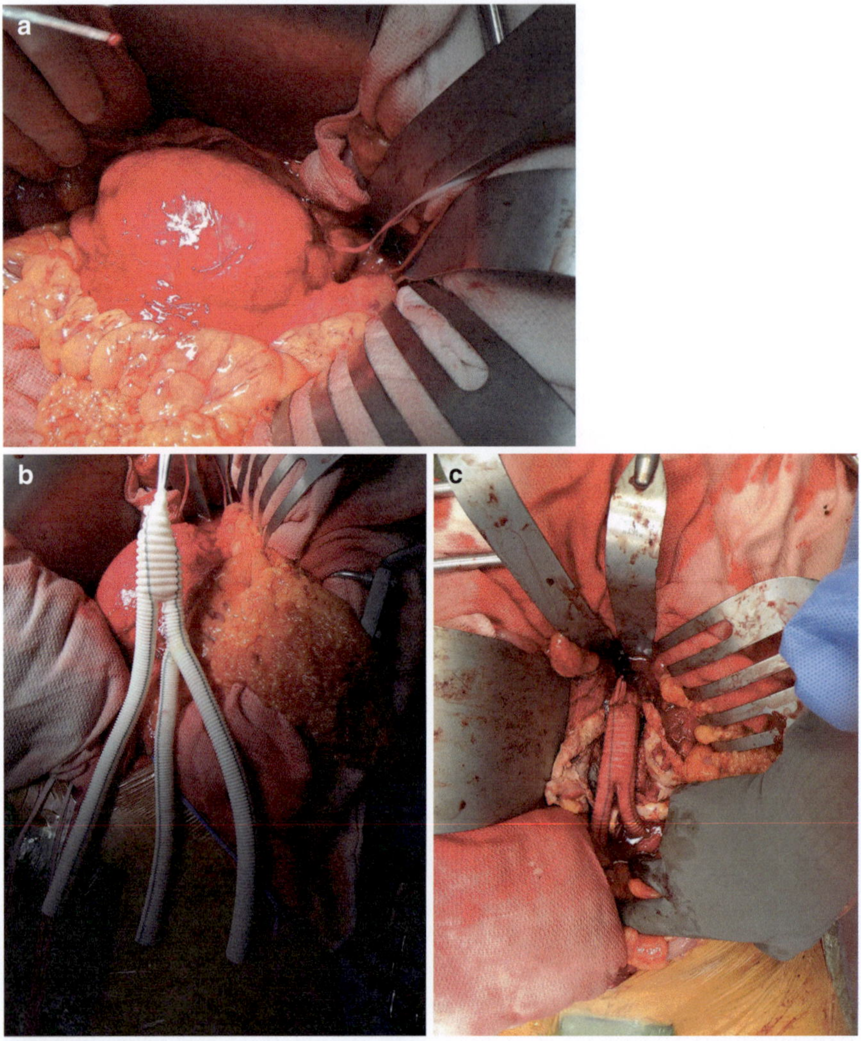

Fig. 7.2 Example of Open Abdominal Aortic Aneurysm Repair. (**a**) Large infrarenal abdominal aortic aneurysm (AAA) with iliac artery involvement. (**b**) Bespoke Dacron graft created to incorporate repair of the AAA with preservation of hypogastric perfusion. (**c**) Completion of open repair of AAA

Method of repair can be broadly categorized as open or endovascular. The traditional open aneurysmorrphy (OR) consisted of proximal and distal control of the aorta and/or iliac vessels above and below the aneurysm followed by replacement of the aorta by direct anastomosis of a prosthetic graft (Fig. 7.2). Approach to the aorta can be accomplished by both transperitoneal and retroperitoneal approaches. This operation is well studied and provides a durable repair with initial operative mortality of 2–3% in most modern series. There is a fair amount of recovery time and the initial stress of the operation carries a risk of peri-operative cardiac and pulmonary complications.

In 1999, the first Endovascular stent graft was FDA approved to allow for relining of the aorta from a femoral approach known as endovascular aortic repair (EVAR) (Fig. 7.3). We are now on the fourth generation of stent grafts and several different constructs are available in regards to graft configurations, materials and delivery systems which have greatly improved the percutaneous delivery and intra-operative success of deployment. These cases can be routinely done under regional or local anesthetic with significant decrease in operative time and patient recovery. The operative mortality for contemporary EVAR is <2% with significantly improved cardiac, GI and pulmonary morbidity compared to OR [14].

The relative safety of EVAR has greatly expanded the pool of patients who are candidates for intervention. Since AAA typically occurs later in life, many patients were previously prohibitive cardiac or pulmonary risks for OR. In fact, approximately 75% of infrarenal AAA in the US are now repaired via EVAR [15]. However, it is important to remember that Endovascular relining does not allow for ligation of the branch vessels of the native aorta (lumbar, sacral, accessory renal and inferior mesenteric) and these can caused continued perfusion of the AAA after repair, a condition known as endoleak. In addition, the EVAR devices require a component of normal aorta and iliac vessels above and below the aneurysm to achieve steal. Several factors can compromise the seal zones including inadequate length, calcium, thrombus and angulation in the area of seal. As the patient continues to age,

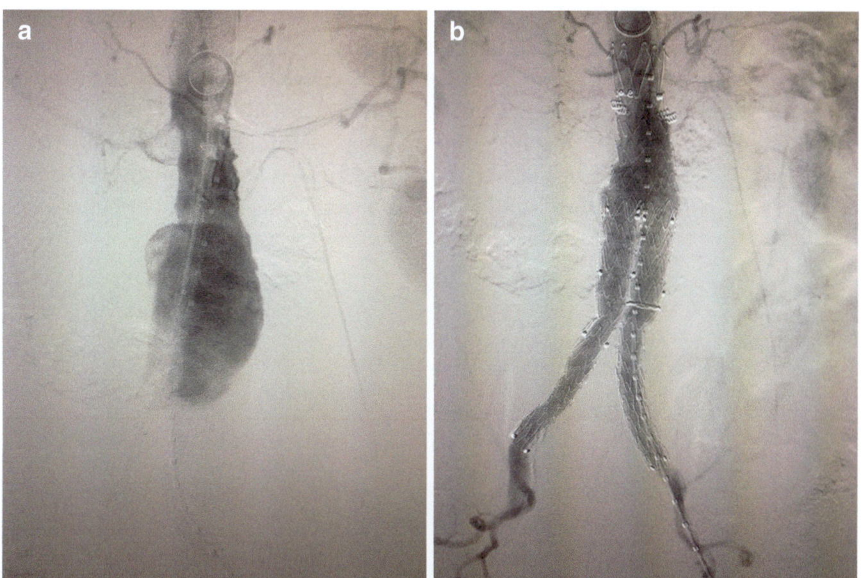

Fig. 7.3 Example of Endovascular Aneurysm Repair (EVAR). (**a**) Angiogram demonstrating abdominal aortic aneurysm (AAA) prior to EVAR. (**b**) Same patient with exclusion of AAA using EVAR graft and endoanchors to secure proximal seal

the outward force of the stent holding the graft in place can cause dilation and failure of the seal. Because of these phenomena, there is a significantly higher need to re-intervene on patients who have their AAA repaired via EVAR and after 8 years, the durability of EVAR suffers compared to OR [16]. As such, Vascular surgeons must have an understanding of both the anatomical restraints of the device placement as well as the patient's overall medical fitness and life expectancy to choose the optimal repair for the individual patient.

Modern EVAR is ever expanding to incorporate fenestrations or branches so that the renal, mesenteric and arch vessels can be incorporated in EVAR. Eventually, technology and refinement of technique should allow for total aortic repair with endovascular technique. In addition to AAA, Vascular surgeons also perform open repair of thoracic-abdominal aneurysm (TAAA), endovascular repair of thoracic aorta (TEVAR) and treatment of aortic dissections. These procedures are of increased complexity and mainly confined to tertiary care centers.

7.2.4 Carotid Artery Stenosis

Disease of the carotid artery is another vascular condition that spans several specialties, and a basic understanding of the etiology/treatment of carotid atherosclerosis is warranted for all practitioners. The role of carotid atherosclerosis in the development of stroke has been well understood for almost 80 years [17]. Due to aberrant hemodynamic forces created by the carotid bifurcation, there is a predilection of plaque formation at the proximal internal carotid artery (ICA) (Fig. 7.4). The risk factors for carotid disease are similar to all atherosclerotic conditions, again with a strong prevalence in any time smokers, hypertension and hyperlipidemia.

Unfortunately, there is much confusion about the etiology of carotid based strokes which clouds work up and appropriate referral. As the carotid artery narrows due to plaque burden, the flow within the ICA becomes increasingly turbulent, thus

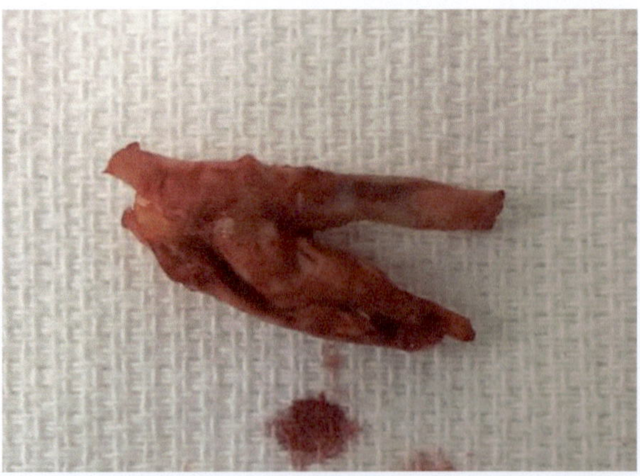

Fig. 7.4 Carotid Plaque. Demonstration of successful plaque removal to prevent stroke using carotid endarterectomy

the increase risk with higher degree of stenosis. This can lead to both thrombus formation as well as abnormal shear forces along the existing plaque. This milieu results in the embolus of plaque/thrombus particles into the cerebral circulation [18]. If small enough, these emboli can cause temporary occlusion of cerebral branches in the ophthalmic or middle cerebral artery territory known as transient ischemic attacks (TIA). The TIA symptoms should be of short duration (usually a matter of minutes but no more than 24 h) and completely resolve. Neurologic deficits lasting longer than 24 h are classified as stroke.

A careful history and physical can help delineate the difference between carotid based events and other neurologic deficits such as vertigo, seizures, dizziness or syncopal episodes. This is critical to focus the work up and guide treatment recommendations as prompt recognition of TIA or stroke can prevent further neurologic damage. As it is exceedingly rare to have bilateral symptomatic carotid plaques, carotid disease is typically unilateral in presentation. Based upon the cerebral territory at risk, the presenting symptoms may be amaurosis fugax, aphasia, dysarthria, unilateral facial asymmetry, or upper/lower extremity parathesias or hemiparesis.

Much like AAA, carotid artery atherosclerosis is also a condition which may warrant intervention in asymptomatic patients to prevent neurologic events. Several landmark RCT were performed in the twentieth century helped define recommendations for carotid treatment and can be found in the suggest readings attached. For symptomatic disease, the threshold to recommend intervention to prevent further neurologic injury is relatively low for most patients. In the North American Symptomatic Carotid Endarterectomy Trial (NASCET) [19], patients with TIA or stroke and ipsilateral carotid lesion of >50% proven on angiographic imaging were shown to have a risk reduction in subsequent stroke from 26 to 9% over 2 years.

Prophylactic carotid intervention has a much higher number needed to treat to realize a benefit in stroke prevention as modern medical therapy—smoking cessation, lipid management and anti platelet agents—has made the risk of carotid embolus much less. However, it is generally accepted that in patients of good operative risk and a >5 year life expectancy, appropriate and safe carotid intervention can result in a reduction of stroke over 5 years from 11 to 6% [20].

Given the devastating effects of stroke on patients, families and population health, it is fortunate that several well studied interventions exist to prevent stroke. The gold standard of treatment is carotid endarterectomy (CEA). Contemporary series of CEA demonstrate that in experienced hands, the operative risk of stroke is <3% and disabling myocardial infarction (MI) or death of <3% as well. Transfemoral carotid stenting (TFCAS) has been developed as a less invasive option to treat carotid lesions and is more easily accomplished under local anesthesia. However, by definition, a TFCAS requires wire and device passage across the aortic arch, common carotid artery (CCA) and the unstable plaque itself before the stent can be deployed to trap the embolic debris. As such, in even the most rigorous trials of TFCAS, the intraoperative stroke risk is double that of CEA. However, this can be offset by a reduction in the operative MI risk of half with equivalent death [21]. Thus, it is critical that the health care team involved in the care of carotid patients appropriately assess the individual patients overall risk of procedure to determine the appropriate procedure. In general, TFCAS should be reserved for those patients with medical co-morbidities making an operative approach prohibitive or in certain anatomic situations—history of neck radiation, reoperative carotid field, presence of tracheal stoma, contralateral vocal cord deficit, or high carotid bifurcation—which may carry an increased risk for CEA.

A newer procedure is emerging that may combine the best of both procedures. A transcarotid artery stent (TCAR) has been studied in recent patient safety and registry data that has reduced the risk of stroke with stenting to the level of CEA [22, 23]. This procedure is conducted via a small cutdown on the proximal CCA and initiation of a flow reversal state in the carotid circulation before engaging the plaque with wires and stent. Further expansion of this technique is being studied and provides a safe alternative to patients at high risk for both CEA and TFCAS.

7.2.5 Venous Insufficiency/Thrombosis

A significant number of patient complaints/referrals are generated due to varicose veins (VV). While not a limb threatening condition alone, VV can be a sign of underlying venous pathology that may warrant treatment. Fortunately, the overwhelming majority of VV are cosmetic in nature and can be treated with reassurance or simple compression garments.

Patients with underlying venous valvular insufficiency can have a myriad of limb complaints such as heaviness, swelling, and fatigue. A clue to an underlying venous cause of these complaints is that they will occur with increasing activity/dependence of the limb throughout the day and will alleviate with rest and elevation. In the worst manifestation of venous insufficiency, patients can progress to have venous stasis changes to the limb and develop pain, discoloration, and wounds due to the breakdown of hemoglobin within the static limb. Any concerns for possible venous stasis warrant referral to a dedicated vein clinic run by a board certified Vascular surgeon for appropriate testing and treatment recommendations [24].

Increasingly, Vascular surgeons are being involved in the care of deep venous thrombosis (DVT). Patients with acute DVT can have dramatic symptoms related to swelling and pain. As with all thrombotic care, immediate initiation of anticoagulation (AC), combined with elevation and compression of the affected limb is paramount. Prompt imaging with venous duplex ultrasound (DUS) should be performed in all cases of suspected DVT. Because of the degree of acute disability, it is tempting to recommend interventional treatment of DVT. However, several RCT have demonstrated no long term benefit to intervention therapy over AC and compression. Two large RCT have demonstrated that in younger, active patients, there is benefit to clearance of acute DVT in the more proximal venous system (ilio-caval DVT) [25, 26]. If there is any question of extent of DVT proximal to the common femoral vein, immediate consultation with a Vascular surgeon is necessary to delineate the need for urgent intervention. The most dramatic presentation of acute DVT is phlegmasia cerulea dolens which is a surgical emergency due to the risk of limb loss from nerve compression and ischemia secondary to severe venous HTN in the limb.

7.2.6 *Hemo-Dialysis Access*

Creation and maintenance of dialysis access is a core component of many Vascular surgery practices. It can be an attractive practice model to some surgeons who have a need for more lenient work/life balance as the majority of these cases are semi-elective and routinely outpatient in nature. The three major modes of hemo-dialysis access are arterio-venous fistula (AVF), arterio-venous graft (AVG) or catheter placement.

The gold standard of dialysis access is the creation of upper extremity AVF. The connection of a peripheral vein to artery through surgical anastomosis promotes hypertrophy of the venous outflow and ultimately high enough flow rates to allow for dialysis in a reasonable time period. The advantages of AVF are prolonged patency and less infectious complications. In patients with inadequate peripheral veins suitable for access, a prosthetic graft can be tunneled sub-cutaneously between a peripheral artery and more central vein to achieve the same result. Catheter dialysis should be used as a temporary bridge to another surgical access as the attendant infectious complications or injury to central venous structures is too high to warrant permanent use in all but the extreme of cases [27].

7.2.7 *Miscellaneous Vascular Conditions*

Vascular surgeons are fortunate to have the ability to treat many other pathologies which are too infrequent to warrant discussion here. The gamut of a robust Vascular surgery practice may also include spine exposure for orthopedic spinal hardware placement, treatment of visceral or peripheral aneurysms, mesenteric occlusive disease, thoracic outlet syndrome (TOS), and treatment of non-atherosclerotic conditions such as arteritis, fibro-muscular dysplasia, and various compression syndromes.

7.3 Pros/Cons of Vascular Training Paradigms

Vascular surgery is a relatively new specialty with the first certificates of special recognition in Vascular surgery being issued in 1982 followed by the requirement of a Vascular fellowship after general surgery training in 1989. As the breadth of the specialty continued to evolve, catalyzed by the rise in endovascular therapy, early specialization in vascular surgery was approved by the American Board of Surgery (ABS) in 2004 followed quickly by the primary certificate in Vascular Surgery in

2007. This primary designation has resulted in the ability to offer a direct residency in Vascular surgery (known as Integrated Vascular Residency IVR) encompassing a primary match into IVR from medical school and a 5 year curriculum which allows for Board Certification by the Vascular Surgery Board (VSB) of the ABS [28]. As of the 2023 match, 93 residency spots were offered into IVR [29]. These trainees will be board certified in Vascular surgery only as compared to the traditional general surgery + 2 year Vascular surgery fellowship(5 + 2) who are eligible for double board certification.

Both training paradigms have produced successful and productive vascular surgeons. The 5 + 2 fellowship match offered 136 positions for appointment in 2023 as well [30]. The most obvious advantage of the IVR is 2 less years of surgical training and the attendant additional financial burden of those years in repaying student debt and working at lower wages. In reviewing our institutional data over the first decade of graduating both 5 + 2 and IVR trainees simultaneously, the only major difference in vascular training is that our IVR graduate with approximately 3 times the number of peripheral vascular diagnostic and therapeutic endovascular procedures compared to the 5 + 2 fellows. Otherwise, there is no statistical difference in the performance of all the other core procedures defined by the ACGME Program requirements [31].

Selection of the best training paradigm for a career in Vascular surgery requires the applicant to make an honest assessment of their career goals, practice setting expectations, and personal financial needs. The practice of Vascular surgery has become so broad and integral to most major health care systems, that the need for double board certification and general surgery skills is nearing obsolete. Obviously, if the applicant desires living and working in a more rural setting where access to care is scarce, a double certification in general surgery and Vascular would be appealing. Further, for those who are considering a career in Vascular surgery but are not convinced at the time of medical school graduation that they may not wish to work in a different discipline, the 5 + 2 program is still a viable option for training. Otherwise, we have had excellent success in graduation, board pass rates, and job placement with the IVR.

7.4 Conclusion

The specialty of Vascular surgery is one of the most exciting surgical sub-specialties due to the ability to operate on almost all anatomic locations and offer the most tailored care for a patient from medical to surgical to minimally invasive procedures. Further, the Vascular surgeon develops a life long rapport with patients and provides life and limb-saving care. This has proven to be a rewarding aspect of surgery almost unique among the surgical disciplines. Further, even for those medical students who ultimately choose another field of practice, a fundamental understanding of the basic principles of vascular surgery will make them a better physician and advocate for their patients.

Appendix. Resources and Suggested Readings/Videos

Handbook of Patient Care in Vascular Disease by Todd Rasmussen:

- Good overview of clinical vascular surgery for medical students
- Compact and fits in your white coat pocket; great to read for clinic or during down-time
  - Login info: https://bookshelf.vitalsource.com/#/
  - Username: stanfordvascsubi@gmail.com
  - Password: Arterial2!

***Advanced Surgical Recall* by Lorne Blackbourne**:

- The vascular surgery chapter is short (~20 pages), includes the most commonly asked questions in vascular surgery cases
- Also covers the most commonly asked questions in general surgery cases

***Atlas of Vascular Surgery and Endovascular Therapy: Anatomy and Technique* by Elliot L. Chaikof and Richard P. Cambria**:

- Review Chaps. 1–5, which are quite short, but provide an excellent overview of *endovascular procedures*

***Rutherford's Vascular Surgery, 9th Edition* by Anton N. Sidawy, Bruce A. Perler**:

- *The vascular surgery textbook*
- Often available online through university libraries

***Vascular and Endovascular Surgery E-book* by Wesley S. Moore, "*Anatomy and Surgical Exposure of Vascular System*" chapter by Jeffrey Ballard**:

- 20-page detailed summary of most common vascular exposures—not as detailed as Valentine's but good for quick review before the case

***Anatomic Exposures in Vascular Surgery* by Gary G. Wind and R. James Valentine**:

- This is a great source for reviewing relevant anatomy for upcoming cases

Gore's Vascular/Endovascular Surgery Combat Manual:

- Good "pocket book" for reviewing major concepts between the cases or during down-time on the floor
- Available online (PDF) https://www.goremedical.com/combat-manual

Landmark Vascular Surgery Clinical Trials: https://vimeopro.com/user11267838/didactic-lectures/video/228501446

- 30 min lecture by Dr. Orion summarizing the major carotid, AAA, bypass vs endo and thrombolysis trials (would watch multiple times)

- Please see the "Essential Articles in General Surgery" chapter on important vascular papers
- Know the size at which we repair aneurysms in different parts of the body and why (rupture vs thrombosis vs embolization)

Society for Vascular Surgery Guidelines:

- Lastly, for advanced learning, SVS has guidelines for AAA, CLI, WIfI score, blunt traumatic thoracic aortic injury, and management of LSA available at the links below, as well as through the SVS app (Apple/Android app store):
- https://vascular.org/research-quality/guidelines-and-reporting-standards/clinical-practiceguidelines
- **CLTI**
  - https://www.sciencedirect.com/science/article/abs/pii/S0741521419303210
- **AAA**
  - https://www.jvascsurg.org/article/S0741-5214(17)32369-8/fulltext
- **PAD—asymptomatic & claudication**
  - https://www.jvascsurg.org/article/S0741-5214%2814%2902284-8/fulltext
- **WIfI score**
  - https://www.jvascsurg.org/article/S0741-5214%2813%2901515-2/fulltext
- **Blunt thoracic**
  - https://www.jvascsurg.org/article/S0741-5214%2810%2901924-5/fulltext
- **Management of LSA**
  - https://www.jvascsurg.org/article/S0741-5214%2809%2901823-0/fulltext
- **Reporting standards for type B aortic dissections**
  - https://www.jvascsurg.org/article/S0741-5214(19)32649-7/pdf
- **Descending Thoracic Aorta Diseases**
  - https://www.ejves.com/article/S1078-5884(16)30178-2/fulltext

***Clinical Scenarios in Vascular Surgery* by Gilbert R. Upchurch Jr. and Peter K. Henke**

- More advanced textbook, helpful for oral board preparation

Audible Bleeding Podcasts

- The vascular surgery podcast, based out of the Vascular Surgery Fellowship Program at New York Presbyterian
- Features interviews from leaders in the field, VSITE exam review, and updates in guidelines/clinical practice
- https://www.audiblebleeding.com/

choosevascular.com

- Website maintained by major national vascular societies to help guide potential students and residents on a career choice in vascular surgery

Video Resources

Suturing	https://www.youtube.com/channel/UC-0GEHkDCHhI7ankr6HjWfw
End to side anastomosis and patch angioplasty	https://www.youtube.com/playlist?list=PLIBTkGxZozxo5SQdkBkrOtD8TBohkQun
Subcuticular stitch for skin closures	https://www.youtube.com/watch?v=IkX5zMyCV1s&t=283s
Sheath removal	https://www.youtube.com/watch?v=dSyZWCDG7U8
Ultrasound-guided femoral access	https://www.youtube.com/watch?v=45Rs90giA8E
Transradial access	https://www.youtube.com/watch?v=8PNzEcvtnkI
Direct puncture of vascular lesions	https://www.youtube.com/watch?v=F-POH4lpX0I
Ultrasound-guided jugular access	https://www.youtube.com/watch?v=UvPc2c_hE9g
Carotid subclavian bypass with TEVAR	https://www.youtube.com/watch?v=0SXQwJG4LDI
Carotid-carotid subclavian bypass	https://www.youtube.com/watch?v=wzHmnIuVgDw
Carotid endarterectomy (Full)	https://www.youtube.com/watch?v=AWXCpRJAN8M
Carotid endarterectomy part 1	https://www.youtube.com/watch?v=wZ8PzhwmSXQ
Carotid endarterectomy part 2	https://www.youtube.com/watch?v=E_wWpRKBy4w
Aorta to right carotid bypass	https://www.youtube.com/watch?v=7LIrcSM7_Ic
Temporal artery biopsy	https://www.youtube.com/watch?v=zzYRhSfVSBk
Open repair of carotid artery pseudoaneurysm	https://www.youtube.com/watch?v=xuvCsWb6_YE
Superficial femoral artery to dorsalis pedis artery bypass	https://www.youtube.com/watch?v=QXjsre0kP4k
Left common femoral artery to anterior tibial artery bypass using PTFE graft	https://www.youtube.com/watch?v=xG2aF-vNSr4
Left femoral to peroneal bypass by reversed ipsilateral great saphenous vein	https://www.youtube.com/watch?v=z9T9DZB6C0g
Posterior approach right popliteal artery aneurysm repair	https://www.youtube.com/watch?v=gaGcnYtKWhk
Popliteal aneurysm and fistula	https://www.youtube.com/watch?v=hXV_fGcjdl4
Obturator bypass	https://www.youtube.com/watch?v=G4FF-9JOV90

Aorto iliac PTFE graft (Cadaver)	https://www.youtube.com/watch?v=2RQb29QhFRQ
Exposing right iliac artery for a distal anastomosis: aortoiliac bypass	https://www.youtube.com/watch?v=NmODIdojDas
Exposing left iliac artery for a distal anastomosis: aortoiliac bypass	https://www.youtube.com/watch?v=XEJbPA6Hdvg
Open aorta: completed aortoiliac	https://www.youtube.com/watch?v=GnG0WoOLvHY
Right visceral rotation	https://www.youtube.com/watch?v=DPxiDYzJwcY
Left visceral rotation	https://www.youtube.com/watch?v=KVuMiAuw5zc
Aorta to superior	https://www.youtube.com/watch?v=xPNDY2ki_Z0
Mesenteric artery and hepatic artery bypass	
Aortic exposure at hiatus (Cadaver)	https://www.youtube.com/watch?v=dK_KeRv4DKo
SMA exposure, thromboembolectomy, patch angioplasty and retrograde stenting	https://www.youtube.com/watch?v=4vyx9LmJCkA
SMA aneurysm—Open surgical repair	https://www.youtube.com/watch?v=OuK4hgofDjQ
SMA stenting	https://www.youtube.com/watch?v=-4PXsMu8d9M
Iliac to SMA bypass ringed ePTFE	https://www.youtube.com/watch?v=g9F0BIXvFeU
SMA embolectomy	https://www.youtube.com/watch?v=5Bv_8xPTgPU
Open repair of renal artery aneurysm in solitary kidney	https://www.youtube.com/watch?v=PF5RYg6V4Gk
TEVAR of contained rupture descending thoracic aorta	https://www.youtube.com/watch?v=Hlhezm-a9E4
Thoracic endovascular repair of rapidly expanding false lumen of chronic type III aortic dissection	https://www.youtube.com/watch?v=jGkLTCVEQ_I
Ascending aortic debranching	https://www.youtube.com/watch?v=y76-6SsCA-E
Endovascular treatment of iatrogenic subclavian arteriovenous fistula	https://www.youtube.com/watch?v=J0CvTwIrQuU
Thoracoabdominal exposure (Cavader)	https://www.youtube.com/watch?v=HEL0o7dbM_g
Open IVC filter removal	https://www.youtube.com/watch?v=GCz2L-hgHp0
Left iliofemoral DVT thrombectomy using INARI ClotTriever	https://www.youtube.com/watch?v=NjlQZuBkFAQ
Left innominate vein bypass	https://www.youtube.com/watch?v=U4mpl1W7w4M
Endovenous laser treatment (EVLT) of the greater saphenous vein	https://www.youtube.com/watch?v=WGW8BUKp76g

Mechanochemical endovenous ablation (MOCA) of the greater saphenous vein	https://www.youtube.com/watch?v=cKzT1k3Ib8k
SVC replacement	https://www.youtube.com/watch?v=2lVauaz5DY0
Leiomyosarcoma of IVC	https://www.youtube.com/watch?v=yZQKtldcG-8
Thoracic outlet syndrome	
First rib resection using an infraclavicular anterior approach	https://www.youtube.com/watch?v=cEEpEC3yTew
Creation of radiocephalic fistula	https://www.youtube.com/watch?v=JGJzKRkrzYg
Right upper extremity infected arteriovenous fistula excision	https://www.youtube.com/watch?v=eBBb2rgkjtE
Right upper extremity arteriovenous fistula revision	https://www.youtube.com/watch?v=CNEPhctwY28
Left upper extremity brachiobasilic arteriovenous fistula creation	https://www.youtube.com/watch?v=Rn5dO8_-8eo
Arteriovenous fistula (AVF) superficialization	https://www.youtube.com/watch?v=G7VG1NgVg-8
Hero graft placement	https://www.youtube.com/watch?v=soSHOvSqzlY
Tunneled dialysis catheter placement	https://www.youtube.com/watch?v=nSe4Gceg11w
Tunneled dialysis catheter removal after inadvertent placement in carotid	https://www.youtube.com/watch?v=MWptbmuzEXQ
Cephalic arch reconstruction	https://www.youtube.com/watch?v=2uSJYa8l9VE
Left cephalic vein turndown	https://www.youtube.com/watch?v=pfvxvJdcte8

References

1. Chaikof EL, Dalman RL, Eskandari MK, Jackson BM, Lee WA, Mansour MA, Mastracci TM, Mell M, Murad MH, Nguyen LL, Oderich GS, Patel MS, Schermerhorn ML, Starnes BW. The Society for Vascular Surgery practice guidelines on the care of patients with an abdominal aortic aneurysm. J Vasc Surg. 2018;67(1):2–77.e2. https://doi.org/10.1016/j.jvs.2017.10.044. PMID: 29268916.
2. Lin PH, Chandra FA, Shapiro FE, Osman BM, Urman RD, Ahn SS. The need for accreditation of office-based interventional vascular centers. Ann Vasc Surg. 2017;38:332–8. https://doi.org/10.1016/j.avsg.2016.06.010. Epub 2016 Aug 20. PMID: 27554695.
3. Jain KM, Munn J, Rummel M, Vaddineni S, Longton C. Future of vascular surgery is in the office. J Vasc Surg. 2010;51(2):509–13; discussion 513–4. PMID: 20141969. https://doi.org/10.1016/j.jvs.2009.09.056.
4. U.S. Department of Health and Human Services, Health Resources and Services Administration, National Center for Health Workforce Analysis. National and regional projections of supply and demand for surgical specialty practitioners: 2013–2025. Rockville; 2016.
5. Armstrong DW, Tobin C, Matangi MF. The accuracy of the physical examination for the detection of lower extremity peripheral arterial disease. Can J Cardiol. 2010;26(10):e346–50. https://doi.org/10.1016/s0828-282x(10)70467-0. PMID: 21165366; PMCID: PMC3006105.

6. Hemamalini MHN. Variations in the origin, course and branching pattern of dorsalis pedis artery with clinical significance. Sci Rep. 2021;11(1):1448. https://doi.org/10.1038/s41598-020-80555-z. PMID: 33446776; PMCID: PMC7809105.
7. Armstrong DG, Tan TW, Boulton AJM, Bus SA. Diabetic foot ulcers: a review. JAMA. 2023;330(1):62–75. https://doi.org/10.1001/jama.2023.10578. PMID: 37395769; PMCID: PMC10723802.
8. Adler AI, Erqou S, Lima TA, Robinson AH. Association between glycated haemoglobin and the risk of lower extremity amputation in patients with diabetes mellitus-review and meta-analysis. Diabetologia. 2010;53(5):840–9. https://doi.org/10.1007/s00125-009-1638-7. Epub 2010 Feb 3. PMID: 20127309.
9. Norgren L, Hiatt WR, Dormandy JA, Nehler MR, Harris KA, Fowkes FG, TASC II Working Group. Inter-society consensus for the management of peripheral arterial disease (TASC II). J Vasc Surg. 2007;45 Suppl S:S5–S67. https://doi.org/10.1016/j.jvs.2006.12.037. PMID: 17223489.
10. McDermott MM. Exercise training for intermittent claudication. J Vasc Surg. 2017;66(5):1612–20. https://doi.org/10.1016/j.jvs.2017.05.111. Epub 2017 Sep 2. PMID: 28874320; PMCID: PMC5747296.
11. Takagi H, Umemoto T, ALICE (All-Literature Investigation of Cardiovascular Evidence) Group. Diabetes and abdominal aortic aneurysm growth. Angiology. 2016;67(6):513–25. https://doi.org/10.1177/0003319715602414. Epub 2015 Aug 25. PMID: 26311742.
12. Powell JT, Greenhalgh RM, Ruckley CV, Fowkes FG. The UK small aneurysm trial. Ann N Y Acad Sci. 1996;800:249–51. https://doi.org/10.1111/j.1749-6632.1996.tb33320.x. PMID: 8959003.
13. Lederle FA, Johnson GR, Wilson SE, Chute EP, Littooy FN, Bandyk D, Krupski WC, Barone GW, Acher CW, Ballard DJ. Prevalence and associations of abdominal aortic aneurysm detected through screening. Aneurysm Detection and Management (ADAM) Veterans Affairs Cooperative Study Group. Ann Intern Med. 1997;126(6):441–9. https://doi.org/10.7326/0003-4819-126-6-199703150-00004. PMID: 9072929.
14. Luebke T, Brunkwall J. Risk-adjusted meta-analysis of 30-day mortality of endovascular versus open repair for ruptured abdominal aortic aneurysms. Ann Vasc Surg. 2015;29(4):845–63. https://doi.org/10.1016/j.avsg.2014.12.014. Epub 2015 Feb 26. PMID: 25725271.
15. Dua A, Kuy S, Lee CJ, Upchurch GR Jr, Desai SS. Epidemiology of aortic aneurysm repair in the United States from 2000 to 2010. J Vasc Surg. 2014;59(6):1512–7. https://doi.org/10.1016/j.jvs.2014.01.007. Epub 2014 Feb 20. PMID: 24560865.
16. Schermerhorn ML, Buck DB, O'Malley AJ, Curran T, McCallum JC, Darling J, Landon BE. Long-term outcomes of abdominal aortic aneurysm in the medicare population. N Engl J Med. 2015;373(4):328–38. https://doi.org/10.1056/NEJMoa1405778. PMID: 26200979; PMCID: PMC4532303.
17. Gurdjian ES, Webster JE, Martin FA. The place of the carotid bifurcation in the production of the stroke syndrome. Trans Am Neurol Assoc. 1955–1956;(80th Meeting):198–201. PMID: 13312043.
18. Zarins CK, Giddens DP, Bharadvaj BK, Sottiurai VS, Mabon RF, Glagov S. Carotid bifurcation atherosclerosis. Quantitative correlation of plaque localization with flow velocity profiles and wall shear stress. Circ Res. 1983;53(4):502–14. https://doi.org/10.1161/01.res.53.4.502. PMID: 6627609.
19. Barnett HJ, Taylor DW, Eliasziw M, Fox AJ, Ferguson GG, Haynes RB, Rankin RN, Clagett GP, Hachinski VC, Sackett DL, Thorpe KE, Meldrum HE, Spence JD. Benefit of carotid endarterectomy in patients with symptomatic moderate or severe stenosis. North American Symptomatic Carotid Endarterectomy Trial Collaborators. N Engl J Med. 1998;339(20):1415–25. https://doi.org/10.1056/NEJM199811123392002. PMID: 9811916.
20. Endarterectomy for asymptomatic carotid artery stenosis. Executive Committee for the Asymptomatic Carotid Atherosclerosis Study. JAMA. 1995;273(18):1421–1428. PMID: 7723155.

21. Brott TG, Hobson RW 2nd, Howard G, Roubin GS, Clark WM, Brooks W, Mackey A, Hill MD, Leimgruber PP, Sheffet AJ, Howard VJ, Moore WS, Voeks JH, Hopkins LN, Cutlip DE, Cohen DJ, Popma JJ, Ferguson RD, Cohen SN, Blackshear JL, Silver FL, Mohr JP, Lal BK, Meschia JF, CREST Investigators. Stenting versus endarterectomy for treatment of carotid-artery stenosis. N Engl J Med. 2010;363(1):11–23. https://doi.org/10.1056/NEJMoa0912321. Epub 2010 May 26. Erratum in: N Engl J Med. 2010 Jul 29;363(5):498. Erratum in: N Engl J Med. 2010 Jul 8;363(2):198. PMID: 20505173; PMCID: PMC2932446.
22. Kwolek CJ, Jaff MR, Leal JI, Hopkins LN, Shah RM, Hanover TM, Macdonald S, Cambria RP. Results of the ROADSTER multicenter trial of transcarotid stenting with dynamic flow reversal. J Vasc Surg. 2015;62(5):1227–34. https://doi.org/10.1016/j.jvs.2015.04.460. PMID: 26506270.
23. Kashyap VS, So KL, Schneider PA, Rathore R, Pham T, Motaganahalli RL, Massop DW, Foteh MI, Eckstein HH, Jim J, Leal Lorenzo JI, Melton JG. One-year outcomes after transcarotid artery revascularization (TCAR) in the ROADSTER 2 trial. J Vasc Surg. 2022;76(2):466–473.e1. https://doi.org/10.1016/j.jvs.2022.03.872. Epub 2022 Apr 2. PMID: 35381327.
24. Masuda E, Ozsvath K, Vossler J, Woo K, Kistner R, Lurie F, Monahan D, Brown W, Labropoulos N, Dalsing M, Khilnani N, Wakefield T, Gloviczki P. The 2020 appropriate use criteria for chronic lower extremity venous disease of the American Venous Forum, the Society for Vascular Surgery, the American Vein and Lymphatic Society, and the Society of Interventional Radiology. J Vasc Surg Venous Lymphat Disord. 2020;8(4):505–525.e4. https://doi.org/10.1016/j.jvsv.2020.02.001. Epub 2020 Mar 3. PMID: 32139328.
25. Enden T, Haig Y, Kløw NE, Slagsvold CE, Sandvik L, Ghanima W, Hafsahl G, Holme PA, Holmen LO, Njaastad AM, Sandbæk G, Sandset PM, CaVenT Study Group. Long-term outcome after additional catheter-directed thrombolysis versus standard treatment for acute iliofemoral deep vein thrombosis (the CaVenT study): a randomised controlled trial. Lancet. 2012;379(9810):31–8. https://doi.org/10.1016/S0140-6736(11)61753-4. Epub 2011 Dec 13. PMID: 22172244.
26. Magnuson EA, Chinnakondepalli K, Vilain K, Kearon C, Julian JA, Kahn SR, Goldhaber SZ, Jaff MR, Kindzelski AL, Herman K, Brady PS, Sharma K, Black CM, Vedantham S, Cohen DJ. Cost-effectiveness of pharmacomechanical catheter-directed thrombolysis versus standard anticoagulation in patients with proximal deep vein thrombosis: results from the ATTRACT trial. Circ Cardiovasc Qual Outcomes. 2019;12(10):e005659. https://doi.org/10.1161/CIRCOUTCOMES.119.005659. Epub 2019 Oct 8. PMID: 31592728; PMCID: PMC6788761.
27. Rayner HC, Besarab A, Brown WW, Disney A, Saito A, Pisoni RL. Vascular access results from the Dialysis Outcomes and Practice Patterns Study (DOPPS): performance against Kidney Disease Outcomes Quality Initiative (K/DOQI) clinical practice guidelines. Am J Kidney Dis. 2004;44(5 Suppl 2):22–6. https://doi.org/10.1053/j.ajkd.2004.08.007. PMID: 15486870.
28. Mills JL Sr. Vascular surgery training in the United States: a half-century of evolution. J Vasc Surg. 2008;48(6 Suppl):90S–7S; discussion 97S. PMID: 19084755. https://doi.org/10.1016/j.jvs.2008.07.090.
29. National Resident Matching Program. Results and data: 2023 main residency match®. Washington, DC: National Resident Matching Program; 2023.
30. National Resident Matching Program. Results and data: specialties matching service 2023 appointment year. Washington, DC: National Resident Matching Program; 2023.
31. ACGME ADS system. https://apps.acgme.org/connect/.

Chapter 8
So you Want to Be a Cardiothoracic Surgeon?

Islam Hasasna, Paul Rothenberg, and J. W. Awori Hayanga

Abstract Cardiothoracic surgery is an exciting and fulfilling career. There are several pathways from medical school to specialized (and subspecialized) fellowship training to consider. Here, we discuss these options as well as key recommendations to embrace opportunities for career advancement and academic growth within the field.

8.1 Introduction

The world of cardiothoracic surgery proffers a wealth of life and career experience. It is, admittedly, a long and difficult road to choose and requires careful thought and consideration. As a medical student considering going into this specialty, you can expect there will be an equal mix of challenge, adversity, and fulfillment, coupled with the opportunity to make a profound impact on the lives of your patients. The pathway from medical school to specialized fellowship training in cardiothoracic surgery proffers a variety of options for career advancement and academic growth and it is an equal responsibility to yourself and the family that the obligations of career and family are balanced with equal emphasis.

I. Hasasna
West Virginia School of Osteopathic Medicine, Lewisburg, WV, USA
e-mail: ihasasna@osteo.wvsom.edu

P. Rothenberg
West Virginia University, Morgantown, WV, USA

WVU Heart and Vascular Institute, Morgantown, WV, USA
e-mail: paul.rothenberg@hsc.wvu.edu

J. W. Awori Hayanga (✉)
Division of Thoracic Surgery, Department of Cardiovascular and Thoracic Surgery, Morgantown, WV, USA
e-mail: jeremiah.hayanga@wvumedicine.org

A. Gillis, C. B. Aarons (eds.), *A How To Guide For Medical Students*, Success in Academic Surgery, https://doi.org/10.1007/978-3-031-66011-5_8

8.2 Lay the Foundation in Medical School

Your journey toward becoming a cardiothoracic surgeon begins in medical school. Here, you will acquire the knowledge and skills necessary to excel in surgical practice while laying the groundwork for future specialization. This is also the time to identify the key mentors and sponsors that will support your career and goals for the long and short term. Key steps during this phase include:

- **Core Clerkships**: Choose rotations that will expose you to the various surgical specialties, including general surgery, cardiology, and cardiac and thoracic surgery, to gain exposure to different aspects of patient care. These experiences may help you better define goals and subspecialties.
- **Research and Scholarly Activities**: Engage in research projects related to cardiothoracic surgery, aim to co-author and publish papers, and present research findings at conferences to deepen your understanding of the field and contribute to medical knowledge and evidence-based clinical practice.
- **Extracurricular Involvement**: Enroll in surgical interest groups, participate in volunteer opportunities (both local and international), and seek mentorship from cardiothoracic surgeons to expand your knowledge and network. A mentor advocates for you in daily and ongoing ventures, meets with you, and provides career guidance in your presence. A sponsor advocates for you and supports your career in your absence, your voice in the arenas to which you do not yet have ready access but in which you are being discussed.

8.3 The Accreditation Council for Graduate Medical Education (ACGME) Training Pathway

After graduating from medical school, you will embark on a structured training pathway designed to prepare you for a career in cardiothoracic surgery. This pathway may include:

8.3.1 (Traditional Five Plus 2) General Surgery Residency

Traditionally, aspiring cardiothoracic surgeons complete a general surgery residency before pursuing specialized training. This residency program typically lasts 5–7 years and provides a broad foundation in surgical principles, patient management, and perioperative care. During this time, residents gain exposure to various surgical subspecialties and develop essential skills in surgical decision-making and technical proficiency. In the fourth year, residents apply for a residency position in cardiothoracic surgery. The clinical training for cardiothoracic surgery takes between 2 and 3 years. After completing the training successfully, residents can apply for certification from both the American Board of Surgery and the American Board of Thoracic Surgery. Some residency programs offer academic time during which the residents spend time doing research and often acquire advanced (masters) degrees in public health or clinical investigation. These opportunities may even involve grant funding through the National Institutes of Health (NIH) for example through the Training Grant (T32) process. These proffer substantial advantage in the highly competitive application for federal funding at later stages in career development.

8.3.2 *Integrated Cardiothoracic Surgery Residency*

Alternatively, the integrated cardiothoracic surgery residency offers an accelerated pathway, combining general surgery and cardiothoracic surgery training into a single program spanning 6 years. These integrated programs provide early more comprehensive exposure to the specialty, comprehensive education, and early hands-on experience in both specialties, preparing residents for the unique challenges of their chosen field. After completing an integrated residency, residents are eligible to become certified by the American Board of Thoracic Surgery, but not by the American Board of Surgery.

8.4 Subspecialty Training

Following residency training, cardiothoracic surgeons choose to pursue additional fellowship training to further specialize in specific areas within the field depending on whether they have chosen cardiac or thoracic tracks. These typically last one year and most are not ACGME affiliated. Some common subspecialties include:

8.4.1 *Transplantation Fellowship*

A transplantation fellowship focuses on the surgical management of heart and lung transplantation, including donor evaluation, organ procurement, surgical implantation, and postoperative care. Fellows gain expertise in managing transplant patients and coordinating multidisciplinary care teams to optimize outcomes.

8.4.2 Mechanical Support Fellowship

Mechanical support fellowships emphasize the use of ventricular assist devices (VADs) and extracorporeal membrane oxygenation (ECMO) to support patients with end-stage heart or lung failure. Fellows learn to manage device implantation, perioperative care, and long-term management of patients requiring mechanical circulatory support.

8.4.3 Thoracic Oncology Fellowship

A thoracic oncology fellowship focuses on the diagnosis and management of thoracic malignancies, including lung cancer, esophageal cancer, and mediastinal tumors. Fellows gain expertise in minimally invasive and robotic-assisted surgical techniques, as well as multimodal approaches to cancer treatment, including chemotherapy, radiation therapy, and immunotherapy.

8.4.4 Aortic Surgery Fellowship

An aortic surgery fellowship specializes in the diagnosis and treatment of aortic diseases, including aneurysms, dissections, and connective tissue disorders. Fellows receive comprehensive training in open and endovascular aortic surgery, as well as complex aortic root and arch reconstruction techniques.

8.4.5 Tracheal Surgery Fellowship

A tracheal surgery fellowship focuses on the management of complex tracheal and airway disorders, including stenosis, tumors, and traumatic injuries. Fellows gain expertise in tracheal reconstruction techniques, including resection, stenting, and anastomosis.

8.5 The Matching Process

When applying for medical training, most programs require the Electronic Residency Application Service (ERAS) application. Programs may occasionally use individual application forms. Each program sets its own criteria for eligibility and interview selection. After the application and interview process, the National Resident

Matching Program (NRMP) registration system uses the Registration, Ranking, and Results (R3) system to match applicants. Applicants submit rank order lists based on their true preferences through the R3 system. The NRMP then runs the matching algorithm to match applicants to their most preferred ranked choices, ensuring the best possible match. Once matched, candidates and programs enter into a binding commitment. If a candidate is not matched, they can participate in the Supplemental Offer and Acceptance Program (SOAP). To participate in the Fellowship Match, candidates must have completed the required training, meet Accrediation Council for Graduate Medical Education (ACGME®) standards for entry into graduate medical education (GME), and fulfill additional eligibility requirements from the sponsoring institution. A similar process is used to apply for CT Surgery fellowship positions in the PGY 4 year of residency.

8.6 Career Options: Private Practice vs. Academic

Upon completing fellowship training, cardiothoracic surgeons have the option to pursue careers in private practice or academic medicine. In private practice, surgeons may work in community hospitals or specialized surgical centers, providing comprehensive care to patients with cardiothoracic conditions. Private practice requires an appreciation of market forces, competition, and business management in a way that does not feature prominently in academic practice. In academic medicine, surgeons may join academic medical centers, teaching hospitals, or research institutions, where they can engage in clinical practice, research, and education. These positions often include training residents and following an academic tenure track that involves progression through assistant, associate, and full professor status.

8.7 Advanced Training: MBA and MPH

For cardiothoracic surgeons interested in expanding their skill sets and career opportunities, pursuing additional training in business administration (MBA) or public health (MPH) can be invaluable. An MBA provides insight into healthcare management, financial planning, and strategic decision-making, while an MPH offers expertise in public health policy, epidemiology, and population health management. These additional credentials can enhance leadership abilities, facilitate interdisciplinary collaboration, and open doors to executive positions in healthcare organizations.

8.8 Academic Growth and Grant Funding

For cardiothoracic surgeons interested in academic research and innovation, pursuing opportunities for academic growth and grant funding is essential. Engaging in scholarly activities, such as conducting clinical trials, publishing scientific papers, and presenting at national conferences, can enhance your academic profile and attract funding from government agencies, private foundations, and industry sponsors. Securing grant funding allows you to pursue cutting-edge research projects, develop innovative surgical techniques, and advance the field of cardiothoracic surgery.

8.9 Chart: Training Pathway Overview

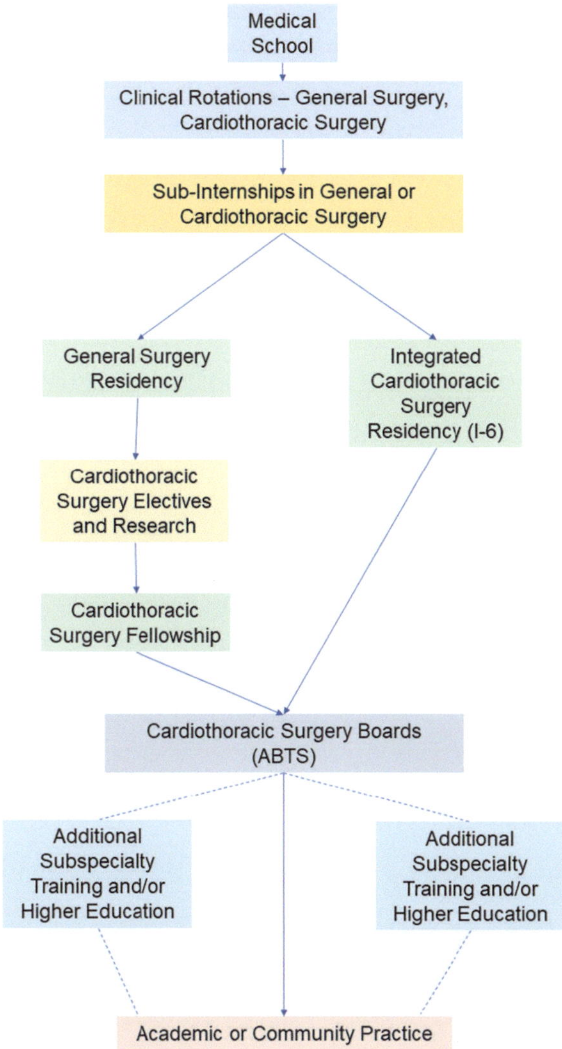

8.10 Conclusion

Becoming a cardiothoracic surgeon is a rewarding and fulfilling journey that requires dedication, perseverance, and a commitment to lifelong learning. By following a structured training pathway, pursuing subspecialty training, and embracing opportunities for career advancement and academic growth, you can embark on a fulfilling career dedicated to saving lives, advancing medical knowledge, and shaping the future of cardiothoracic surgery.

In conclusion, embrace the journey, seize every opportunity for learning and growth, and embark on a career dedicated to excellence in cardiothoracic surgery.

Chapter 9
Maximizing the Clinical Years in Medical School: A Fourth Year Student's Perspective Preparing for Surgical Training

Noah Tocci and Kennedy Jensen

Abstract The clinical years of medical school lay the foundation for the remainder of one's career in surgery. Maximizing this time provides an advantage when entering residency. Establishing systems and routines during these years for highly effective growth and learning will pay dividends during rotations and beyond as students move forward in their training. This chapter outlines several strategies for success both inside and outside of the hospital during clinical rotations and sub-internships.

9.1 Introduction

The clinical years of medical school will be some of the most challenging and rewarding times during your medical school career. As you make your transition from the classroom to the wards, you will be challenged to apply the didactic knowledge base you have established during your pre-clinical years to patients in front of you, all while integrating yourself into the unfamiliar clinical space with a variety of team structures. These challenges provide an enormous growth opportunity and set the stage for the remainder of your career as a surgeon and healthcare provider. Being intentional about maximizing your clinical time, both in the hospital and outside of the hospital, will set you apart while on your rotations. Furthermore, the habits you establish and the mindset you bring to bear on this formative time will provide you an advantage when transitioning to residency, as it establishes a strong foundation that you carry with you throughout the journey of surgical training.

N. Tocci
Department of Surgery, Cleveland, OH, USA
e-mail: toccin@ccf.org

K. Jensen (✉)
Department of Surgery, Salt Lake City, UT, USA
e-mail: Kennedy.E.Jensen@hsc.utah.edu

A. Gillis, C. B. Aarons (eds.), *A How To Guide For Medical Students*, Success in Academic Surgery, https://doi.org/10.1007/978-3-031-66011-5_9

The following chapter will describe strategies, systems, and habits to help you succeed as a medical student during clerkships, subinternships, and beyond. The chapter is divided into three sections: *Clerkships, Sub-Internships, and Off the Wards*. There is a great deal of overlap in the applicability of the recommendations within these sections, but they are organized as such for the sake of clarity. Keep in mind that this chapter is written from the perspective of two fourth year medical students, and what we offer are suggestions rather than prescriptions. Each medical student has individualized priorities and goals, and therefore, there is no one-size-fits-all when it comes to navigating a medical student's approach to a future career in surgery. That being said, we feel that the following strategies contributed significantly to our success and we hope you find them useful.

9.2 Clerkships

Clerkship rotations are one of the most valuable learning experiences of a medical education. Never again in your career will you be completely immersed in different medical specialties every month. These rotations will provide you with exposure to different patient populations, give you appreciation for different specialties, and establish a well-rounded foundation of medical knowledge that is essential for all surgeons. It is an incredible privilege to learn in a variety of clinical spaces, and each clerkship should serve as an opportunity to help you become the surgeon and physician you want to be.

Each clerkship rotation will have its own explicit established curriculum and specific learning goals. For example, you will be expected to master the core principles of heart failure management while on your internal medicine rotation, while suturing and managing early postoperative patients will be key objectives of your surgical rotation. However, your clinical time will also expose you to the so-called "hidden curriculum" of clinical medical education [1]. Beyond learning the basics to your core clerkship rotations, your rotations will expose you to a variety of clinical settings, team structures, leadership styles and aspects of multidisciplinary, interprofessional care. By experiencing diverse approaches to interpersonal dynamics and patient care, medical students have the opportunity to learn and grow well beyond the confines of curricular structure.

The variety of opportunities during your clinical time can be engaging and at other times overwhelming, particularly when juggling preparation for shelf examinations, extracurricular commitments, and family or personal responsibilities. Here, we recommend some approaches for time spent both inside and outside of the hospital that have helped other students maximize their clerkship experiences and feel well prepared when it comes time for exams.

9.2.1 Learning on the Wards: Making the Most of your Time in the Hospital

Particularly on early clerkship rotations, learning on the wards may feel chaotic and piecemeal at best. Unlike most traditional preclinical medical education, which has discrete time set for didactic lectures or small group guided learning, in the clinical space there are rarely scheduled learning objectives for a given day or week. Clinical medicine is fluid and dynamic. Learning for medical students, residents and even attendings happens in real time, as well as during your "off hours." While there might be chalk-talks given during your rotation, or impromptu discussions over a challenging topic, most clinical time is spent caring for patients and documenting this care. Therefore, it is imperative to push yourself to take ownership of your education and be intentional about your learning goals. You will be the one to set these learning objectives as you navigate your clinical rotations. The skills of building your own mini curriculum and learning goals are what establish you as an adult learner, and will pay off both in the short-term (exam scores, rotation feedback, etc.), and long-term (established good practice habits that will benefit patient care, initiating a growth-oriented mindset that will carry on throughout your career). While this can be challenging and demanding, this is something you owe to yourself along this journey through surgical training, as well as for your future patients.

9.2.2 Goal Setting

In order to maximize your time during the seeming chaos of clinical medicine, use goal setting to your advantage. Spend a few minutes before every rotation to write down your overarching goals for the clerkship. Include both content goals (i.e. master the workup for an acid base disturbance) and skill-based goals (i.e. practice placing a peripheral IV). As you continue to advance and improve your knowledge base and comfort in the clinical space, also establish some nonclinical competencies (professionalism, interpersonal and communication skills, and self-reflection) you hope to achieve as these have been shown to correlate with future success in residency and are highly valued by residency programs [2, 3].

While making the initial list of goals is great, draw from and add to this list throughout your rotation to constantly further your education as you gain more skills and knowledge. Use the same exercise, at a smaller scale, on a weekly and daily basis. While each person has their own approach to making goals—excel spreadsheets, notebooks, outlining them as SMART goals (Specific, Measurable, Achievable, Realistic and Time-limited)—the method is less important than the practice. Having the committed practice of establishing your goals will provide a guide for future growth and an inspiring retrospective log of how much you have achieved over the course of your clinical time.

When setting your goals, it can be challenging to know where to start. Identifying your knowledge gaps and creating a realistic plan to fill in those gaps requires time and self-reflection. In thinking about your learning goals, make sure that you are conscious about how you will aim to obtain these goals, and what resources you will need to achieve them. One helpful model in thinking about achieving learning goals in medical education is the Challenge Point Framework [4]. Guadagnoli et al. describes this framework and its usefulness in medical education as tasks are placed on a continuum of the benefit obtained from achieving the learning goal and the level of challenge required to complete this task (Fig. 9.1). There is an optimal space where the learning benefit remains high and the challenge facilitates skill retention, while not diminishing the educational benefit due to undue stress associated with the task. This can be a helpful model when trying to organize your goals during a clerkship. As you continue to progress in your knowledge-base or technical ability, your threshold for challenge will inherently change, and goals must be constantly adjusted as you change positions along the learning curve.

Creating more intentionality around your learning on the wards and generating concrete learning objectives will help you focus and get more out of your time on service. Additionally, you will frequently be asked by the attending or resident on your team what you want to get out of a rotation. Showing that you have taken the time to think about what you hope to achieve will show preparedness, maturity, and readiness for growth, all of which are essential in becoming a contributing member of your clinical team.

9.2.3 Accountability

At a smaller scale, use your clinical experiences to generate learning goals for you to take home. Given that most of the time spent in the clinical space will be focused on providing clinical care, aim to identify three things every day that you want to read more about. This should be separate from, and in addition to, the time you spend studying for shelf exams. Let your patients be your guide; learn about their problems and the rationale behind their management. This is especially true if you see a medical comorbidity on their problem list that is not the focus of their hospitalization. This is a great way to broaden your knowledge base and stimulate your curiosity.

Hold yourself accountable for this learning, whether you can spare five minutes or thirty. Use resources that match your learning style. Doing this daily will help you feel more prepared for rounds. It may feel scattered at first, but this type of learning compounds; starting early will serve you well as you go forward in your medical career. Each time you need to revisit a topic, it will allow you to dig into one more layer of depth, and you will retain a broader framework of knowledge to carry forward into the future. Furthermore, this exercise of consistently reading about a few new things will serve you well long after your rotations, in residency and beyond.

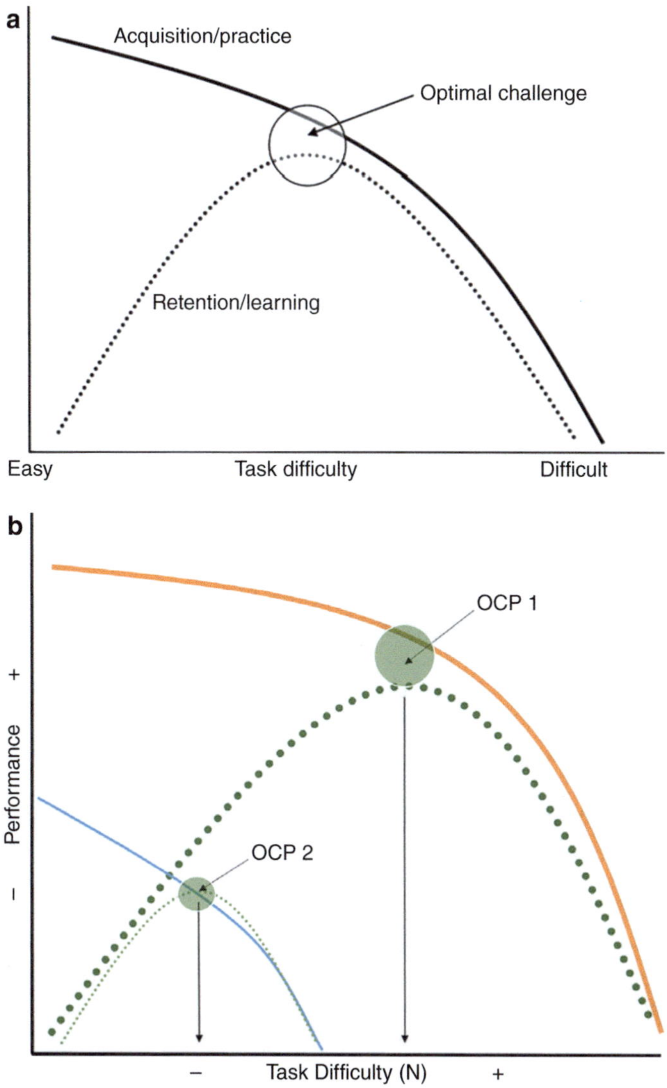

Fig. 9.1 Challenge point framework schematic illustrating how optimal challenge of a given task can provide retention of learning. In both A and B, the X axis demonstrates task difficulty, with the Y axis representing performance on a task. The dashed-lined arc represents retention and learning of the skill. (**a**) Maximum learning occurs at the "Optimal Challenge Point," where the task is difficult enough to be engaging but not so challenging that it becomes unobtainable. (**b**) Growth over time, as the change from Optimal Challenge Point 1 (OCP 1) to Optimal Challenge Point 2 (OCP 2) demonstrates the continuum across which skill acquisition changes based on where learners find themselves on the learning curve, outlining a natural progression of graded difficulty required to progress along skill acquisition. (Schematic used with permission from Dr. Mark Guadagnoli)

Given the time constraints of clinical medicine, it is possible that team members will prepare quick talks on a disease or the management of a condition and give an impromptu discussion on it. This is an outstanding learning opportunity. If a member of the team asks you to prepare a 'chalk talk' for a topic, use it as a chance to shine. While it can feel daunting or a nuisance at times, developing the skills to prepare a quick talk and extract salient teaching points on a challenging topic will further your learning transfer to other aspects of your academic career (i.e. oral presentations, discussion of new research).

9.2.4 Immersion in Rotations

Recognizing your knowledge gaps and striving to fill them is part of a larger mindset which is perhaps the most valuable piece of advice we can offer: go all in on each of your clerkship rotations. Even if you have already decided on a future career in surgery, treat every rotation as if it is your one chance to learn everything about that field that you possibly can. This will certainly pay off in your clerkship evaluations and for your future patients. Outside of the OR, surgeons are doctors. Though the best surgeons consult appropriately, they manage a wide variety of medical problems independently and you will undoubtedly manage patients with many of the nonsurgical conditions you encounter during your clerkships. Additionally, having the basic understanding of who to turn to and when to turn to someone for help comes with a broad knowledge base and familiarity with your own limitations. This is essential to becoming a good resident as well as a good surgeon. Rotations are likely the last time you will be immersed in another specialty and have dedicated time to learn about it; make the most of it. Keep your mindset undifferentiated, take ownership over your patients, and show up to each rotation as if it might be your future path. This will help your patients directly when you know how to assist in their care and provide holistic quality care. This will also help your patients indirectly as you are able to speak the language necessary for effective, high-quality multidisciplinary care coordination.

9.2.5 Establishing Expectations While on a Rotation

In addition to setting your own goals and objectives on a rotation, it is also important to check in with your team regarding their expectations of you and discern what they hope you will gain from the rotation. Each rotation will have specific expectations for medical students that are established by the rotation leadership. Beyond that, the senior resident or attending education lead for the service will also have expectations on how you will integrate into the team structure. Make sure you reach out to this person before the rotation and, if possible, have a discussion about expectations with your own personal learning objectives ready. This will help clarify what the team will want and need from you, and how you can be a helpful member of the team who advances patient care. This will also establish what you can do to be prepared and set yourself up to succeed and get the most out of the rotation.

9.2.6 Feedback

Feedback is an invaluable tool for personal and professional growth during clinical rotations. Approach feedback as a constructive learning opportunity and a pathway to refining your clinical skills rather than a critique. Cultivate a growth-oriented mindset to accelerate your progress; focus on areas for improvement and avoid viewing advice as reflections on your potential ability [4, 5]. Remember that each feedback exchange is composed of two components: how it is delivered, and how it is received. If you receive feedback that is extremely constructive and productive but you fail to act upon it, then the feedback loses its value. Separate your emotional response to the initial feedback and remind yourself that the feedback is intended to help you improve.

Try to initiate conversations with your preceptors and supervisors, expressing your genuine interest in improvement. Remember, feedback often starts with self-assessment on your performance, so be prepared to reflect on how you performed and what you think you need to improve on. Use your own self-reflection of your performance to guide the feedback discussion. If you believe you need to improve in one area and your preceptor thinks you should focus on another, that is valuable information. Feedback can help drive a new set of goals and objectives and steer you on the path of continual improvement. The self-reflection and proactiveness of asking for feedback demonstrates self-awareness and eagerness for improvement, both of which are characteristics of a mature learner and are essential for a growth mindset.

While you may be eager to understand how you are doing, be thoughtful about the timing of these conversations. Take the schedule and additional time commitments of your preceptors into account, and be mindful of the time and energy it takes to give feedback. Always read the room; asking someone for feedback when a patient is clinically deteriorating or during a critical portion of a case is not the best time to get focused feedback. Be proactive and considerate when choosing when to request feedback.

Be specific in your requests for feedback, focusing on particular aspects of your performance or areas in which you want to improve. If you are given an opportunity to demonstrate action on prior feedback, circle back with the preceptor and ask about how you have improved and what you could continue to work on.

Finally, cultivate an attitude of open mindedness and gratitude even in the face of feedback you may disagree with. Seek to find the helpful pieces of what is said and use those to help you continue to grow and evolve as a future surgeon. While hearing blunt feedback is hard, the practice of self-awareness in those situations and mindfulness promote grit and resilience. With the right mindset and self-talk, the prospect of tough feedback can be transformed into an opportunity to grow and demonstrate improvement the next time you find yourself in that situation or work with that preceptor.

9.3 Excelling on the Surgery Clerkship

9.3.1 Rounds

For medical students interested in surgery, excelling on the surgery clerkship will help set you apart from your peers and establish a foundation for success on your future subinternships. While all of the general principles of clerkship performance still apply, there are a few differences that set the surgery clerkship apart. Rounds will likely start earlier in the morning, will be faster paced than rounds on other services, and may occur more than once a day depending on the service and patients. Be extremely observant during your time on rounds and see what your residents do. Keen observation will allow you to get up to speed quickly, understand the pace of rounds, and know what to focus your presentations on.

Integrating into the flow of rounds is essential to make you an active participant rather than mere observer. Arrive early with plenty of time to pre-round on your patients. For medical students, pre-rounds typically include looking through your patient's chart to gather objective data as well as going to physically see the patient to gather subjective data and perform a physical exam. When chart-checking, in addition to gathering relevant data (lab results, scans, vitals, intake and outputs, etc.), it is important to understand the details of the patient's care for the preceding 24 hours and its contribution to the arc of their overall hospital course. The methodology of chart checking is very individualized and service-specific, and describing how to do so is beyond the scope of this section. However, it is always a good idea to ask your teammates how they look through a chart to understand the pertinent parts of a patient's history for that particular service.

When pre-rounding on a patient, your goal is to get a sense of how the past 24 hours have gone for them including pain control, progress towards discharge milestones (voiding, eating, ambulating, discharge needs and supplies secured), and symptoms relevant to their pre- and post-operative diagnoses. Nursing staff are great allies, both as a medical student and during residency. When you are pre-rounding, asking a nurse's perspective of how the past shift has gone and any concerns they have about the patient can be a great way to close care gaps. While your residents likely will not physically go see patients before rounding as a team, this is an important opportunity for you to provide information about the patient to the team that they otherwise might not know. Your residents will not be able to spend as much time hearing directly from the patient. This will benefit your learning, as patient stories assist in learner retention, morale, as well as improve patient experience.

During rounds, keep your presentations concise and center the overall theme of your presentation around the patient's perioperative course. Be ready to participate in bedside patient care activities including dressing changes, drain management, and suture or staple removal. This requires anticipation; having the necessary supplies on hand will help you assist with these tasks and continue the flow of rounds.

9.3.2 The Operating Room

Perhaps the greatest distinguishing feature of the Surgery Clerkship is experience in the operating room. The operating room is a unique environment with a steep learning curve; sterility and aseptic technique, team dynamics, closed-loop communication, and technical skills all present new challenges. During your first experiences in the operating room, it can be difficult to know how best to be involved and not be in the way. When in doubt, ask. For the most part, people would much prefer you ask permission than for forgiveness. This applies to how best to stay sterile, how to get gowned and gloved, what is clean vs dirty in a case etc. That being said, everyone has had a "first time" in the OR, and mistakes happen. If a mistake is made, it can be fixed as long as you speak up so that others can help you, and the operating room can continue the task at hand. Once you get more comfortable with your surroundings, and all of the dynamics in the operating room, you will see all of the intricate work it takes to ensure an operation runs smoothly and safely.

Before you step into the operating room, there is plenty that can be learned ahead of time to optimize your experience intraoperatively. Before the case starts, your preparation should focus on the patient and the procedure. With regards to the patient, you should understand their history, similarly to how you would gather information for patients in clinic or on rounds. Know their past medical history, past surgical history, medications (anticoagulation, or immunosuppressives), allergies (if they have an antibiotic, contrast, or adhesive allergy that might affect how a patient is managed during a surgery), as well as the relevant work up to date (labs, imaging, diagnostic testing, etc.). The patient's work up will be driven by the pathophysiology of the disease, and it is a great way to expand your knowledge base, recognize patterns, and develop frameworks for common disease processes. Though this may seem like a lot of information, framing it as a larger narrative that answers the question "How did this patient get to the operating room?" will help you remember key details. This strategy acts as a memory hook for key information and also helps maintain the perspective that the patient underneath the drapes is a person with their own story.

The second aspect of preparation for the operating room is learning about the procedure itself. First, understanding what surgery the patient is having is all contextualized by their history and workup, as described above, so above all else, know the patient. Second, it will be helpful to read about the indications, contraindications, alternatives (other surgical approaches or less invasive measures), and possible complications of the procedure. Along with this comes knowing the basic steps of the procedure. Helpful methods to understand a procedure can include reading about it, watching annotated videos, attempting to write the steps out yourself, and drawing your own pictures. While the steps are an essential part of understanding the procedure, having a good grasp of the anatomy is principally important, as it drives the reasoning behind the steps of the procedure. Think of the anatomy layer by layer within each step. Anatomical and surgical atlases are very helpful.

Once you have a good grasp of the patient and the procedure, the next aspect is how to effectively participate in the operating room. While it can feel like a lot of observing, there are invaluable ways for you to be involved in the surgery. Helping the patient get positioned and prepared for surgery is key. It will allow for a smooth transition in the case and will not go unnoticed by the OR staff. Take each opportunity you have to be hands-on with a patient; if a patient needs a foley placed, ask to help place one. If the anesthesia staff is willing, observe intubation, IV access and line placement, and be involved when appropriate. Assisting in patient comfort is another large impact that students can have. Going into surgery can feel overwhelming and vulnerable for patients. Making sure to keep a patient warm with blankets, talking with them or explaining what is going on around them, and keeping them modest and covered when possible are ways that students can positively impact patient care.

While the case is underway, your role may feel relatively limited at times but is often quite important. Retraction is a common medical student role, and while this may not be the most thrilling part of the case, it is essential and integral to the case moving forward. The same is true for driving a laparoscopic/thoracoscopic camera. Maintaining exposure and a clear view of the operative field are critical and often under appreciated. When invited, palpate key structures or excised specimens, and appreciate complex anatomy as residents and attendings talk through essential aspects of the case. As you become more comfortable with the staff and the procedure, it can be appropriate to anticipate portions of the operation such as getting the suture scissors ready when a stitch or tie is used, or using the suction for smoke evacuation or fluid clearance. You can also offer to bring specimens down to the pathology lab if there is a need for frozen sampling. This is also a great learning experience to see the other side of what happens from specimens extracted during surgery. Oftentimes the pathologist and pathology lab technicians are eager to show you the process and it can be a valuable learning opportunity. All of these are good ways to ensure you are active during a case, and integrated into the team.

When the case is wrapping up, closure can become your moment to shine. Ensuring you have practiced tying square knots, running subcuticular stitches, or deep dermal stitches for laparoscopic port sites can be a great way to show off your technical skills. Take pride in closing incisions and remind yourself that the closure of the incision is often the only indication to the patient that the surgery occurred. If you are working on a closure with a resident, it is a great time to have them observe your technical skills and provide feedback, as well as debriefing questions that arose during the case.

Once the case is complete and closure is done, help clean up any bodily fluid or irrigation that got around the drapes during the surgery, move the patient off the operating table into a hospital bed, get them warm blankets for recovery, and go with them to post anesthesia care unit (PACU). Pay close attention to resident sign-out in PACU. Sign-out may vary depending on the culture of the institution, but it typically includes a one-liner about the patient, what operation was done, if there were any complications, and then any instructions for the recovery team such as post operative labs, or discharge instructions if it is a same day surgery. Listening to these sign-outs can be helpful for your learning, and try to practice in your head what you would want to sign-out to a recovery nurse after a patient's surgery. Additionally, post operative checks on your patient will further your learning and provide continuity of care. The clinical status of surgical patients often evolves quickly, and taking ownership of that patient by making time to check on them as if you were the one primarily responsible for their overall care is a practice and mind-set that will serve you well.

9.3.3 Evaluation

Though each institution has its own system for student evaluation, your performance on both your surgery clerkship and subinternships are considered an important component of your residency application package. Asking for frequent feedback will be helpful for improving throughout your rotations so that your final evaluations are not a surprise. Though there may be a tendency to fixate on your technical performance in the OR, keep in mind that your evaluation will be based more heavily on your work ethic, contributions as a team member, knowledge base, and preparation for cases.

While this section has largely focused on succeeding during your rotation, just know that success takes on many different forms. Additionally, getting Honors during your rotation does not mean that you will or will not be successful as you progress through your training. Continue to focus on the holistic picture of ensuring you are learning and staying active in patient care, and the "grades" and comments on your performance will be sure to follow.

9.3.4 Studying During Clinical Years: Honing your Study Strategy in your Limited Time

It will rarely feel like you have sufficient time during clinical years, so maximizing the limited time you have becomes essential. There are a few strategies that can help you study effectively and efficiently.

Do your best to find a system that works for you and stick to it. This may differ from what works for your classmates; what matters is that you have identified what is effective for you and that you practice it consistently. When designing your routine, draw on the systems you developed during preclinical years. Now is not the time to reinvent the wheel; while you may need to make slight changes or accommodations to your approach, do not try to start from scratch. If practice questions have worked for you before, continue using practice questions; if flashcards are how you learn best, continue to use flashcards. Although you should be dedicating time to reading more about what you've encountered in the hospital, when it comes to studying material for clerkships and the U.S.M.L.E. Step 2 exam, use the strategies that have worked for you in the past.

During clinical rotations, time limitations will make it even more important that you stay organized. Use a study schedule and set concrete goals for what you plan to accomplish on a daily basis. Use habits to your advantage. Showing up consistently will give you better results in the long run than studying for hours in the week leading up to the exam. While you should stick with your plan and schedule each day, recognize that the way you achieve your daily study goal may need to remain flexible. For example, if you are consistently finishing clinic later in the day, and need to prepare for the following day right after, you may need to shift some studying to the morning or find additional pockets of time to fit some studying in. It is okay to pick up a topic or a question block and have to revisit it later in the day. Being able to balance going from studying to other tasks simulates life as a resident and will hone your skills of refocusing on important tasks at hand.

9.4 Subinternships

Subinternships differ from clerkships primarily in the amount of responsibility you are awarded and expectations for your performance. The primary objective is for you to gain more experience in your field of choice and grow to function at the level of an intern. When surveying program directors on the largest opportunities for medical student growth, the majority chose sub-internships as a challenging clinical experience that provides students an opportunity for development [2, 6]. Concretely, this usually entails following a larger portion of the patients on the service's list, being prepared to present patients in the morning, writing progress notes, taking care of floor work (pulling drains, dressing changes, following up on afternoon labs), and taking a more active role in the operating room if given the chance. While subinternships might be more floor-based work, get excited at the opportunity to make an impact on your service and know the ins-and-outs of your patients' care. Strive to lighten the load of the intern on service and be a set of helping hands whenever needed. Each day will present its own challenges; take it all in stride and find more ways that you can aid the team in a learner-appropriate fashion.

Although there are typically no formal examinations, continue to invest time reading and studying on a daily basis. Rather than practice questions or flashcards, this will likely take the form of prepping for cases in the OR and clinic or reading more about the pathology of your patients.

Subinternships at other institutions, commonly referred to as "away rotations," represent an important opportunity for fourth year medical students to explore potential residency programs. In many ways, these rotations represent an extended interview at a program of interest. By working directly with residents and faculty at another institution, participating in an away rotation is the most straightforward way to provide a potential program with a sense of how good a fit you may be. Away rotations are also an invaluable opportunity for you to assess if the program would serve your individual goals and career objectives. There is no better way to see a program from the inside and get a sense of its values and culture. When rotating at a different program you will be exposed to the inner workings of the program. Resident-resident, resident-staff and staff-staff interactions are all good things to keep an eye on that might only become apparent while on your sub-internship. Additionally, seeing the case volume and case-mix provides valuable insight into the type of environment you hope to train in.

During an away rotation, you should be intentional about getting to know faculty members at that institution. Though it is essential that you remain a good team player and do your part helping with work on the floor, remember that attendings will play a large role in evaluating you and whether they want you to be a part of their training program. Furthermore, even if you realize that you are not interested in the program, opportunities come through people. Away rotations are a chance to broaden your network of connections. Meet as many faculty and residents as you can; you never know when you may stumble across a future mentor, appealing career path, or interesting research endeavor.

One logistical consideration to keep in mind is the financial burden of participating in away rotations. Particularly when it comes to housing and transportation, away rotations can be financially taxing. Try to plan ahead and work with financial aid to ensure you've taken out adequate student loans. Some students sublet their housing at their home institution to offset the cost of a short-term rental in another city, but this requires proactive coordination.

9.5 Off the Wards

9.5.1 Extracurriculars—The Broader View

While your clinical time will be busy and filled with work that centers on your rotations, life outside of the hospital continues as well. During your clinical years, extracurricular activities will necessarily take a backseat. However, you should continue to engage in enrichment outside of your clinical education that motivates and inspires you and makes you feel more like a complete person. It is essential that you evaluate your commitments critically prior to starting your clerkship rotations. You will have less unscheduled time than the preclinical portion of your education, and it is easy to overestimate the amount you will be able to accomplish. As is touched on in the upcoming section, Extracurriculars—The Broader View, keep in mind that the quality and depth with which you engage in activities outside your formal education is more important than the sheer number of responsibilities you choose to take on. Err on the side of minimizing the number of extracurricular obligations you have before starting rotations so that you can focus on your clinical learning and responsibilities.

9.5.2 Research

For medical students interested in a future career in academic surgery, engaging meaningfully in research will contribute to your professional development, deepen your understanding of the field, strengthen your application to residency, and provide exposure to valuable mentors. However, particularly during clinical years, balancing extracurricular research and clinical responsibilities is challenging and requires thoughtful organization, clear communication, and careful time management.

The initiation into research can come organically, or through thoughtful outreach. Whether you choose to speak with professors after didactic sessions, set up meetings with clinical faculty members to discuss their research, or simply reach out via email to staff whose work interests you, you will likely need to put yourself out there to find good opportunities. Additionally, upper class medical students might be able to provide guidance and hand off projects that they have found fruitful. While wet lab research is a traditional path, there are a multitude of alternatives (translational research, clinical outcomes, medical/surgical education, healthcare delivery science, quality improvement, health equity, etc.). Seek out the research questions that are most interesting to you; the type of research you do matters less than what you will get out of it.

When considering your research options, be very honest with yourself and your mentor. Will the benefit of being involved in the work translate to time well spent on the project? Consider the ease of publishing the work, the content of the work (is it in your field of interest), the learning potential of the content, and the mentor relationship that would spring from this experience. There is no way to answer these questions with certainty, but think through these aspects when choosing a research project. Also, when in a research project, work with your research mentors to establish clear priorities and realistic schedules to accomplish your research goals. As much as possible, build flexibility and adaptability into those timelines, recognizing that your clinical demands will fluctuate.

9.5.3 Volunteering

Taking time to volunteer outside of your normal academic routine can be very fulfilling. Volunteer opportunities often allow time to slow down, connect with a specific patient population or community that means a lot to you, and recharge your emotional battery. Volunteering your time to help and support others can also give you a refreshed perspective of why you chose to pursue medicine. As stated above, ensure that your volunteering opportunities are meaningful to you and that you are conscious about your time constraints when making commitments.

9.5.4 Leadership Opportunities

Finding opportunities to lead during your medical education will serve as a foundation for leadership as a surgeon. Leadership skills are essential as a surgeon, both inside and outside of the operating room. Within the OR, the surgeon must orchestrate the coordinated movements of numerous team members to ensure a procedure runs efficiently. Outside of the OR, surgeons lead multidisciplinary teams in providing quality care for patients, conducting research, and guiding department-level and hospital-wide administrative initiatives. Therefore, it is important to find opportunities that will help nurture the leadership skills necessary to become the future surgeon leader you hope to become.

Investments compound over time. Whenever possible, stick with the organizations or initiatives you joined early in your medical school career and continue to grow as a leader within that structure. Seek out opportunities that will allow you to grow and learn new ways to communicate and interact with others. There are a multitude of leadership styles, and although surgery often connotes a more forward, controlling style, this is not always the most effective. The Multifactorial Leadership Questionnaire created by Bass and Avolio separate leadership styles into two categories, Transactional and Transformational [7]. A Transactional leadership style is a task-oriented approach in which the leader assigns team members responsibilities and determines team goals and outcomes that should be achieved. There are many pros and cons related to transactional leadership, as it can facilitate task completion, but it can also facilitate team member burnout. A Transformational leadership style works on the basis of influencing team members towards a collective goal. The emphasis is typically placed on a more Socratic method to heighten the performance of the surrounding team members while working to develop the individualized skills of those members [7]. A Transformational leadership approach has been shown to improve team cohesion, facilitate free flowing communication, and establish a culture of improvement. Building a culture where all team members are compelled to speak up for the common mission of delivering high quality care to the patient inside and outside of the OR will ultimately improve patient outcomes [7].

9.5.5 Mentorship

Mentorship represents a critical component of a career in academic surgery, and you should continue to invest in these relationships throughout your clinical education. Be intentional about investing in formal mentorship relationships that can provide career guidance. Good mentors will be the most valuable resource in helping you navigate a difficult path. You are often unaware of what you do not know until you gather more contextual learning or perspective; this is where mentors truly make their impact on budding surgeons. A mentor who is willing to tease out your blind spots and find opportunities to bridge a knowledge or perception gap is someone who is truly invested in your growth and development. Mentors are essential in the development of trainees becoming self-directed learners who will optimize their experiences. There are many turns in this journey that require guidance. From the undergraduate medical education path, residency applications, to the ultimate decision of pursuing a surgical subspecialty, the opportunities for mentors' involvement are nearly endless.

Find role models in the clinical environment who you admire and choose the aspects of their practice style that you want to emulate as a physician. You can learn and grow from every practitioner you interact with; be perceptive as to what you want to take with you and what you want to leave behind. While most of this section has focused on mentorship in the clinical and professional space, when appropriate, mentors can be critical to navigating collisions between personal and professional life challenges as well.

9.5.6 Balance, Community and Connection

In addition to creating systems to help you succeed academically on your rotations, be thoughtful in building personal systems that provide enough balance to keep things sustainable for you. Keep the components of your life that are essential to your well-being sacred. In addition to carving out time for loved-ones outside of medicine, many students find peer connection invaluable during clinical years [8, 9]. Few individuals will understand the trials and frustrations of your clinical education as well as your classmates and fellow students who have shared those experiences. Lean on your community when you need to, and support your peers when they are struggling. It is easy to get caught up in all there is to complete along your journey through surgical training, but keep in mind this is less about the destination and more about the experience of navigating your own path. Just as it is essential for you to study and work hard on your rotations, it is equally important to take a breath and enjoy the people and activities that help recharge you emotionally. Taking time to care for yourself will make you a better form of you and therefore a better surgeon.

9.6 Conclusion

The clinical years of your medical education will be some of the most exhausting and fulfilling. Continue to push yourself for growth within the clinical and non-clinical spaces, with mentors serving to guide you along your path. Nurturing the right systems, mindset, and preparation will help you make the most of this invaluable learning experience. Enjoy this path of developing into the surgeon you hope to become, and use each opportunity as a way to grow personally and professionally.

References

1. Hafferty FW, Franks R. The hidden curriculum, ethics teaching, and the structure of medical education. Acad Med. 1994;69(11):861–71.
2. Lyss-Lerman P, Teherani A, Aagaard E, Loeser H, Cooke M, Harper GM. What training is needed in the fourth year of medical school? Views of residency program directors. Acad Med. 2009;84(7):823–9.
3. Langdale LA, Schaad D, Wipf J, Marshall S, Vontver L, Scott CS. Preparing graduates for the first year of residency: are medical schools meeting the need? Acad Med. 2003;78(1):39–44.
4. Guadagnoli M, Morin MP, Dubrowski A. The application of the challenge point framework in medical education. Med Educ. 2012;46(5):447–53.
5. Dweck CS. Mindset: the new psychology of success. Random House; 2006.
6. Avolio BJ, Bass BM. Multifactor leadership questionnaire (TM). Menlo Park: Mind Garden; 2004.
7. Hu YY, Parker SH, Lipsitz SR, Arriaga AF, Peyre SE, Corso KA, Roth EM, Yule SJ, Greenberg CC. Surgeons' leadership styles and team behavior in the operating room. J Am Coll Surg. 2016;222(1):41–51.
8. Abrams MP, Salzman J, Espina Rey A, Daly K. Impact of providing peer support on medical students' empathy, self-efficacy, and mental health stigma. Int J Environ Res Public Health. 2022;19(9):5135.
9. Malau-Aduli BS, Roche P, Adu M, Jones K, Alele F, Drovandi A. Perceptions and processes influencing the transition of medical students from pre-clinical to clinical training. BMC Med Educ. 2020;20(1):1–3.

Part II
Navigating the Residency Application Process

Chapter 10
Developing a Competitive Residency Application

Jessica Zagory, Vikas Dudeja, and Tania K. Arora

Abstract Applications to surgical residency can seem like an arms race. It can be overwhelming trying to assess whether your application is competitive. Mentors and program directors (PD) are a helpful resource, and medical students should meet with them once the decision is made to pursue a surgical specialty. Ideally, you will have experiences and accomplishments from your pre-clinical years that will enhance your application; however, we see many successful applicants who realize late in their third year that they want to pursue a surgical career and need to bolster their curriculum vitae (CV) in a short amount of time.

Fortunately, there is no one-size-fits-all or "ideal" applicant to surgery, and programs screen and select residents based on factors that may be biased (Lipman JM, J Grad Med Educ. 15:652–668, 2023). As challenging as it may be, try not to compare yourself to your peers. Focus on your strengths, what makes you unique, what you will contribute to a program, and what you can do before the application is due. The current chapter will give you guidance to help you become the best applicant you can be. Here, we outline a framework that can organize your approach to developing a competitive residency application for a future in academic surgery.

J. Zagory
Louisiana State University Health New Orleans, Children's Hospital New Orleans, New Orleans, LA, USA
e-mail: jzagor@lsuhsc.edu

V. Dudeja (✉) · T. K. Arora
Division of Surgical Oncology, Department of Surgery, Birmingham, AL, USA
e-mail: vdudeja@uabmc.edu; tkarora@uabmc.edu

A. Gillis, C. B. Aarons (eds.), *A How To Guide For Medical Students*, Success in Academic Surgery, https://doi.org/10.1007/978-3-031-66011-5_10

10.1 Develop an Outline

Congratulations on deciding on a career in surgery! Whether you are in your first year of medical school or near the end of third year, starting by creating a timeline can help organize tasks and to ensure that your application is submitted on time. A common approach is to work backwards from the Electronic Residency Application System (ERAS) review date, which is typically at the end of September. We encourage you to read carefully through "Applying to Residencies with the ERAS System" on the Association of American Medical Colleges (AAMC) website (https://students-residents.aamc.org/applying-residencies-eras/applying-residencies-eras-system). If you are applying to a non-ERAS residency (ophthalmology and plastic surgery in the San Francisco Match or the American Urological Association for urology residency), the same information is available on their respective websites.

As applicant numbers and the number of programs applied to per applicant increase, it becomes increasingly important to have a complete application submitted by the review date. This date is when residency programs may begin reviewing MyERAS applications and Medical School Performance Evaluations (MSPE) in the Program Director's WorkStation (PDWS). A program may utilize the completeness of your application as a filter to interview as it can be a surrogate for your ability to be timely with tasks. Therefore, having a complete application is crucial to maximize your interview invites, and completing the application after PD has begun to download applications may cause you to lose the opportunity to be screened for an interview.

Admittedly, all aspects of your application are not solely within your control. Letters of recommendation (LOR) from mentors, PDs, and chairs are also considered as part of your application on the PDWS. As this is also a very busy time for surgeons who are likely writing multiple LOR, giving a 2- to 4-week buffer for them can be helpful. Provide letter writers with as much information as possible (draft of your personal statement, CV, USMLE statements, unofficial transcripts). Some will need to get to know you in a short period of time. Additionally, some mentors may ask you to write a "dream letter of recommendation." However, even if they don't, this is your opportunity to reflect on your strengths, highlight any patient interactions or experiences on service, and make sure that there are some personal points to the LOR. This should be seen as an opportunity rather than doing the work for your letter writer. Ultimately, a personal goal of having your application and LOR *uploaded 1 week early* will minimize last minute stressors.

10.2 Get Feedback on your Competitiveness

A review of surgical residency application cycles from 2017 to 2021 showed that the mean number of applications per applicant increased 32% during this period [1]. As more applicants cast a wider net, meeting with mentors and gathering advice on where to apply and interview will decrease your cost and effort. It is a good idea to keep a few concepts in mind:

- Schedule a meeting with the PD/Associate PD (APD) once you have committed to a surgical career, and again over the summer before your fourth year.
- Be prepared for this meeting. Have your CV and personal statement drafts available for review. Be ready to discuss why you are choosing surgery and what your career goals may be.
- Develop insight into what type of learning environment may be best for you. This may include size of program, type of hospital setting, geographic area, university versus community setting, and number of and type of fellowships at the institution.

Your mentors may give you feedback on areas in your application that may not be as strong as other areas. Consider in the time you have left what meaningful additions you can add to make yourself more competitive. These efforts should ideally be areas where you genuinely have passion; however, this is not always possible to do on a short timeline. Ask if there are opportunities for abstract or manuscript submissions such as invited reviews, posters of case reports, or research projects, attending surgery meetings (especially if they are local) even if you are not presenting, or participating in a committee. If scientific research is not your passion, consider non-peer reviewed publications. Many surgical societies (Association for Academic Surgeons (AAS), Association of Women Surgeons (AWS)) have blogs, tweet chats, committee activities and other opportunities as well that can enhance your CV and network. Surgical organizations, including the AAS, AWS, American College of Surgeons (ACS), Association for Surgical Education (ASE), all have formal service pathways for medical students to be involved. Consideration and admission for these positions does vary from a simple sign up and membership, to a more robust application and screening process. These committee roles are an important way to differentiate yourself, build a group of peer and faculty mentors outside your institution while you work on valuable work that aligns with your interests (workshops, manuscripts, community outreach, etc.).

10.3 Additional Educational or Training Opportunities

Some students pursue a dual degree (Masters in Public Health, Masters in Business Administration, Ph.D.) concurrently or in addition to their medical degree. Although these degrees can be valuable, they should not be pursued if it detracts from your medical education or if you do not envision it fitting into your future career plans.

As the bar seemingly becomes higher for applications, an increasing number of students are taking an additional year between their third and fourth years of medical school for a dedicated research year. Again, we recommend discussing this with your mentor or PD prior to making this decision. You want to ensure that this year will be productive and successful; picking the right research mentor is crucial.

Finally, each year that your medical education is prolonged outside the standard 4 years must be accounted for during medical school licensing and credentialing.

10.4 Putting Together your Application

The ERAS application is organized into sections. A good rule is to have your CV formatted in the same way so that you can copy it straight to the ERAS website when the application opens in June. It is generally accepted that honors and activities from undergraduate studies are included; high school is typically left off. Starting your CV early in medical school and keeping it updated regularly will help ensure that you don't forget poster presentations, volunteer activities, or awards.

10.4.1 Experiences

Starting with the 2023–2024 cycle, your work, research, and volunteer experiences are consolidated and limited to 10 experiences. Which experiences and how to organize them may depend on your CV. Some applicants choose to list each research project separately by publication; others list all their research under the principal investigator they worked with to leave room for other experiences such as volunteering or teaching. If you are a non-traditional applicant, this is a great opportunity to highlight your work, education, or other experiences you had prior to medical school. Don't underestimate your experiences; examine what values and traits they exemplify. For example, consider if your positions enhanced communication skills, leadership, demonstrated resilience, reliability or demonstrated your work ethic. Most programs may not consider away rotations as something that should be listed here. If you have questions about individual experiences, we recommend discussing this with your PD.

10.4.2 Letters

A strong LOR from a respected faculty member can go a long way for an application; conversely, a mediocre or weak letter may be detrimental. Do not wait until the need for a letter arises. The advice of your surgical faculty, specifically surgical education leadership cannot come early enough or often. While in clerkship, network with surgery interest group students and faculty. Ask fourth year students, matched or applying to surgery about what they would have done differently. If the desire for surgery starts later, sit down with the PD to get realistic advice. When considering who to approach for a recommendation, the ideal letter writer is one who knows you well and can speak to your abilities and potential as a future academic surgeon, is well respected or has a leadership position within your department, and has agreed to write a *strong* LOR. However, getting 3–4 letters from people who satisfy these characteristics is not always possible. Therefore, having a diverse set of letters from faculty who know you well, in addition to a chair or PD who may not have worked directly with you but can attest to your potential, will be helpful to those who are reviewing your application.

There is always the question of whether a letter from a non-surgeon is acceptable. These should be discussed on a case-by-case basis with someone like your PD or APD. A community primary care doctor who you rotated with for a week in the summer as part of an externship may not be able to comment on your future in surgery; however, your lab principal investigator will be able to support your ability to become a surgeon-scientist.

Most letter writers will expect you to either discuss the request for a LOR with you at the completion of their clinical rotation or via email. Try to identify potential letter writers in advance of your clerkship or acting internship. This will allow you to proactively send them information about you and let you ask about their expectations of you. Not all programs require PD or chair letters. Specific program requirements are often found on their residency website or the AMA FRIEDA™ website (FREIDA™ AMA Residency & Fellowship Programs Database (ama-assn.org)). FRIEDA has a number of application tools and allows for comparison of programs. You may be asked to set a meeting to discuss your application; you should schedule this through their administrative assistant if they have one. Ask what you should bring to the meeting in addition to a copy of your CV and a draft of your personal statement. If it is early in your third year and you have not started your personal statement, be prepared to talk about yourself and what experiences have been formative for you.

Multiple studies since the 1980's have demonstrated gender and racial bias found in letters of recommendation [2, 3]. While many surgical faculty receive bias training and education, you can provide your letter writer with gender-neutral prompts that can help strengthen your letter.

As mentioned previously, some mentors will ask you to write your own LOR. This should be treated as a generous opportunity to have control over the one aspect of your application that is dependent on someone else! If you are not sure where to start, ask if your mentor would be willing to share a sample LOR with the previous applicant's identifiers removed.

Some programs still require a Chair letter. This can be difficult as most medical students do not get a lot of face time with the Chair clinically. It is important to approach a meeting with the Chair prepared with your CV. The Chair's administrative assistant can be a very helpful resource and you may consider asking the assistant for materials you are expected to bring to this meeting.

10.4.3 Personal Statement

This is often the most dreaded aspect of ERAS. Most of us do not like writing about ourselves! Additionally, feedback on the personal statement is the most variable and conflicting set of opinions that one can receive. Often, your personal statement can be perceived as either "too personal" or "too bland". Ultimately, the PD or application reviewer should get an idea of who you are and what values drive you toward future goals after reading your personal statement.

There are 2–3 models of writing that are commonly utilized in a personal statement for surgical residency. These include story-telling through a notable patient or life experience versus a thesis. Most PDs see the personal statement as a way for us to get to know you before we invite you to the interview, but it should not be a rambling narrative. The typical personal statement has the following components: the reason you want to become a surgeon (personal experience, family or friend who had a surgical disease, an experience in the operating room or with a patient that drew you in), what you have accomplished thus far (leadership, research, volunteer activities), what you hope to do in residency, and your future goals as an academic surgeon. These personal statements are typically no longer than 1 page. Avoid the mistake of leaving too much room on the page. The statement is an opportunity to highlight your strengths with specific examples, paint a vision of your future in surgery and your contributions to a program and the profession.

However, not all of us have a compelling life story or an exciting case we got to be a part of during our clinical rotation. Not every book on the best seller list is a thriller. Being genuine about your interest in surgery and what you hope to accomplish in your career can still make for an excellent personal statement. If you do have a meaningful story to tell, make sure that the story is told concisely and illustrates a point. Don't leave it to the reader to come to a conclusion about what the story says about you.

One of the common pitfalls that applicants fall into is to make up an extraordinary case—you could be asked about it at your interview, so you don't want to be caught in a lie. There are also topics that you may want to avoid, such as taking sides on a divisive issue. Although medicine and politics are intertwined, and advocating for our patients can sometimes be political, your personal statement should be respectful of a broad audience. If in doubt, discuss it with your PD/APD or a trusted mentor.

Ultimately, your personal statement can also allow the reader to get to know you outside of what is already on your ERAS application. Selling yourself is not always an easy or comfortable task, but you should strive to write a statement that makes the reader want to meet you. Be positive, talk about the things that make you proud or excited, and put your best version on paper.

If you have any deficiencies in your application, challenging experiences, or failures, the personal statement is a good place to explain any gaps or weaknesses. If you had a difficult adjustment to medical school and your grades reflect that, this would be a good place to note it and show how you have improved during your clinical rotations. Perhaps you decided on a surgical career late; explain how you switched from doing primary care outreach work to surgical research, but also that you learned valuable skills and lessons from your time working in these clinics. PDs do not expect every applicant to have a perfect resume, owning setbacks, providing honest explanations, and showing how you overcame difficulties can show more about your character.

Recognize that it is normal to have multiple drafts of this statement, so it is advisable to start early and get feedback from individuals that know you well and those that don't. While presenting your statement to multiple individuals may be time consuming and get you multiple opinions that can be confusing, it can reveal blind spots and lead to a better finished product.

10.4.4 Signals and the Supplemental Section

Signals and the supplemental section are relatively new parts of the residency application that allows the medical student to show interest in geography, institution, or training environment of urban versus rural and expand on meaningful experiences. For the 2023–2024 cycle, applicants were still limited to 5 signals in general surgery, whereas specialties such as orthopedics or urology allow up to 30 signals [4]. These other subspecialties utilize signals as a filter; some programs will not invite an applicant to interview unless they signaled that program. Currently, general surgery residency programs utilize signals with variable weight [5, 6]. As this process is still in evolution, reference the Association for Progran Directors in Surgery (APDS) website and the PD at your institution for the latest updates on the number of signals and how programs intend to use them. For more information see Chap. 7.

10.4.5 Scores and Transcripts

Since the transition to pass/fail grading for the United States Medical Licensing Examination (USMLE) Step 1 exam in 2022, there has been increasing importance set on Step 2 as a screening tool [7, 8]. The weight Step 2 carries is even greater as medical schools also transition to either a pass/fail system or no longer provide class rank. Programs vary on score minimums. These can be referenced in the program website or FRIEDA™. Submission of scores after the programs download applications can lead to omission of your application from their screening process. Always alert programs if your scores or transcripts are delayed but recognize that time and bandwidth may not allow some programs to increase the number of applications they are screening.

Since 2017, the implementation of holistic review has become more ubiquitous. The Association of American Medical Colleges (AAMC) has encouraged this method of admissions to mitigate bias and promote equity [9]. These strategies include decreasing the emphasis on scores and increasing the attributes and background of the applicant. While many programs have decreased their score minimums and the emphasis on grades, they are a measure of academic performance and will still remain as a part of the screening process.

10.5 Choosing the Right Set of Programs

The number and type of programs that you apply to will be tailored to your personal and professional ambitions and barriers. Consider how wide a net you can cast geographically. Perhaps being in a region of the country will afford you proximity to family or friends for 5–7 years of training. If your academic pursuits include applying to a competitive fellowship or becoming a surgeon-scientist, look for programs with a proven track record and faculty that have had success in funding and publication. Online calculators can give you rough estimates of how many programs to apply to and your overall chances of matching, but use these with caution [10]. Objective advice from a trusted mentor who knows the match patterns for the peers that graduated over the last several years will likely offer you a realistic picture of your relative standing. In 2022, AAMC data reflects that the average number of programs applied to per applicant was 60. In 2024 the average is 70 applications per candidate (ERAS® Statistics | AAMC). While the number of applicants has remained stable, the number of applications per applicant has continued to rise since 2018 when this figure was 39 [11]. This rise is likely multifactorial but does translate to additional costs for the applicant. Total costs for applicants have been offset by the advent of virtual interviewing which started in 2020, but these costs will fluctuate as many programs are including in person visits.

It is important to have a set of programs that is realistic to your desires, abilities, and track record. Seek advice on what programs will be 'dream-schools', reasonable and 'safety'. If you receive feedback that your chances of matching are low, do not lose faith. Use the opportunity to practice interviewing and then consider a host of alternatives. Some applicants seek out a preliminary residency positions through the Supplemental Offer and Acceptance Program (SOAP) or in addition to categorical positions. Others will look for a year of research or activities to bolster their CV. Occasionally, not matching is an opportunity to reflect and consider another specialty. Remember, your journey will end in success and need not match anyone else's. Further, having a backup plan is not a sign of weakness. Preparation is essential to achievement.

10.6 Advice for Special Groups

Certain groups have historically been disadvantaged and/or challenged in successful residency matching into categorical positions in surgery. Those groups include Doctors of Osteopathic Medicine (DO), US and Non-US International Medical Graduates (IMG), Underrepresented in Medicine (URiM), preliminary residents, those applying to more than one specialty, and those who are couples matching. Individuals seeking a more competitive residency program should consider acting internships, writing personalized letters to the program indicating their specific interests and qualifications. For many categories, data are collected by the NRMP, but selected data is available online. The match rates for MD seniors and DO seniors in general surgery categorical spots in 2023 was 5.7% and 3.6% respectively [12]. IMG match rate in 2023 was 2.1%. Match data by race is not found on the NRMP website. Couples match data is not broken down by specialty.

As programs work towards becoming more inclusive (more comfortable with COMLEX scores, greater implementation of holistic review), these disparities should improve. Some programs still require that DO applicants submit USMLE scores, but greater attention is being given to this topic by PDs and the APDS. IMG's should try where possible to have letter writers emphasize their clinical acumen, familiarity with the electronic medical record, ability to establish rapport with patients and fluency in English. These are frequently encountered concerns amongst surgical faculty.

Applicants from historically excluded groups such as Black, Hispanic, LGBTQA+, and other backgrounds often do not have the benefit of finding mentors who look like or have life experiences similar to them [13]. Identity and Affinity groups such as the Society of Black Academic Surgeons (SBAS), Society of Asian Academic Surgeons, Latino Surgical Society, and Out Surgeons are an excellent resource for students from underrepresented backgrounds for networking and seeking advice [14]. Surgeons within SBAS performed a nationwide multicenter study using ERAS data to look at rates of application, matriculation, and graduation from general surgery programs, and found that underrepresentation at every stage persists for Black physicians, with Black male surgeons especially affected [15]. Even though Asian Americans are not underrepresented within medical school, residency, and in junior surgeon ranks, they are not promoted to leadership positions at the same rate and continue to experience unique challenges [16, 17]. URiM are still absent from many academic surgery centers, many where racial minorities and other vulnerable patients obtain their care; therefore, part of eliminating health care disparities requires that patients have access to surgeons who share a cultural or ethnic background with them [18].

The 2022–2023 data from the AAMC notes that the proportion of active residents in General Surgery who are Native Hawaiian/Pacific Islander, American Indian/Alaska Native, Black/African American, or Hispanic/Latino/Spanish Origin are 0.4%, 0.7%, 6.4% and 9%, respectively [19]. Very little data exists on LGBTQ+ applicants. Minority applicants should consider the messaging, branding, commitment to DEI by activities, and success of previous minority residents when assessing the program. While programs are not allowed to ask applicants about their gender, race, sexual orientation, or religion, this can be tactfully brought up by the applicant to evaluate the program's ability to provide a supportive environment.

10.7 Conclusion

In summary, preparing your best residency application begins with a timeline. Audit parts of the application and get advice and feedback on each section and your selection of programs. Getting the invitation to interview is the first of many milestones to securing your future career in academic surgery.

References

1. Singh NP, Boyd CJ. Rapidly increasing number and cost of residency applications in surgery. Am Surg. 2023;89:5729–36.
2. Newkirk-Turner BL, Hudson TK. Do no harm: graduate admissions letters of recommendation and unconscious bias. Perspect ASHA Special Interest Groups. 2022;7:463–475.
3. Khan S, et al. Gender bias in reference letters for residency and academic medicine: a systematic review. Postgrad Med J. 2023;99(1170):272–8.
4. Breeding T, et al. Virtual signaling and emerging trends in its use across surgical specialties. Am Surg. 2024;90:1740–3. https://doi.org/10.1177/00031348241227207.
5. LaFemina J, et al. The relationship between program and applicant characteristics with applicant program signals in the 2022 residency recruitment cycle: findings from three specialties. Acad Med. 2023;99:430–6. https://doi.org/10.1097/ACM.0000000000005586.
6. Rosenblatt AE, et al. Impact of preference signals on interview selection across multiple residency specialties and programs. J Grad Med Educ. 2023;15:702–10.
7. Khalil S, et al. The importance of USMLE step 2 on the screening and selection of applicants for general surgery residency positions. Heliyon. 2023;9:e17486.
8. Berk GA, et al. The next step: replacing step 1 as a metric for residency application. Laryngoscope Investig Otolaryngol. 2022;7:1756–61.
9. AAMC. Holistic review. 2021. https://www.aamc.org/services/member-capacity-building/holistic-review. Accessed 12 Feb 2024.
10. Residency match calculator: your chances | BeMo® (bemoacademicconsulting.com, Charting Outcomes™: Characteristics of Applicants who Match to Their Preferred Specialty | NRMP).
11. AAMC. ERAS statistics. 2022. https://www.aamc.org/data-reports/interactive-data/eras-statistics-data. Accessed 12 Feb 2024.
12. 2023-Main-Match-Results-and-Data-Book-FINAL.pdf (nrmp.org). Accessed 12 Feb 2024.
13. Morris-Wiseman LF, Cañez C, Romero Arenas MA, Hsu C-H, Nfonsam VN. Race, gender, and international medical graduates: leadership trends in academic surgical societies. J Surg Res. 2022;270:430–6.
14. Wang TS, et al. Proceedings from the advances in surgery channel diversity, equity, and inclusion series: lessons learned from Asian academic surgeons. J Surg Res. 2022;278:14–30.
15. Keshinro A, et al. Examination of intersectionality and the pipeline for black academic surgeons. JAMA Surg. 2022;157:327–34.

16. Nakayama DK. Asian Americans in leadership positions in academic surgery. Ann Surg. 2012;255:583–8.
17. Kuo LE, Chu DI, Gao T, Brahmbhatt TS, Wang TS. Asian American and Pacific islander experiences and challenges in academic surgery. Am J Surg. 2022;223:211–3.
18. Butler PD, Longaker MT, Britt LD. Major deficit in the number of underrepresented minority academic surgeons persists. Ann Surg. 2008;248:704–11.
19. Table B5. Number of active MD residents, by race/ethnicity (alone or in combination) and GME specialty | AAMC. Accessed 12 Feb 2024.
20. Lipman JM, et al. A systematic review of metrics utilized in the selection and prediction of future performance of residents in the United States. J Grad Med Educ. 2023;15:652–68.

Chapter 11
Navigating the Residency Application Process: Understanding the Updates to the Recruitment Process

Hayley Reddington and Jennifer LaFemina

Abstract Residency recruitment is a continuum of events spanning application submission, review, interview offer and completion, rank list submission and finally, the match of applicants and programs. Since its inception, the continuum has evolved, recently experiencing marked change in light of observed challenges including but not limited to those associated with ballooning application numbers, COVID-19 implications, and inequities. The recent innovations in recruitment are discussed with this in mind. Holistic review, preference signaling, secondary assessment, single release periods for first round interview invitations, and virtual interviews are a few of the recent innovations that have been implemented. These and others—their impetus, available data, and future directions—will be explored throughout this chapter.

11.1 Overview of the Recruitment Cycle Process

The residency application process spans several critical events, starting with the application submission, followed by the program's application review, interview invitation, interviews, and rank list creation and submission by both applicants and programs, and ultimately the matching of candidates and programs (Fig. 11.1).

Most commonly and for most specialties, applicants submit applications to training programs through the Association of American Medical Colleges' (AAMC) Electronic Residency Application Service, or ERAS. Some specialties have more recently moved from a single application platform to a wider variety of options. Plastic and Reconstructive Surgery (PRS) programs have encouraged programs to utilize the Plastic Surgery Common Application (PSCA); currently, PRS programs can use PSCA, ERAS, or both [1]. Additionally, in light of some of the challenges

H. Reddington · J. LaFemina (✉)
Department of Surgery, University of Massachusetts Chan Medical School, Worcester, MA, USA
e-mail: Hayley.Reddington@umassmemorial.org; Jennifer.LaFemina@umassmemorial.org

A. Gillis, C. B. Aarons (eds.), *A How To Guide For Medical Students*, Success in Academic Surgery, https://doi.org/10.1007/978-3-031-66011-5_11

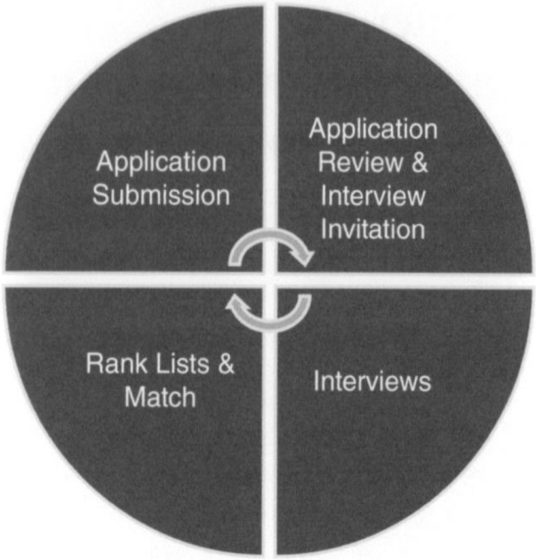

Fig. 11.1 Cycle of resident recruitment process

through the cycle (discussed in detail in the next section), including barriers to holistic review and rising application numbers and cost, Obstetrics and Gynecology (OBGYN) has announced that the specialty's training programs will use a specialty-specific application system, ResidencyCAS in place of ERAS in the 2024–2025 cycle [2]. With this new platform, the cost of applying will align to the number of signals allowed by the specialty (see below), which is anticipated to reduce application costs. At this time, applicants who primarily apply in OBGYN but who will also apply to other specialties ("dual appliers") or need to enter the Supplemental Offer and Acceptance Program (SOAP; see below) will also need to submit applications via ERAS. To address rising costs, ERAS has recently announced a new, simplified fee schedule for the 2025 ERAS Application Season [3].

After interviews, programs and applicants submit their preferred rank lists to the matching service utilized by the specialty. The most commonly used service is the National Resident Matching Program (NRMP), which runs the matching algorithm for the majority of residency specialties [4]. SF Match is utilized by Ophthalmology and Plastic Surgery, along with a number of fellowship programs; the American Urological Association oversees the Urology Match [5, 6].

Some applicants will unsuccessfully secure a position through the matches, and these applicants will most commonly take part in SOAP. This NRMP program allows programs a uniform, open market means of offering unfilled positions to partial or unmatched applicants. Historically, applications are submitted by applicants via ERAS, and the process that occurs during Match week [7]. Challenges and potential future directions, including the proposed two-phase Match, are summarized later in this chapter.

11.2 Challenges in Recruitment

Throughout the residency application process, there are challenges faced by both applicants and residency programs as both groups seek a successful recruitment season (Table 11.1). Initially, during application submission, these challenges are primarily centered around ballooning application numbers, driven by the fear of being unmatched and the application to multiple specialties ("dual appliers"), among other considerations.

The sheer number of applications is a challenge to both applicants and programs, and application numbers are discordant from what would be expected for a successful match [8]. The 2023 NRMP Applicant Survey, which is self-reported, indicates United States (US) MD, US DO, and other applicant types, including international medical graduates (IMGs), submitted an average of 68.5, 66.5, and 133.5 applications in a successful cycle; unsuccessful candidates submitted an even greater number [9]. ERAS 2023 data demonstrates that US MD graduates (public school)

Table 11.1 Modern challenges and innovations in resident recruitment process

Phase of recruitment process	Challenge	Proposed innovation
Application submission	• Rising application numbers • Rising application costs • Dual appliers	• Multiple application submission platforms • New ERAS fee structure
Applicant review & interview invitation	• Limitations on communicating value-alignment • Limitations on program identification of mutual interest/values • Barriers to holistic review • Interview "hoarding" • Reduced number of interview cancellations	• Holistic review • Secondary assessment • Preference signals • Geographic preferences • Single first-round interview release period • Required 48 h response time by applicants • Interview invitations are equal to number of slots available
Interviews	• Inability for applicants to assess "goodness of fit" in virtual cycles • Inability of programs to highlight key attributes in an in-person visit • Inequitable cost barriers associated with in-person interviews	• Uniform and transparently communicated interview platforms that align to principles of equity
Rank lists & matching	• Compressed SOAP timeline	• Two-phase match
Overall	• Limited modern data correlating applicant traits and match outcomes • Inequities in recruitment	• Unification of data between application, interview, and match • Implicit bias training

submitted an average of 73.8 applications, US DO candidates submitted 92.0, and IMG submitted 144.4 [10]. These data consistently reflect a discordance of applications submitted by different applicant groups, which possibly reflects challenges some groups may face successfully matching into particular specialties as well as the ongoing need for transparent guidance about firm, program-specific requirements.

To understand the scope from the program perspective, the NRMP 2022 Program Director Survey indicated that General Surgery programs received 1064 applications to fill a quota of 6 residency spots, representing a 177-fold greater number of applications received than positions available [11]. AAMC data reflects similarly high, and rising, total application numbers across specialties: application numbers rose to an average number of 1058 applications through ERAS 2021, though in the last two cycles (2022 and 2023), numbers are showing a downtrend, possibly reflecting the innovations that have been implemented [10].

The volume of applications poses several obstacles for both applicants and programs. First, it inhibits the ability of the applicants to demonstrate unique attributes and communicate shared values. Similarly, programs are challenged to appreciate this value alignment. Further, rising costs associated with applying, ranking, and interviewing have increased the financial burden on applicants in a manner than can expose inequities in the process [12]. A recent paper demonstrated a 32% total increase in ERAS applications to surgical specialties from 2017 to 2021. This translated to an increased application cost of $329 per applicant, which equated to an almost $8 million increase in application cost over the time period.

Transitioning to the interview period, applicant interview practices align to that of the game theory concept of the "prisoner's dilemma": individuals over-interview with the goal of reducing the likelihood of an unsuccessful match though this can reduce interview availability for the larger population [13, 14]. Interview "hoarding" (i.e., the disproportionate accumulation of interviews by interview-rich candidates relative to other candidates, considering the historic number of number of necessary interviews for a successful match) reduces the number of available interviews for interview-poor candidates, which was compounded with the transition to virtual interviews: with the removal of travel and cost barriers, fewer interview cancellations occur [8, 14]. This raises concerns that less competitive applicants may receive a lower number of interviews and have a lower likelihood of a successful match; programs might observe a higher risk of unfilled slots [8]. Capping interviews has been proposed but has not yet been adopted in specialties other than Ophthalmology, which has utilized a single interview scheduling portal to facilitate adherence [15, 16].

An additional major challenge faced by stakeholders are the systemic and individual biases that exist throughout the recruitment process. Many times, these can take the form of implicit bias (i.e. unconscious attitudes or stereotypes that influence decision-making) and can inadvertently seep into the recruitment cycle [17]. The dynamic COVID landscape led to a call to action by organizations, specialties, programs, and applicants, among other stakeholders, to develop innovations that were applicant-centric, did not induce harm, and provided equitable opportunities across diverse applicant groups [18, 19]. Addressing implicit bias requires residency programs to be proactive with education and self-reflection for everyone involved in the process. To guide this, multiple organizations and specialties put forth implicit bias trainings and best practices in recruitment, which remain excellent resources in the evolving landscape. One example is the AAMC webinar training to address implicit bias for residency interviewers to decrease the bias in virtual interviews. [17]

11.3 Innovations in Recruitment

The challenges associated with the surgical residency application process have been met with innovations to enhance the experience for both applicants and programs (Table 11.1). The following section will highlight the impetus and available outcomes on some of the more recent innovations across the continuum. The sections will also outline future directions and potential evolution of these and other possible opportunities.

11.3.1 Holistic Review

The benefits of recruitment of a diverse workforce to programs, departments, and patients has been widely published [20, 21]. However, with the significant number of applications, programs have adopted initial filters to screen applicants for interviews. Many of these filters have relied upon parameters that are known to disadvantage individuals who are underrepresented in medicine (URiM). The United States Medical Licensing Examinations (USMLE) Step 1, until it transitioned to a Pass/Fail grading system, was historically one of the most important criteria on which selection decisions were based [21–29]. However, this same criterion has long been shown to disadvantage URiM and female applicants. Recent 2022 program data shows that only 4% of programs do not consider USMLE in the selection of US MD and IMG applicants when extending interviews, suggesting that other objective data and additional examinations, like USMLE Step 2 and the Comprehensive Osteopathic Medical Licensing Examination (COMLEX) Step 2, may take the place of Step 1 in importance [11].

Holistic review is a comprehensive method that should be applied equitably to all candidates to evaluate the entirety of the individual. It is defined by the AAMC as a method to “take into consideration applicants’ experiences, attributes, and academic metrics as well as the value an applicant would contribute to learning, practice, and teaching” [30]. As such, a number of resources to facilitate holistic review have been set forth. This review increases the proportion of individuals who are historically underrepresented across residences, including but not limited to General Surgery [30, 31].

By 2022, more than 50% of programs report incorporating holistic review, noting benefits of increasing resident diversity, identifying promising applicants, improving value alignment, and supporting the program's mission. It was found to be particularly helpful in evaluating traits such as personal attributes, interest and interprofessional skills, ethics, and professionalism [11]. Challenges though still exist, observed in the 2022 NRMP Program Director Survey, which reported that 76% of responding programs were not familiar with the AAMC model of holistic review [11].

11.3.2 Secondary Applications, Surveys, and Assessments

To gain further information about applicants and mission alignment, some programs have implemented secondary assessments to enhance holistic review processes. These secondary surveys are typically issued after the original primary application submission and can take various forms, including but not limited to program-specific essays or situational judgment tests (SJTs). Attributes of this innovation can include augmented "fit" as applicants can more specifically communicate their perceived program-specific alignment. Further, the added effort and time may reduce the number of applications, as those without significant interest may not complete the additional work required [21, 32].

SJTs are another form of program-specific secondary assessment through which applicants receive scenario-based prompts that assess non-cognitive characteristics [33, 34]. These tests have been developed to help better assess professional and personal attributes that might not be as evident on traditional applications, such as teamwork and nontechnical skills. Early studies have been favorable, showing an increase in interview offer rates to URiM applicants and those who would not have met program-defined traditional USMLE thresholds [33, 34]. SJTs, like other secondary surveys and simulation, require increased applicant and program time and can be prone to biases if language proficiencies and cultural contexts are not considered. Long-term data on the effectiveness of these strategies are limited to date, though single-institution data from one General Surgery program's categorical residents from 2018 to 2022 showed a significantly higher rate of attrition among residents who scored low on the SJT [35].

Incorporation of simulation in the residency application process is not widespread across programs, though the most prominent data on the topic is from the Mayo Clinic, where simulation was first implemented in the 2017–2018 cycle [36]. Potential benefits include the opportunity to obtain an objective measure to assist with ranking, partnered with a correlation of future surgical skill in training [21, 36, 37]. Especially in the context of a virtual interview format, simulation can be difficult to implement and increases cost and assessment time for programs.

To help solve the challenge that secondary surveys aim to address, the AAMC ERAS initiated a pilot study with a voluntary supplemental application (SuppApp) in the 2021 recruitment season, initially including Dermatology, General Surgery, and Internal Medicine residencies [38] The purpose of this was to create a data-driven means of helping applicants share more about themselves and facilitating program holistic review and value alignment [38]. The original SuppApp included past experiences, geographic preferences, and preference signals (see below) [39, 40].

11.3.3 Preference Signaling

Preference signaling was initially designed and implemented in the economics job market and was first implemented in residency recruitment by Otolaryngology in 2020–2021 [41]. At the time of inception, applicants had a limited number of signals to send to programs at the time of application, indicating their particular interest. After the original positive correlation of a signal with an increased interview offer rate in Otolaryngology, preference signals were introduced via the SuppApp to Dermatology, General Surgery, and Internal Medicine in the following year [42].

From an applicant perspective, signaling significantly increased the likelihood of receiving an interview, reflecting that the presence of a preference signal allowed applicants to be noticed by the programs for which they had interest. Additionally, the SuppApp study showed that signals benefited all participating applicant groups (US MD, US DO, and IMG), genders, and groups that were URiM [43]. Reassuringly, the 2021 Applicant Reaction Survey showed that 70% of respondents reported their preference signals reflected their true preferences at the time of application [44]. Programs used signals to support holistic review and identify applicants who may have otherwise been overlooked, sometimes using the signals as a tiebreaker in deciding who to invite to interview [38, 43]. Data also demonstrated that 25% of programs received about 50% of signals [38]. Understanding how different programs, including how signal number receipt impacts interpretation or use of signals, can help to inform future applicants about effective signal distribution.

After initial positive findings in the SuppApp, variations in signaling were introduced in the future cycles. Unlike the original pilot utilizing a small number of signals, some specialties introduced high signals numbers (e.g., Orthopedics, OBGYN) and asymmetric ("two-tier") signaling with gold and silver signals (e.g., OBGYN) [45]. The use of a high number of signals has been proposed as a means of inducing soft application limits and allowing broader distribution of the signals along a larger number of programs for which an applicant has genuine interest [42]. The opposing viewpoint, in favor of low signals, stems from their original use in the economics job market: when signals are scarce, the signals become more credible, and programs can have greater confidence in their value [41]. Additionally, if a program does not receive a signal, it does not mean that an applicant is uninterested; it simply implies they ran out of signals, guarding against the potential for programs to overvalue a signal as a primary determining factor [46]. Preliminary data from the 2023–2024 cycle shows, with the exception of Neurosurgery, a 20–30% reduction in application numbers in specialties that adopted at least 25 signals (Orthopedics, Urology, Otolaryngology, Dermatology); this reduction was larger versus those that continued with low signal numbers [46]. The impact on a successful match are unknown at this time, and data unification across phases of the process is essential to better interpret the impact of signals on applicant placement and inform best signaling practices (high vs low signal numbers, tiered signals, etc.) and future directions, such as the role of a bidirectional or post-interview signaling mechanism.

11.3.4 Geographic Preferences

Both program directors and applicants report that geographic location is an important factor in residency selection [21]. Geographic preferences were first included in the Internal Medicine and Dermatology SuppApp in the 2021–2022 application cycle and were introduced in additional specialties in the following years [47]. The preferences are split into two components: geographic division preferences (i.e., up to three US census divisions) and setting preference (i.e., rural or urban). Available data from the first 2 years of the geographic preference feature suggests there may be value in this feature in residency selection and that most applicants indicated a preference for the location of their permanent address and/or medical school location [47]. Variability with use exists, and the fairness and value added of features remains under study [39, 47].

11.3.5 Single Release Dates for Interviews

To more evenly offer interviews to applicants and reduce disparities between interview-rich and interview-poor candidates, a single release period for the first round of residency interviews has been proposed and recommended by several specialties, first by OBGYN and subsequently in other specialties including but not limited to General Surgery [14, 48]. In this model, the specialty strongly encourages programs to issue the first round of invitations to applicants within a predefined window, followed by rolling offers pending cancellations. Historically, the period after submission can be all-encompassing for applicants, as they anxiously await news of interview invitations. In addition to the stress, the process can compromise education, as applicants are worried about losing an opportunity should they do not immediately respond to an extended invitation. A pre-defined release period can provide structure to this process so that applicants can expect a specific window, easing stress and optimizing education by allowing applicants to pre-plan for period of peak offers. Further, as applicants have a finite time to prioritize the received interviews of most importance, there is greater ability to decline invitations—when they are all received at once—that can be redistributed over the remaining pool of applicants who may have more interest in the program; the result is to reduce interview hoarding and allow a broader distribution of interviews across all candidates [14]. This innovation pairs particularly well with the new NRMP requirement allowing a 48-h response time before programs re-extend the invitation to another candidate and requiring programs to offer interviews equal to the available number of slots available [49].

11.3.6 Virtual Interviews

Due to COVID, there was an abrupt transition to an all-virtual application process for the 2020–2021 cycle. Initial concerns included the sentiment that both applicants and programs would not be able to assess the programs and applicants, respectively, and determine "goodness of fit" with program faculty, residents, and culture/mission. The data collected on the virtual interview process, primarily in qualitative survey format, has shown the virtual platform to have more advantages than disadvantages [50, 51]. One major benefit to applicants is the decreased cost, as applicants previously had to travel and pay for accommodations to attend interviews [51]. This time spent traveling can now be redirected to medical school educational experiences. Overall, applicants have reported sufficient exposure to programs to build their rank lists [50]; from 2021 to 2022, applicants reported an increased desire for virtual interviews and a reduction in desire for in-person interviews [52]. Interestingly, while subsequent years showed an improvement in applicants' feeling that they were able to obtain the necessary information to inform their rank decisions from the virtual platforms, more than 40% still felt it was very challenging to assess culture virtually in 2022 [52]. Nearly 25% of programs also noted concerns that virtual platforms moderately or significantly impacted the ability of programs to showcase highlights, among other disadvantages including but not limited to, the challenge of last minute cancellations [52].

Understanding the benefits in equity that virtual interviews provide, a call for virtual interviews continued in the period following the start of the COVID pandemic. More recently, there is increased dialogue around creating processes that may better align to the goals of applicants and programs while maintaining equity. In the same vein, transparency and bias mitigation about interview conduct, along with a uniform process offered to all candidates, have been recommended [19, 53]. Some specialties, like General Surgery, have set forth innovative ways to navigate these recommendations including the option of a voluntary, post-evaluative in-person site visit after rank list finalization, which allows the applicant the flexibility of visiting the site to assess factors critical for rank decisions, without challenging the principles of equity should travel not be possible [48, 54].

11.3.7 Standardized Letters of Recommendation

Standardized letters of recommendation (SLOR) have been used by Emergency Medicine since implementation in 1997 and have gradually been adopted by other specialties including OBGYN, Otolaryngology, and Orthopedic Surgery [55]. Traditional letters of recommendation (LOR) have been critiqued for their inclusion of implicit bias in the narrative words used to describe an applicant [56, 57]. With LORs playing a central role in the determination of who is granted an interview, the benefits of a SLOR to facilitate time-efficient interpretation, increase interrater reliability, and provide a more objective measure of applicant skills while mitigating gender and racial/ethnic bias have been highlighted [55]. The possibility that SLORs may mitigate this bias is appealing, and the early data from Orthopedics is favorable: the significant differences in the use of standout words in narrative LORs observed by gender and race/ethnicity were mitigated and no longer significant with utilization of SLOR [56].

11.3.8 Two-Phase Match

The SOAP process was originally developed to create an open-market, reliable, and equitable means to Match unmatched candidates during Match week. Applicants learn, on the opening of Match week, if they are or are not fully Matched. With the compressed time schedule, compounded by application numbers, there are rising stressors on the applicants and programs that mimic those described above. For this reason, the NRMP proposed in 2022 a two-phase Main Residency Match, which would include two complete Match processes within the Main Match timelines with the elimination of SOAP [58, 59]. After an initial call for comment, the proposal did not move forward, though a goal of ongoing dialogue about future directions to improve the Match week experience was prioritized.

11.4 Additional Future Directions

The recruitment cycle is undergoing a particularly dynamic period, with innovations that stretch widely across the continuum, ignited by a myriad of challenges that came to the forefront during the start of the COVID pandemic. Additionally, with advances in technology, there is interest in how artificial intelligence (AI) can be implemented in the recruitment process. The potential possibilities are endless in terms of application screening, keyword matching to screen program websites for value alignment, virtual interview analysis, predictive algorithms, and language processing technology to optimize holistic candidate evaluation [60]. It is important to remember that AI in recruitment will only be as good as the data on which the model is trained, and awareness of potentially propagating biases must be prioritized [61]. Regardless of the innovation, ongoing attention to data and the assurance of processes that are equitable are essential.

References

1. American Council of Academic Plastic Surgeons—Applying to plastic surgery [Internet]. [cited 2024 Jan 20]. https://acaplasticsurgeons.org/PSCA/.
2. New Dedicated Residency Application Platform for Obstetrics and Gynecology—Association of Professors of Gynecology & Obstetrics—APGO [Internet]. [cited 2024 Jan 20]. https://apgo.org/page/rrrapplicationplatform.
3. AAMC [Internet]. [cited 2024 Jan 20]. AAMC establishes new fee structure for 2025 ERAS residency application season. https://www.aamc.org/news/press-releases/aamc-establishes-new-fee-structure-2025-eras-residency-application-season.
4. Roth AE. The origins, history, and design of the resident match. JAMA. 2003;289(7):909–12.
5. Specialties—SF Match—Residency and Fellowship Matching Services [Internet]. [cited 2024 Jan 20]. https://www.sfmatch.org/specialties.
6. Urology and Specialty Matches—American Urological Association [Internet]. [cited 2024 Jan 20]. https://www.auanet.org/meetings-and-education/for-residents/urology-and-specialty-matches.
7. NRMP [Internet]. [cited 2024 Jan 20]. SOAP. https://www.nrmp.org/residency-applicants/soap/.
8. Carmody JB, Rosman IS, Carlson JC. Application fever: reviewing the causes, costs, and cures for residency application inflation. Cureus. 2021;13(3):e13804.
9. NRMP [Internet]. [cited 2024 Jan 20]. Charting Outcomes™: Applicant Survey Results, 2023 Main Residency Match®. https://www.nrmp.org/match-data-analytics/interactive-tools/charting-outcomes-applicant-survey-results-main-residency-match/.
10. AAMC. Download [Internet]. AAMC; 2023. https://www.aamc.org/media/39341/download.
11. Results of the 2022 NRMP program director survey [Internet]. 2022. https://www.nrmp.org/wp-content/uploads/2022/09/PD-Survey-Report-2022_FINALrev.pdf.
12. Singh NP, Boyd CJ. Rapidly increasing number and cost of residency applications in surgery. Am Surg. 2023;89(12):5729–36.
13. Weissbart SJ, Hall SJ, Fultz BR, Stock JA. The urology match as a prisoner's dilemma: a game theory perspective. Urology. 2013;82(4):791–8.
14. Santos-Parker KS, Hammoud MM, Winkel AF, Marzano D, Frank S, Franz P, et al. Distributions of residency interviews with the implementation of virtual interviews and standardization of interview offer dates. J Surg Educ. 2022;79(5):1105–12.
15. Morgan HK, Winkel AF, Standiford T, Muñoz R, Strand EA, Marzano DA, et al. The case for capping residency interviews. J Surg Educ. 2021;78(3):755–62.
16. AAMC [Internet]. [cited 2024 Jan 7]. Applying to residency is stressful. Here's how experts hope to change that. https://www.aamc.org/news/applying-residency-stressful-here-s-how-experts-hope-change.
17. AAMC [Internet]. [cited 2024 Jan 7]. Unconscious bias resources for health professionals. https://www.aamc.org/about-us/equity-diversity-inclusion/unconscious-bias-training.
18. Dao AT, Garcia MM, Correa R, Gay LJ, Wininger DA, Sweet M, et al. AAIM recommendations to promote equity and inclusion in the internal medicine residency interview process. Am J Med. 2022;135(12):1509–1516.e1.
19. Spritz D, Dent D, Lovell E, McCausland J, Wininger D. OPDA interview standards for the 2022-2023 Residency and Fellowship Application Season [Internet]. 2022. https://cmss.org/wp-content/uploads/2022/08/OPDA-Interview-Standards-statement-7.29.2022-final.pdf.

20. LaFemina J, Rosenkranz KM, Aarons CB, Abdelfattah K, Choi J, Collier KT, et al. Outcomes of the 2021-2022 APDS general surgery recruitment process recommendations. J Surg Educ. 2023;80(6):767–75.
21. Tidwell J, Yudien M, Rutledge H, Terhune KP, LaFemina J, Aarons CB. Reshaping residency recruitment: achieving alignment between applicants and programs in surgery. J Surg Educ. 2022;79(3):643–54.
22. Green M, Jones P, Thomas JX. Selection criteria for residency: results of a national program directors survey. Acad Med. 2009;84(3):362–7.
23. Gorouhi F, Alikhan A, Rezaei A, Fazel N. Dermatology residency selection criteria with an emphasis on program characteristics: a National Program Director Survey. Dermatol Res Pract. 2014;2014:e692760.
24. Makdisi G, Takeuchi T, Rodriguez J, Rucinski J, Wise L. How we select our residents—a survey of selection criteria in general surgery residents. J Surg Educ. 2011;68(1):67–72.
25. Stain SC, Hiatt JR, Ata A, Ashley SW, Roggin KK, Potts JR, et al. Characteristics of highly ranked applicants to general surgery residency programs. JAMA Surg. 2013;148(5):413–7.
26. Morris DB, Gruppuso PA, McGee HA, Murillo AL, Grover A, Adashi EY. Diversity of the national medical student body—four decades of inequities. N Engl J Med. 2021;384(17): 1661–8.
27. Edmond MB, Deschenes JL, Eckler M, Wenzel RP. Racial bias in using USMLE step 1 scores to grant internal medicine residency interviews. Acad Med. 2001;76(12):1253–6.
28. Jarman BT, Kallies KJ, Joshi ART, Smink DS, Sarosi GA, Chang L, et al. Underrepresented minorities are underrepresented among general surgery applicants selected to interview. J Surg Educ. 2019;76(6):e15–23.
29. Rubright JD, Jodoin M, Barone MA. Examining demographics, prior academic performance, and United States medical licensing examination scores. Acad Med. 2019;94(3):364–70.
30. AAMC [Internet]. [cited 2024 Jan 20]. Holistic review. https://www.aamc.org/services/member-capacity-building/holistic-review.
31. Nehemiah A, Roberts SE, Song Y, Kelz RR, Butler PD, Morris JB, et al. Looking beyond the numbers: increasing diversity and inclusion through holistic review in general surgery recruitment. J Surg Educ. 2021;78(3):763–9.
32. Puscas L, Esclamado R. Use of a secondary essay in the residency application process. JAMA Otolaryngol Neck Surg. 2015;141(7):591.
33. Takacs EB, Tracy CR. Evaluating the whole applicant: use of situational judgment testing and personality testing to address disparities in resident selection. Curr Urol Rep. 2022;23(11):309–18.
34. Gardner AK, Cavanaugh KJ, Willis RE, Dunkin BJ. Can better selection tools help us achieve our diversity goals in postgraduate medical education? Comparing use of USMLE step 1 scores and situational judgment tests at 7 surgical residencies. Acad Med. 2020;95(5):751–7.
35. Willis RE, Kempenich JW, Patnaik R, Dent DL. Identifying potential attrition during the residency applicant screening process using a situational judgment test. J Surg Educ. 2022;79(6):e103–8.
36. AlJamal Y, Prabhakar N, Rivera M, McKenzie T, Stulak J, Heller S, et al. A simulation-based selection process for trying to identify medical students who will become outstanding general surgery residents. Am J Surg. 2020;220(1):76–82.
37. Moore EJ, Price DL, Van Abel KM, Carlson ML. Still under the microscope: can a surgical aptitude test predict otolaryngology resident performance? Laryngoscope. 2015;125(2):E57–61.
38. AAMC [Internet]. [cited 2024 Jan 7]. Supplemental ERAS application data and reports. https://www.aamc.org/data-reports/students-residents/report/supplemental-eras-application-data-and-reports.
39. Mavilia M. AAMC supplemental ERAS® application: key findings from the 2022 application cycle; 2022
40. Gillespie L. Supplemental ERAS® 2022-2023 application cycle: results of the Program Director Reaction Survey; 2023

41. Cawley J, Roth A, Siegfried J, Coles P, Levine P, Niederle M. The job market for new economists: a market design perspective. J Econ Perspect. 2010;24:187–206.
42. Pletcher SD, Chang CWD, Thorne MC, Malekzadeh S. The otolaryngology residency program preference signaling experience. Acad Med. 2022;97(5):664–8.
43. Rosenblatt AE, LaFemina J, Sood L, Choi J, Serfin J, Naemi B, et al. Impact of preference signals on interview selection across multiple residency specialties and programs. J Grad Med Educ. 2023;15(6):702–10.
44. 2021 AAMC supplemental ERAS® application: final results of the applicant reaction survey [Internet]. AAMC; 2022. https://www.aamc.org/media/58051/download.
45. Students & Residents [Internet]. [cited 2024 Jan 21]. Program signals overview for residency applicants. https://students-residents.aamc.org/applying-residencies-eras/publication-chapters/program-signals-overview-residency-applicants.
46. AAMC [Internet]. [cited 2024 Jan 21]. Preliminary program signaling data and their impact on residency selection. https://www.aamc.org/services/eras-institutions/program-signaling-data.
47. AAMC [Internet]. 2023. Supplemental ERAS® 2022–2023 application cycle: evaluation of geographic preferences. https://www.aamc.org/media/64501/download.
48. APDS Task Force. APDS task force general surgery application and interview recommendations for 2023-2024 recruitment cycle [Internet]. AAMC. https://students-residents.aamc.org/media/13466/download.
49. Match participation agreement for programs [Internet]. NRMP; 2023. https://www.nrmp.org/wp-content/uploads/2023/12/2024-MPA-Main-Match-Program-2.pdf.
50. Quinn KM, Runge LT, Parrado RH, Streck CJ, Abbott AM, Talley CL. General surgery applicants report the impact of virtual interviews on their rank list and match. Global Surg Educ. 2022;1(1):65.
51. Domingo A, Rdesinski RE, Stenson A, Aylor M, Sullenbarger J, Hatfield J, et al. Virtual residency interviews: applicant perceptions regarding virtual interview effectiveness, advantages, and barriers. J Grad Med Educ. 2022;14(2):224–8.
52. Virtual experience and holistic review in the transition to residency: an examination of the 2021 and 2022 main residency matches [Internet]. NRMP; 2022. https://www.nrmp.org/wp-content/uploads/2022/07/2022-Virtual-Exper-Research-Brief_Final.pdf.
53. Match code of conduct for programs [Internet]. NRMP; 2022. https://www.nrmp.org/wp-content/uploads/2023/08/NRMP-Match-Code-of-Conduct_Programs.pdf.
54. O'Connor AB, Blatt AE, Fletcher KE, Martin SK, Rasnake MS, Uthlaut BS, et al. Multicenter study of optional in-person visits to residency programs after virtual interviews. J Grad Med Educ. 2023;15(6):692–701.
55. Tavarez MM, Baghdassarian A, Bailey J, Caglar D, Eckerle M, Fang A, et al. A call to action for standardizing letters of recommendation. J Grad Med Educ. 2022;14(6):642–6.
56. Powers A, Gerull KM, Rothman R, Klein SA, Wright RW, Dy CJ. Race- and gender-based differences in descriptions of applicants in the letters of recommendation for orthopaedic surgery residency. JB JS Open Access. 2020;5(3):e20.00023.
57. Grimm LJ, Redmond RA, Campbell JC, Rosette AS. Gender and racial bias in radiology residency letters of recommendation. J Am Coll Radiol. 2020;17(1 Pt A):64–71.
58. NRMP [Internet]. 2022 [cited 2024 Jan 7]. NRMP® call for public comment regarding consideration of a two-phase main residency match. https://www.nrmp.org/about/news/2022/08/nrmp-call-for-public-comment-regarding-consideration-of-a-two-phase-main-residency-match/.
59. NRMP [Internet]. 2022 [cited 2024 Jan 21]. Decision of the NRMP® board of directors regarding the proposal for a two-phase match. https://www.nrmp.org/about/news/2022/10/decision-of-the-nrmp-board-of-directors-regarding-the-proposal-for-a-two-phase-match/.
60. John AS, Kavic SM. Leveraging artificial intelligence for resident recruitment: can the dream of holistic review be realized? Artif Intell Surg. 2022;2(4):195–206.
61. Leung TI, Sagar A, Shroff S, Henry TL. Can AI mitigate bias in writing letters of recommendation? JMIR Med Educ. 2023;9(1):e51494.

Chapter 12
Navigating the Residency Application Process: Preparing for Both Virtual and In-Person Residency Interviews

Deanna L. Palenzuela Rothman and Sophia K. McKinley

Abstract The interview plays a pivotal role in resident selection from both applicant and program perspectives. We advise applicants to begin with self-reflection, aligning personal goals with program characteristics, and preparing for different interview scenarios. Mock interviews are an essential component of practice and confidence building for both virtual and in-person formats. Professionalism is important in both attire and demeanor, along with etiquette for pre-interview socials and interactions with program staff. For virtual interviews specifically, we recommend creating a professional, distraction-free environment, conducting technology trials, and optimizing the online interview setup. Post-interview, applicants are advised to send thank-you notes, use personal networks to gain additional program insights, and consider second looks for a better understanding of the program. Overall, thoughtful preparation can significantly enhance an applicant's performance during the interview process.

12.1 Introduction

The residency interview is a pivotal component of the application process for both the applicant and residency program. Program directors have cited the interview as the most important factor in determining resident selection [1–3]. From a program perspective, the interview allows for the assessment of non-cognitive factors, such as interpersonal skills, communication, and interest in the field [1–3]. Similarly, the interviews allow the applicants to interact with the program director and residents to help determine their general "fit" in the program [1, 4, 5]. The landscape of residency interviews underwent a significant shift due to the SARS-CoV-2 (COVID-19) pandemic. The conventional in-person format swiftly pivoted to a virtual, web-based setup in 2020 to adhere to social distancing mandates and travel restrictions

D. L. Palenzuela Rothman (✉) · S. K. McKinley
Department of Surgery, Massachusetts General Hospital, Boston, MA, USA
e-mail: DPALENZUELA@mgh.harvard.edu; skmckinley@mgh.harvard.edu

A. Gillis, C. B. Aarons (eds.), *A How To Guide For Medical Students*, Success in Academic Surgery, https://doi.org/10.1007/978-3-031-66011-5_12

imposed by institutions. Despite the relaxation of distancing norms, virtual interviews have remained prevalent in the realm of residency applications. This shift has presented advantages such as cost reduction, widened recruitment opportunities, and minimized disruption to clinical duties [6–10]. However, it has also introduced fresh challenges, requiring applicants to adapt to new interview protocols and evaluate programs without having visited the hospital campuses [9–11]. The aim of this chapter is to provide applicants with guidance on how to best prepare for interview process, whether in-person or virtual, so that they can confidently put forth their strongest performance.

Preparing for effective interviewing begins long before the first interview day. While many residency interviews have remained virtual, some are now transitioning back to in-person. Therefore, students should be prepared to encounter either scenario. Regardless of the interview format, pre-interview preparation should focus on self-reflection and preparing to answer interview questions. For virtual interviews, this is also the time to begin creating an optimal physical space for interviewing [12–15].

12.2 Self-reflection

The initial stage of interview preparation involves deep introspection. We urge candidates to challenge themselves, reflecting on their identity and desired career path. In this self-reflection phase, candidates should carefully examine their resumes. Each entry could trigger interview questions, so candidates should be able to confidently discuss all activities and accolades. We suggest weaving questions about values and career direction into practice interviews. With this in mind, candidates should reflect on specific accomplishments or aspects of themselves they want to showcase during the interview. Irrespective of the interview format, a clear grasp of their goals empowers applicants to communicate effectively, therefore displaying maturity and thoughtfulness. We have previously published a list of example self-reflection questions as a reference for applicants to consider prior to their interviews [15].

Once an applicant has defined their personal goals, the next step involves assessing program characteristics that align with their aspirations. For instance, candidates with a research inclination may seek out academic programs that have the resources to nurture their scholarly pursuits, while applicants interested in education may favor centers offering diverse teaching opportunities. Several other factors, such as international rotations, location, and lifestyle during residency, can significantly influence a candidate's program selection. To prepare for interviews, we recommend applicants create a list of specific questions tailored to each program, ideally derived from thorough exploration of the residency program's website. This approach not only bridges the informational gap inherent in virtual interviews but also equips candidates with insightful questions when the inevitable "what questions do you have?" arises. This proactive approach once again serves to demonstrate the applicant's maturity and thoughtfulness.

12.3 Mock Interviews

We highly recommend applicants engage in mock interviews as part of the preparation process. Participating in simulated interviews enables candidates to gain confidence for the actual event by practicing potential questions [16]. It is advisable for candidates to rehearse responses to frequently asked questions about their future career objectives, individual strengths and weaknesses, and hobbies. While the nature of most interviews will be conversational, one may encounter the high-pressure tactic of "stress interview" questions. Such questions might probe ethical dilemmas or assess the candidate's capacity for problem-solving. The intent behind these inquiries is often not to find the "correct" answer but rather to understand the applicant's core values and approach to decision-making. We recommend applicants practice the habit of reflecting before answering, as opposed to offering immediate responses. Admitting "I don't know" is acceptable, but it's advantageous to also discuss how one would navigate unknown situations or seek further clarification. Additionally, applicants should purposefully seek mock interviews in both a virtual and in-person format to feel comfortable in either setting.

Often, medical schools will offer mock interviews for students to practice with academic advisors. However, if the applicant's school doesn't offer this opportunity, or they would like additional practice, there are other avenues to explore. Many academic societies, such as the Association of American Medical Colleges (AAMC), offer resources with common interview questions for students to begin crafting their responses independently [17]. Surgical societies often also offer additional, surgery-specific, resources. For example, the American College of Surgeons offers mock interviews as part of their medical student curriculum during the annual Clinical Conference in addition to multiple online resources for interview preparation [18]. We would also recommend practicing with a trusted surgical educator or mentor. Having a mock interview with a mentor allows for the applicant to practice questions one-on-one, while also providing the opportunity for individualized feedback and debriefing afterwards.

12.4 Making the Best First Impression

Before interviews have begun is also the best time for the applicant to begin thinking about how to make a strong first impression. Often, the key to the first impression is maintaining a high standard of professionalism. One display of applicant professionalism is their choice of interview attire. The attire should be comfortable, yet business professional. For men, this means a suit, dress shirt with a tie, and formal dress shoes. For women, this could be a pant suit or skirt with a conservative blouse. T shirts, jeans, sneakers, and short skirts should be avoided. While attire can be used to subtly reflect the individual applicant's personality, we would recommend avoiding flashy items or bright colors that can be distracting for the interviewer. Trying on the chosen interview attire ahead of time allows for the applicant to confirm their clothing looks polished and well-tailored. In an interview setting, it's important to portray professionalism and maturity by smiling, articulating responses clearly, holding steady eye contact, sitting up straight, and engaging attentively. It is also beneficial to minimize any distracting movements, such as fidgeting with hair, clothing, or glasses. Another advantage of mock interviews is the ability to trial potential interview attire and practice interview etiquette.

12.5 In-Person Considerations

There are certain unique aspects of the in-person interview format that are important to note in preparation for the interview day.

12.5.1 Pre-interview Social

Traditionally, the interview activities begin with a pre-interview social. These socials are typically hosted by the residency program at a nearby restaurant or bar and designed to be specifically for residents and applicants. While it is not required to attend, this is often the best time for applicants to meet residents and get a sense of residency life within that program. These pre-interview socials are usually less formal; however, it is important to remember that any interaction with the residency program can be used to evaluate an applicant [14]. With that in mind, there are certain best practices to maintain during these socials [14]. Business casual attire is usually recommended unless otherwise specified by the program. For men, this can be slacks or khakis with a dress shirt and nice shoes, while women should opt for a nice blouse with dress pants or skirt, or a work-appropriate dress. While these settings are usually informal, T shirts, jeans, sneakers, or revealing attire should still be avoided. Of note, the residents may be coming from the hospital after their shift and therefore may be in scrubs; however, this does not reflect the attire expected of the applicants. There often is alcohol available at these events, however, we would recommend drinking with discretion. Having too much to drink could reflect poorly on an applicant, as well as impact their sleep for the following interview day. The social is a great time to ask residents about their experiences thus far but avoid contentious or controversial topics. Lastly, it is important to keep an eye on the clock; be sure to allow time for a good night's sleep to be ready for the interview the next day.

12.5.2 What to Bring

When preparing for the in-person interview, planning what to bring for the day is an important consideration. Programs usually provide pamphlets or other reading material with additional program information, so it is helpful to have some place to store everything. Usually, men will bring a leather binder or small briefcase, while women usually opt for a professional purse or tote. These carrying cases are also perfect for storing a notebook to jot down thoughts from the day, keeping prepared questions, and holding an extra resume copy, just in case. In addition to the previously mentioned attire considerations, applicants should also select comfortable, professional shoes. In-person interview days often involve a tour of the hospital campus, so applicants should be prepared to walk varying distances.

12.5.3 On the Interview Day

We previously touched on interview etiquette, however, there are a few additional points to make in preparation for in-person interviews. First, we would recommend applicants practice their handshake. While this may seem like a small detail, a firm handshake with eye contact portrays confidence and sets a strong opening tone to an interview. Secondly, applicants encounter many different people during the interview day. These include residents, staff, and faculty. Even outside of the formal interviews, applicants should be aware that every interaction matters. To that end, it is important to be courteous and respectful with everyone encountered.

12.6 Virtual Considerations

While interview preparation is similar for both in person and virtual interviews, there are additional factors to consider in advanced of virtual interviews [12–15].

12.6.1 The Interview Environment

Creating the right setting for a virtual interview is a critical aspect that should not be overlooked. The space where the interview will take place needs to be both professional in appearance and conducive to comfort, which will help the interviewee perform at their best. Applicants should seek out a secluded area that promises quietness and is safeguarded against potential disruptions. With that in mind, they should steer clear of any location that could be affected by loud noises, like ongoing construction, railways, or heavy traffic. If the applicant's home doesn't offer a suitable spot, they should consider arranging to use an office or similar professional space. To craft an optimal interview environment, consider the following: select a comfortable chair that supports a poised posture, enhance the area with soft, indirect lighting to avoid harsh shadows, and choose a simple, unobtrusive backdrop. Ensuring the camera on the laptop or web device is aligned with their line of sight allows for a natural, direct gaze. This might require placing the computer on textbooks or yoga block to achieve the correct height. Lastly, make sure there is a reliable power source nearby to prevent any unexpected loss of power during the interview.

12.6.2 Technology Trial Run

Prior to the scheduled interview, it is important to acquaint oneself thoroughly with the technological aspects of the virtual interface. Conducting trial runs of the designated software has several benefits, including confirming the compatibility of the computer system, verifying the software has been appropriately updated, and facilitating comfort with the user interface. We recommend applicants engage in a comprehensive rehearsal of their technological setup, the environment of the interview, and their chosen attire with a trusted advisor or peer who can provide constructive criticism on various facets, including the ambiance of the setup, the attire choices, the fidelity of the audio-visual transmission, as well as the overall execution of the mock interview. Simulating the interview conditions can bring to light unanticipated details, such as unstable internet connections, noise disturbances or suboptimal lighting conditions, necessitating preemptive modifications to the interview setting. Additionally, the stability and security of the internet connection is critical; reliance on a network that is utilized concurrently by multiple users or is a public or unsecured server could adversely affect the quality of the video stream. Securing a dedicated and protected network is recommended to ensure uninterrupted communication.

12.6.3 On the Interview Day

Applicants should refer to the provided interview schedule to smartly intersperse breaks for hydration, snacks, and stretching. Before diving into the interview, make sure to have all devices plugged in, silence any possible distractions from other gadgets and browser notifications, and adjust the camera to eye level. Keep a few snacks and water, along with any key notes that may be needed, within easy reach but out of the camera's view. Taking these steps to prime both themselves and their space will allow applicants to start the interview on a strong and confident note.

During the virtual interview, we do not recommend the use of digital backdrops, which can sometimes seem too casual or even block a clear view of the applicant.

For a more engaged conversation, try downsizing the interview window and placing it right below the webcam to mimic eye contact. It may also be helpful to disable the view of one's own video in case a candidate finds it distracting. Applicants should be cautious with the chat feature; double-check messages are going to the right person and remember that the host ends up with a record of all chats after the session. To keep the interviewer's attention on the applicant, the microphone should be muted when not talking during group discussions, and the video should be turned off for visually distracting tasks. Applicants should consider using screenshots to capture key points in presentations. Just make sure the device's screenshot sound is turned off.

12.7 After the Interview

Following a successful interview day, there are a few additional steps we recommend taking to round out the interview experience [15]. After the interview, emailed thank-you notes are typically welcomed by the interviewers and programs. Moreover, we recommend utilizing the contact details provided during the interviews to inquire about any unresolved questions post-interview. Applicants should leverage their personal connections to professionally discuss programs with mentors, professional colleagues, and mutual contacts to acquire deeper insights into the programs of interest. Cultivating personal relationships and networks can facilitate spontaneous and casual dialogues, which may be somewhat constrained in virtual interview settings.

It is important to remember that the interview day is not only about program resident selection, but also about determining whether the program is the right fit for the applicant. For applicants with several interviews, they can often blend together, and details get blurry when the time comes to making a rank list. We therefore recommend taking time immediately after each interview to reflect on overall impressions of each program. What were their strengths? What stood out? What were your overall impressions? Were there any "red flags"? Taking the time after each interview to write down these thoughts will make creating a rank list easier when the time comes.

12.8 Second Looks

Lastly, for virtual interviews, applicants can consider visiting their favorite programs. If resources permit, candidates can address some of the limitations inherent in virtual interviews by visiting certain programs in person after the initial interviews. This allows the applicant to obtain a more tangible understanding of the day-to-day realities of residency, the hospital's atmosphere, the location, and whether the program feels like the right match. However, in an effort to ensure fairness, these follow-up visits are typically organized and led by current residents, which may mean that interaction with program leaders is not always possible or even prohibited. While less common, applicants who participated in in-person interviews can also schedule second looks as a way to learn more about specific programs. All of the advice pertaining to attire and behavior are relevant for second look visits.

Finally, it is important to note that ideally, second look visits would be purely for the benefit of the applicant to learn more about the program. However, the program and applicant rank list certification dates have not yet been staggered, and so there is no guarantee that programs would not use second look information in their selection process.

12.9 Conclusion

There are several steps applicants can take ahead of their interviews to be best prepared for their interview day. Whether the interviews are virtual or in person, taking the time to be thoughtful about interview preparation will reflect positively on the interview day. We hope that by following these interview practices, applicants will be more prepared to present themselves strongly and successfully navigate the interview process.

References

1. Stephenson-Famy A, et al. Use of the interview in resident candidate selection: a review of the literature. J Grad Med Educ. 2015;7(4):539–48.
2. LaGrasso JR, Kennedy DA, Hoehn JG, Ashruf S, Przybyla AM. Selection criteria for the integrated model of plastic surgery residency. Plast Reconstr Surg. 2008;121(3):121e–5e.
3. Makdisi G, Takeuchi T, Rodriguez J, Rucinski J, Wise L. How we select our residents—a survey of selection criteria in general surgery residents. J Surg Educ. 2011;68(1):67–72.
4. Deiorio NM, Yarris LM, Gaines SA. Emergency medicine residency applicant views on the interview day process. Acad Emerg Med. 2009;16(Suppl 2):S67–70.
5. Schlitzkus LL, Schenarts PJ, Schenarts KD. It was the night before the interview: perceptions of resident applicants about the preinterview reception. J Surg Educ. 2013;70(6):750–7.
6. Selvam R, et al. Virtual interviews: less carbon, less bias? J Clim Change Health. 2022;8:100167.
7. Oliffe JL, et al. Zoom interviews: benefits and concessions. Int J Qual Methods. 2021;20:16094069211053522.
8. Dey P, et al. Lessons from the COVID-19 pandemic: the case for virtual residency interviews. Ann Surg Open. 2021;2(3):e077.
9. Anteby R, et al. Challenges of virtual interviewing for surgical fellowships: a qualitative analysis of applicant experiences. Surg Endosc. 2022;36(6):3763–71.
10. Kubi B, Keiler J, Douglas IIA. A game of adaptability: reflecting on the highlights and challenges of applying for surgical residency during the COVID-19 pandemic. Ann Surg. 2021;274(5):e381.
11. Rojas KE, Teshome M, Tevis SE. Unforeseen collateral damage of COVID-19 with the virtualization of fellowship interviews. Ann Surg. 2021;273(6):e271.

12. McKinley SK, et al. Successful virtual interviews: perspectives from recent surgical fellowship applicants and advice for both applicants and programs. Ann Surg. 2021;273(2):e55–9.
13. Lee TC, et al. Pearls and pitfalls of the virtual interview: perspectives from both sides of the camera. J Surg Res. 2021;262:240–3.
14. Olson DP, et al. The residency application abyss: insights and advice. Yale J Biol Med. 2011;84(3):195–202.
15. Palenzuela D, McKinley SK. Successful virtual interviews for surgery residents. Surgery. 2023;174:389–91.
16. McKinley SK, Mullen JT, Phitayakorn R. Prepare students for their surgical residency interviews with a residency workshop. American College of Surgeons. [Internet]. [cited 2024 Jan 14]. https://www.facs.org/for-medical-professionals/news-publications/journals/rise/articles/interview/.
17. Medical school applicant interview preparation guide. AAMC. [Internet]. https://students-residents.aamc.org/medical-school-interviews/publication/medical-school-applicant-interview-preparation-guide/.
18. Medical Student Program. American College of Surgeons. [Internet]. https://www.facs.org/for-medical-professionals/conferences-and-meetings/clinical-congress-2023/education-program/medical-student-program/.

Chapter 13
Navigating the Residency Application Process: A Recent Applicant's Perspective on Choosing a Residency Program

Ofelia Negrete Vasquez

Abstract Choosing a general surgery residency training program is multifactorial and complex. The present chapter attempts to demystify the experience by detailing one recent applicant's journey in navigating the application process as supported by recent literature.

13.1 Introduction

According to current Association of American Medical Colleges data, some 350 institutions sponsor a general surgery residency training program, and this figure will continue to rise in the coming years [1]. Perhaps it goes without saying, but the choice of a general surgery residency program is a major one—with not only direct implications for a critical period in trainee growth, but also pivotal in longitudinally shaping a surgeon's career. Factors which frequently influence choice of residency program include location, perceived quality of life of current residents and reputation, program size and setting, case volume and variety, quality of the training and skills curriculum, and availability of subspecialists in areas of interest [2]. Ultimately, the decision of where to pursue surgical training is one that is unabashedly personal. The present chapter will provide insight into one recent applicant's experience in navigating the general surgery residency application process, drawing from relevant current literature as warranted, in hopes that it may demystify the process for others.

O. Negrete Vasquez (✉)
Department of Surgery, University of Texas Southwestern Medical Center, Dallas, TX, USA
e-mail: Ofelia.NegreteVasquez@UTSouthwestern.edu

A. Gillis, C. B. Aarons (eds.), *A How To Guide For Medical Students*, Success in Academic Surgery, https://doi.org/10.1007/978-3-031-66011-5_13

13.2 Where to Apply

As a fourth-year medical student, the decision of where to apply, and to how many programs, is daunting for several reasons. On one hand, the general surgery applicant pool at large is vastly talented, comprised of many academic and research top performers and future leaders. Consistently, the average number of applications submitted by each applicant has risen dramatically in recent years [3]. By submitting too few applications (so-called "*under-applying*"), there exists a real risk of even a highly qualified applicant being left unmatched. Conversely, greater selectivity when initially choosing programs affords more flexibility in personalizing the common application. Program director perception of applicant interest is an important determinant of interviewee selection [3]. As such, a more refined approach to initial applications may conceivably result in greater interview yield from an applicant's top-choice programs. The choice of where to apply must also be made with information that is often incomplete, as surgery departmental websites have been found to inadequately capture many core aspects of the training experience considered important by prospective applicants [4]. Also of note, program ranking according to reputation does not consistently correlate to rankings according to other objective measures of program quality [5].

In view of these challenges, the value of drawing from the knowledge and experiences of those around you cannot be understated. Mentors (both in general surgery and beyond) who understand your background and priorities are an invaluable sounding board. While most applicants have had direct exposure to a handful of programs (e.g., through away rotations) or fewer, a general surgery mentor may very well have some knowledge about many other institutions through their own training, prior work experience, and professional collaborations. Current residents in your home general surgery program can also provide important insights derived from their medical school and interview experiences.

13.2.1 The "Non-negotiables"

Many applicants use a list of so-called "non-negotiables" to narrow their final list of residency program applications. The author of the present chapter contends that this approach may be highly useful but must be applied selectively. Importantly, applicants will have exposure to many different programs across the interview cycle, whereby their goals and priorities are also likely to evolve with time. We suggest that a candidate focus on a few key variables that would directly affect their ability to succeed personally and/or professionally. Perhaps the most pragmatic consideration is location. Make no mistake about it—general surgery residency is hard [6]. According to one prior survey on attrition among current general surgery residents, support from family and significant others was the single most cited protective factor in the decision to continue with residency [7]. A particular geographic region, or other factors which may adversely affect access to your support system, should strongly be taken into consideration when submitting initial applications.

Beyond a handful of true potential "non-negotiables," the number of programs to which an applicant should apply requires a certain amount of introspection regarding the strength of their candidacy. Admittedly, there will always be some degree of imprecision and unpredictability when thousands of candidates are applying for hundreds of spots. However, characteristics of a highly competitive general surgery residency application have been well defined. As may be expected, factors including academic performance, research involvement and output, and membership in selective professional societies are valued across multiple general surgery program director and faculty surveys [8–10]. Such characteristics are common to both university- and community-based programs [11]. Although data on the downstream effects of the 2022 transition of Step 1 to a pass/fail grading system continue to mature, medical students and program directors alike anticipate that this will confer even greater emphasis on Step 2 Clinical Knowledge scores, research output, and medical school reputation [12–14]. Whether this change actually results in a more holistic review process, as was cited among the primary rationales for a pass/fail grading system, remains poorly characterized [15, 16]. Thus, be it through self-reflection or a trusted mentor capable of providing candid feedback, an applicant's unique personal characteristics are useful in guiding application submissions.

13.2.2 The Virtual Interview Era

The residency interview day offers critical insights into the culture and structure of a general surgery program. While the merits and limitations of continued virtual interviews in the aftermath of the COVID-19 pandemic have been widely debated, virtual interviews are likely to remain commonplace for the foreseeable future. Many applicants report a good sense of exposure to program culture via virtual social "happy hours" and faculty interviews [17, 18]. Following the transition from in-person to virtual interviews, some studies have reported no significant change in the geographical distribution of residency match results, suggesting no difference in the propensity of medical students to pursue residency in a new location [19]. The virtual interview experience also seems to be positively evolving since its inception, with applicants now reporting greater insight into the work environment and professional culture during subsequent application cycles compared to the first season [20]. Interestingly, however, one study of faculty interviewee scores during in-person versus virtual interviews found that virtual interview scores were similar but with less variability, suggesting a greater challenge in detecting subtle differences between candidates [21]. Consistently, from the applicant perspective, it remains a concern as to whether the virtual format allows for enough interpersonal interaction to determine if a program may be a "true fit." [3, 22, 23] Whether recent changes in interview format actually lend to differences in future resident satisfaction, well-being, attrition, and career trajectory merits future study.

13.2.3 Program and Geographic Signaling

A growing number of medical specialties have incorporated preference signaling into their residency application process. In general surgery, preference signaling was introduced during the 2021–2022 application cycle, with a total of 5 program signals allotted to each applicant (current as of the 2023–2024 cycle). General surgery applicants report a wide range of motivations in choosing where to signal, which may include perceived program fit, selective targeting of "reach" or "safety" programs, and geographic preference [24]. As has been shown from prior otolaryngology application cycles (which likewise initially allotted 5 signals per applicant), your chance of receiving an interview invitation is higher at the programs you signal—a phenomenon that is independent of applicant competitiveness [25]. In fact, in the 2021–2022 urology match (which also gave each applicant 5 preference signals), signal status was the most robust predictor of an interview invitation [26]. The strong association between signal status and interview invitation appears consistent across all gender and racial applicant subgroups [27]. Signaling is generally looked upon favorably by applicants and program directors alike because it allows applicants to purposefully demonstrate interest in a specific program [25]. Nevertheless, the direct impact of program signaling on the general surgery residency match remains incompletely characterized, and the extent to which your probability of an interview invitation is decreased at non-signaled programs via a 5-signal application process is unclear.

Of note, program signaling remains in its infancy, and is highly variable across medical specialties with an ever-evolving landscape [24, 28]. At present, many other specialties likewise allow for a small number of preferences per applicant (e.g., 3–5). However, others have transitioned to a larger number of preference signals (e.g., 25–30), or even a two-tiered system of a handful of "gold" signals in addition to a larger number of "silver" signals. As the number of signal preferences per applicant increases, the odds of receiving an interview at signaled vs non-signaled programs appears to further increase, whereby candidates afforded a greater number of signals are less likely to receive an interview at non-signaled programs. For example, in a survey of 2022–2023 orthopedic surgery applicants (30 preference signals per candidate), 56% received interview offers exclusively from programs which they had preference signaled [29]. The chance of receiving an interview was 24.4% at signaled programs versus just 0.92% at non-signaled programs, corresponding to a 26.5 times greater likelihood of an interview invitation with signaling [29]. At these higher signal preference thresholds, some programs may even exclusively interview only those candidates who had signaled their institution [29]. In effect, this signal preference schema indirectly caps the number of interview offers a candidate can receive. Interview and/or application caps have been proposed by several authors as a means of combating inefficiencies in the residency application process as well as the financial strain on applicants [30–32]. However, strict caps have not been put into practice, and statistical models report conflicting effects of these caps on match outcomes, as well as their implications for candidates who may be either more or less competitive according to standard metrics [33–35].

In addition to program signaling, geographic preference signaling has garnered significant interest as part of the residency application process [36]. The 2023–2024 ERAS cycle was the first time that geographic preference data was collected from all applicants [37]. Candidates were allowed to indicate up to 3 geographic regions of interest (or lack of preference) as well as any preference for institution setting (i.e., rural, suburban, or urban). Consistent with the overall pool of residency applicants at large, most general surgery residency applicants indicated 3 geographic preferences (62%) [37]. The next most common approach was to not indicate a geographic preference (25%), while only a minority of applicants listed 2 (6%) or 1 (4%) geographic preference. Most applicants listed "no preference" for institution setting [37]. For all ERAS applicants, the order of geographic preferences was similar among MD, DO and international medical graduates (with 3 geographic regions being the most common approach), although the magnitude of this difference did vary based on some specific factors [37]. Namely, international medical graduates were more likely to report no geographic preference compared to United States MD applicants, while United States DO applicants were more likely to report some geographic preference across many medical specialties [37]. Across several specialties (including general surgery), applicants who self-identified as Hispanic or black were more likely to report no geographic preference compared to white applicants [37]. Applicants who select 'no preference' may truly not prioritize geographic location or, alternatively, commonly also report concern that their application may be overlooked at programs outside of their preselected regions of interest [37].

The above-mentioned differences in geographic preference signaling as a function of applicant background may underlie recent reports of higher interview rates among applicants who submitted at least 1 geographic preference compared to those with no regional preference (internal medicine 2021–2022 application cycle) [38]. Nevertheless, geography does appear to play an important role in the residency application process. In one study of applicants to 6 different specialties (all of which used preference signaling without formal geographic signaling), a preference signal was even more likely to result in an interview if the candidate also had a geographic connection to the institution [39]. Compared to prior application cycles, the association between geographic ties and interview invitations may be even stronger now in the era of virtual interviews [40].

13.3 What Type of Program (Categorical Versus Preliminary)

As a prospective general surgeon, the extent to which you should focus on preliminary position opportunities again centers on the recurring theme of introspection. For appropriate applicants, a preliminary year offers an invaluable platform to acclimate to an institution, refine professional interests, and has been the launching pad for many highly successful surgeons. A recent survey of former preliminary general surgery interns spanning a 25-year period at Mayo Clinic (Rochester, Minnesota) found that most respondents viewed this experience as an overall "strong foundation" for their future career, and 82% reported willingness to repeat their preliminary year experience [41]. The institutional experience of preliminary general surgery residents at the University of Colorado in Denver, characterized by a large annual preliminary resident cohort and strong longitudinal mentorship program, has been described as very positive, with 79% of residents ultimately receiving categorical training positions (including general surgery, surgical subspecialties, and non-surgical specialties) [42]. Preliminary general surgery residents are frequently retained at the institution where they complete their preliminary training [42, 43].

Importantly, however, a preliminary position may also be associated with several unique challenges. In the aforementioned Mayo Clinic survey, a majority of respondents reported significant stress associated with their non-categorical status, while 1-in-3 also reported the perception of implicit comparison versus their categorical general surgery peers to be a negative experience [41]. Further, 40% of respondents noted fewer interview invitations during their second versus first application cycle and, in retrospect, more than half (54%) of respondents may have instead opted for a categorical position at a different institution [41]. In one American Board of Surgery resident survey, non-designated preliminary residents reported an overall less rewarding experience compared to their categorical resident contemporaries, including lower program satisfaction, less collegiality, worse operative experience, and lower commitment to ultimate completion of surgical residency training [44]. Similarly, a recent Society for Improving Medical Professional Learning (SIMPL) data registry analysis found first-year preliminary general surgery residents to have less operative autonomy and less likely to receive operative feedback compared to their categorical resident peers, despite demonstrating similar overall performance in the operating room, conceivably contributing to inferior performance of preliminary versus categorical residents during PGY-2 year [45].

Taken together, a preliminary general surgery position would seem to be a potentially valuable opportunity, with the caveat that not all positions are created equal. Institutional factors predictive of future success in obtaining a categorical residency position include larger residency class size, research infrastructure, and the availability of preliminary PGY-2 positions [46]. Several factors related to applicant background and career aspirations may also influence the ultimate success of a preliminary resident in matriculating into a categorical general surgery position [47]. However, most preliminary candidates likely fare better at an institution which offers structured support and career mentorship specific to preliminary residents [48]. As a candidate for a preliminary general surgery position, it is critical to understand the track record of your predecessors in achieving their intermediate and long-term career goals.

13.4 Program Culture

General surgery residents are faced with a wide array of professional and personal stressors [49, 50]. According to one prior survey, as many as 1-in-5 categorical general surgery residents will leave residency (most often to pursue non-surgical residency) [51]. Resident burnout is multifaceted, driven by both professional and personal factors, and independently associated with many aspects of the organizational and educational environment, workload, social support, and sense of personal satisfaction [52]. In general, as evidenced by the fact that residents from programs with historically high attrition rates are also the most likely to strongly consider leaving residency themselves, program culture is undoubtedly a key determinant of success toward a career in general surgery [7].

Once applications are submitted, interviews begin, and you will start to learn about the intricacies and culture of each program. Program culture means different things to different people but, as your rank list begins to take shape, culture should be a priority. Relationships at work are critical to the well-being of a general surgery resident (both positively and negatively) [53]. Among general surgery trainees, a sense of social belonging is positively associated with well-being, and inversely associated with a desire to leave residency [54]. In fact, work conditions on specific rotations—even more so than excessive work hours—are a frequently cited cause for residents to seriously consider leaving a general surgery training program [7]. The relationship between senior and junior residents in particular has been shown to have a direct effect on the well-being of junior residents [55]. Resident socialization with attending physicians, as well as perception that they can turn to their attendings with problems, are significant predictors of overall residency satisfaction [56]. Positive reinforcement from more senior physicians can also help with progression of learning, operative ability, and advancement in surgical training [57]. In addition, program culture affects trainee response to medical errors, as well as their ability to constructively learn from mistakes [58].

Beyond relationships with peers and faculty, job satisfaction among general surgery residents is directly related to a perception of organizational support [59]. There exists significant variability in how program directors solicit information, engage in, and respond to issues regarding resident wellness [60]. To that end, mixed-methods survey data has identified program responsiveness as a significant predictor of general surgery resident wellness [61]. Common themes among those who leave general surgery residency include a perception that their education is not prioritized, negative interactions with leadership, and non-responsiveness to personal and/or program concerns [62].

Applicants should also consider the extent to which their program affords the opportunity for a healthy work-life balance. Burnout rates are directly associated with number of hours worked per week, and reported by 100% of respondents working $\geq$ the ACGME 80 hour-per-week limit [50]. Conversely, the perception of being well rested is a commonly cited protective factor among general surgery residents who complete their residency [7].

13.5 Program Type, Size, and Location

World-class surgical training can be found at both university- and community-based surgical residency programs across the United States. One prior national survey found residents in community programs to be most satisfied with their operative experience (85%) compared to their counterparts in university (73%) or military (62%) programs [63]. Surgical residents in community programs were also more likely to report their opinions valued and found it easy to ask for help from attending physicians [63]. However, current evidence suggests no significant difference in operative autonomy between university- or community-based general surgery residency programs [64]. General surgery residents at university- and community-based programs also experience similar rates of attrition [65]. Training in certain geographic regions has been associated with decreased chief resident confidence in their ability to practice independently after residency, although it remains unclear whether such observations result from differences in training *per se*, or rather from other factors including career choice [66, 67]. Irrespective of training setting, one consistent theme across multiple reports of trainee satisfaction and operative confidence is the importance of case volume, which is also thought to underlie other facility/location-related differences in the trainee experience [63].

Training setting does seem to have an impact on a trainee's future practice setting owing to exposure to different types of faculty role models. A prior survey of new general surgery residency graduates on career selection revealed that most graduates who opted for general surgery practice were significantly influenced to forego subspecialty fellowship by a general surgery mentor [68]. Conversely, exposure to more faculty subspecialists and fellows at a university program likely facilitates greater exploration of various subspecialty career opportunities, which is noteworthy given that career ambitions among incoming PGY-1 general surgery residents are highly labile and seldom predictive of ultimate career path [69]. (Several studies have reported the presence of a fellowship program to have a net benefit on the general surgery resident training experience with minimal impact on resident case volume [70–72].) Additionally, many general surgery residents will perform more cases in their intended fellowship choice compared to their peers, suggesting an opportunity for some level of pre-fellowship specialization during residency [73]. Importantly, the vast majority of both those pursuing general practice as well as fellowship are highly satisfied with their career choice [68].

13.6 Research

According to one recent review of United States general surgery residency programs, nearly 60% were found to offer dedicated research time (ranging from 1–4 years), while dedicated research time was a requirement of 12% of programs [74]. Dedicated research time is generally more common at large, university-based, and fellowship-affiliated institutions [75]. Overall, more than 1-in-3 general surgery residents extend their training by 1–2 years for research [76].

There are several potential advantages to a dedicated research experience during general surgery residency. One prior survey of surgery trainees found that a large proportion of those who took research time subsequently went on to become funded investigators [77]. Some programs allow trainees to pursue another advanced degree (e.g., MPH, MBA, or PhD) during their dedicated research time, which may also be effective in preparing for a career in academic surgery [78]. Many trainees consider this period to be very formative with respect to professional development, career exploration, and cultivating mentorship [79].

Importantly, however, general surgery residents report a broad range of motivations for pursuing dedicated research time. While many residents are encouraged for academic and professional reasons, some residents are instead motivated by burnout, or the perception of insufficient research support or mentorship within the traditional residency structure [79]. In fact, in one survey of several hundred PGY-3 clinical and dedicated research residents, those out on research were less likely to perceive their program as a "good fit," and were also less likely to consider their program to have approachable faculty or an adequate support system [75].

Thus, far more important than a dedicated research period in and of itself is the resident's motivation for pursuing this experience and, by extension, how they choose to use this time. Among surgical trainees who partake in dedicated research time, subsequent grant funding is significantly associated with the actual number of manuscripts authored during this period [77]. Moreover, if research time is pursued, it often carries an expectation of research productivity (be it explicit or implicit). While direct literature from research-year residents is sparse, one prior survey of program directors and applicants on dedicated research time after medical school (e.g., to strengthen a residency application) found a median of 2.5 (interquartile range 2–3) publications and median 2 (interquartile range 2–3) publications per year to be considered "academically productive" [80]. For trainees with future fellowship and/or academic aspirations, it thus stands to reason that research output below this threshold during a dedicated research period may invite new questions regarding their capacity for academic productivity.

Applicants must also understand the implications of dedicated research time for their own career as well as for their program. Dedicated research time has major financial implications on resident and programs alike, including an estimated net opportunity cost in excess of $1 million on future career earnings [81]. Candidates interested in research time must also be aware of funding, which is highly variable across institutions, and may include departmental funds and institutional training grants, or alternatively require individual grants from other professional societies [76]. One prior survey of new general surgery residency program graduates found taking dedicated research year(s) to be independently associated with decreased confidence in performing several open surgical procedures [66]. Although the nature of survey data precludes cause-and-effect analysis, it is important to consider how dedicated research time may or may not affect your progression as a surgical trainee.

13.7 Additional Considerations

This section touches upon additional features of residency programs which merit consideration during the application process. These factors may be of high importance to select applicants with specific needs or certain career aspirations. However, for most applicants, these will be of secondary importance to program location, culture and setting, and research requirement/duration.

13.7.1 Departmental and Institutional Infrastructure

Both directly and indirectly, residency program coordinators are highly influential in shaping a resident's day-to-day experience, and are a well-described source of social support across multiple medical specialty training programs [82, 83]. The presence of advanced practice providers is generally viewed to have a positive impact on the general surgery resident training experience, as it may streamline care and decrease physician workload, although the exact role of advanced practice providers may be somewhat variable [84–88]. Effective partnership with clinical support staff has also been shown to have a significant positive effect on general surgery education and wellness [89].

13.7.2 Robotics Curriculum

A growing number of general surgery residency programs are offering greater breadth and depth of robotic surgery experience [90]. However there remains no formal or standardized curriculum, and current exposure remains highly variable in terms of composition, credentialing, and case tracking, and thus likely in resident competency [91]. This has led to growing interest in a formal robotics curriculum, including early operative exposure and robust simulation training, during surgical residency [92]. A recent survey of general surgery program directors found that most respondents agree on the importance of robotics exposure as a core residency requirement and 83% reported a net benefit associated with robotic training [93]. Compared to community-based programs, university programs may offer greater trainee exposure to robotics, although robotic surgery continues to gain widespread traction among general surgeons in all settings [93, 94].

13.7.3 ABSITE Preparation

The American Board of Surgery In-Training Examination (ABSITE), while originally designed as a medical knowledge assessment without tangible implications, is now being used in some instances for resident evaluation and fellowship selection [95]. Among general surgery residents, a regular study schedule throughout the year (opposed to a focused curriculum closer to the test date) is related to higher ABSITE scores (as well as less burnout) [96]. General surgery program directors report a wide range of strategies for preparing trainees for this exam [95]. Most program directors report ABSITE scores to be a "low priority" or "not a priority." [95] However, different programs may have different attitudes toward ABSITE, as well as the implications of a resident's performance. It would be reasonable to expect that a program which places greater emphasis on trainee performance also have the resources in place to help them succeed. This may include an academic stipend, protected study time, or department-funded question banks and review courses.

13.7.4 Global Health

Approximately one-third of general surgery residency programs offer international experiences for current residents, typically during PGY3 or PGY4 years, most often based in either Central and South America or Africa [97]. Such opportunities may involve clinical experiences, research, or a combination of both [98]. However, the duration of such opportunities typically lasts 1–4 weeks, and the primary source of funding is variable, potentially requiring a sizable personal contribution [97]. This may be of particular importance to candidates with specific global health career aspirations.

13.7.5 Practice Readiness

Despite established patient safety and quality improvement curricula in general surgery residency programs, many residents feel unprepared to lead quality improvement initiatives, participate in patient safety measures, and provide cost-conscious care [99]. According to one survey of general surgery residency program directors, fewer than half of residency programs offer an autonomous general surgery outpatient experience, and only one-in-four programs offer some type of practice management curriculum [100]. An increasing number of programs are instead fulfilling these requirements with emergency/acute care surgery rotations at a program's main teaching hospital, which do notably positively contribute to case volume and operative experience [100, 101]. Nevertheless, the availability of an autonomous outpatient experience and/or practice management curriculum may be of interest to applicants with an inclination for independent practice after residency [100]. A chief resident service, wherein the chief resident is designated with operative, call, and administrative responsibilities as to parallel a trainee's first year experience after graduation, may indeed be highly effective in promoting resident autonomy [102].

13.8 Integrated Specialty Applicants

General surgery specialty integrated programs are growing in acceptance and popularity [103, 104]. Integrated programs tend to match highly competitive applicants based on relevant predictors of match success [105–107]. However, such applicants also frequently report negative experiences during general surgery interviews, and feel that their application to integrated specialty programs is a detriment to their chance at matching to a general surgery program [108]. Trainees in integrated specialty programs also report concerns about curriculum variability and incohesive integration with traditional general surgery training [109]. Given these unique barriers, integrated program applicants should seek mentorship within their subspecialty of interest and, when possible, also pursue guidance from those specifically familiar with integrated pathways.

13.9 Unique Populations

Growing emphasis is being placed on a holistic general surgery residency application review process [110]. Several initiatives for promoting diversity within general surgery residency programs have been described [111]. However, increasing gender and racial diversity among matriculating medical school cohorts has not consistently translated to greater diversity among general surgery applicants [112]. Women, underrepresented minorities, and individuals who identify as LGBTQ+ face unique challenges during surgical residency which merit additional consideration during the application process.

Women in surgery are more likely to report dissatisfaction with their residency experience compared to their male counterparts [56]. Females surgeons are also more likely to strongly consider leaving residency training and report higher rates of burnout [7, 50]. Underrepresented minorities in general surgery may be more prone to issues with program fit and report greater difficulties in successful integration with faculty and peers [113]. Lower graduation rates also exist among underrepresented minorities in general surgery residency programs [114]. Although available data are sparse, LGBTQ+ surgery residents more often report mistreatment, discrimination, and even suicidality [115].

Women, underrepresented minorities, and LGBTQ+ individuals may have to actively seek program information pertinent to their own training experience. For those interested in childrearing, it is important to recognize that significant heterogeneity exists between program policies on parental leave, childcare services, and resources for breastfeeding [116]. Several barriers inhibiting a program's support of maternal and lactation policies have been described [117]. Unfortunately, parental benefit information for residents is also inconsistently available publicly [118]. Of note, several programs have worked to refine their interview process in recent years by offering informational sessions specifically tailored to resources available for women, underrepresented minorities, and LGBTQ+ individuals, which many candidates find helpful [20]. As efforts to promote diversity among trainees are not necessarily paralleled amongst departmental leadership, candidates may also wish to consider the documented value of finding mentors with shared backgrounds and experiences, particularly as it relates to a future career in academic surgery [119–124].

13.10 Conclusions

Success in the general surgery residency match is predicated on a sound and honest understanding of an applicant's own strengths and weaknesses. Identifying a very select list of program features deemed critical to the applicant, particularly those which directly influence access to social support, may be useful in guiding the applicant's program list. Beyond these "non-negotiables," program culture, in the form of peer and faculty relationships and organizational support, is paramount. Exceptional operative experience may be found at both university and community programs as trainee confidence appears most related to operative case volume. The biggest difference between university- and community-based programs is likely the professional responsibilities of faculty mentors, which may influence a trainee's career trajectory, although graduates pursuing independent practice and fellowship alike report very high rates of professional satisfaction. Many programs offer or require dedicated research time, which may have several academic and professional advantages, but also carries a significant opportunity cost and is sometimes only pursued out of necessity to mitigate burnout. Additional program factors which may be of interest to applicants include robotics curriculum, practice management experience, standardized test prep, global health opportunities, and other institutional resources. Integrated surgery applicants, as well as women, underrepresented minorities, and LGBTQ+ individuals, may also face unique challenges during the application process and likely further benefit from strong mentorship.

References

1. Meagher AD, Beadles CA, Sheldon GF, Charles AG. Opportunities to create new general surgery residency programs to alleviate the shortage of general surgeons. Acad Med. 2016;91(6):833–8. https://doi.org/10.1097/acm.0000000000001005. PubMed PMID: 26606721.
2. Stefanidis D, Miles WS, Greene FL. Factors influencing residency choice of general surgery applicants—how important is the availability of a skills curriculum? J Surg Educ. 2009;66(6):325–9. https://doi.org/10.1016/j.jsurg.2009.06.004. PubMed PMID: 20142129.

3. Naaseh A, de Virgilio C, Nahmias J. General surgery residency match: time for more than a virtual change. J Surg Educ. 2021;78(6):1771–5. https://doi.org/10.1016/j.jsurg.2021.06.003. Epub 2021 July 30. PubMed PMID: 34340955; PMCID: PMC8635495.
4. Hashmi A, Policherla R, Campbell H, Khan FA, Schumaier A, Al-Mufarrej F. How informative are the plastic surgery residency websites to prospective applicants? J Surg Educ. 2017;74(1):74–8. https://doi.org/10.1016/j.jsurg.2016.08.002.
5. Wilson AB, Torbeck LJ, Dunnington GL. Ranking surgical residency programs: reputation survey or outcomes measures? J Surg Educ. 2015;72(6):e243–50. https://doi.org/10.1016/j.jsurg.2015.03.021. Epub 2015 May 14. PubMed PMID: 25980829.
6. Yaow CYL, Mok HT, Ng CH, Devi MK, Iyer S, Chong CS. Difficulties faced by general surgery residents. A qualitative systematic review. J Surg Educ. 2020;77(6):1396–406. https://doi.org/10.1016/j.jsurg.2020.06.003.
7. Gifford E, Galante J, Kaji AH, Nguyen V, Nelson MT, Sidwell RA, Hartranft T, Jarman B, Melcher M, Reeves M, Reid C, Jacobsen GR, Thompson J, Are C, Smith B, Arnell T, Hines OJ, de Virgilio C. Factors associated with general surgery residents' desire to leave residency programs: a multi-institutional study. JAMA Surg. 2014;149(9):948–53. https://doi.org/10.1001/jamasurg.2014.935. PubMed PMID: 25075473.
8. Stain SC, Hiatt JR, Ata A, Ashley SW, Roggin KK, Potts JR, Moore RA, Galante JM, Britt LD, Deveney KE, Ellison EC. Characteristics of highly ranked applicants to general surgery residency programs. JAMA Surg. 2013;148(5):413–7. https://doi.org/10.1001/jamasurg.2013.180. PubMed PMID: 23677403.
9. Iwai Y, Lenze NR, Becnel CM, Mihalic AP, Stitzenberg KB. Evaluation of predictors for successful residency match in general surgery. J Surg Educ. 2022;79(3):579–86. https://doi.org/10.1016/j.jsurg.2021.11.003. Epub 2021 Nov 29. PubMed PMID: 34852956.
10. Makdisi G, Takeuchi T, Rodriguez J, Rucinski J, Wise L. How we select our residents—a survey of selection criteria in general surgery residents. J Surg Educ. 2011;68(1):67–72. https://doi.org/10.1016/j.jsurg.2010.10.003.
11. Jarman BT, Joshi AR, Trickey AW, Dort JM, Kallies KJ, Sidwell RA. Factors and influences that determine the choices of surgery residency applicants. J Surg Educ. 2015;72(6):e163–71. https://doi.org/10.1016/j.jsurg.2015.05.017. Epub 2015 July 2. PubMed PMID: 26143518.
12. Lin LO, Makhoul AT, Hackenberger PN, Ganesh Kumar N, Schoenbrunner AR, Pontell ME, Drolet BC, Janis JE. Implications of pass/fail step 1 scoring: plastic surgery program director and applicant perspective. Plast Reconstr Surg Glob Open. 2020;8(12):e3266. https://doi.org/10.1097/gox.0000000000003266. Epub 2020 Dec 17. PubMed PMID: 33425583; PMCID: PMC7787322.
13. Ganesh Kumar N, Makhoul AT, Pontell ME, Drolet BC. Characterizing the effect of pass/fail U.S. medical licensing examination step 1 scoring in neurosurgery: program directors' perspectives. World Neurosurg. 2020;142:e440–4. https://doi.org/10.1016/j.wneu.2020.07.053.
14. Ozair A, Bhat V, Detchou DKE. The US residency selection process after the United States medical licensing examination step 1 pass/fail change: overview for applicants and educators. JMIR Med Educ. 2023;9:e37069. https://doi.org/10.2196/37069. Epub 2023 Jan 6. PubMed PMID: 36607718; PMCID: PMC9862334.
15. Girard AO, Qiu C, Lake IV, Chen J, Lopez CD, Yang R. US medical student perspectives on the impact of a pass/fail USMLE step 1. J Surg Educ. 2022;79(2):397–408. https://doi.org/10.1016/j.jsurg.2021.09.010.
16. Raborn LN, Janis JE. Current views on the new United States medical licensing examination step 1 pass/fail format: a review of the literature. J Surg Res. 2022;274:31–45. https://doi.org/10.1016/j.jss.2022.01.002. Epub 2022 Feb 1. PubMed PMID: 35121548.
17. Quinn KM, Runge LT, Parrado RH, Streck CJ, Abbott AM, Talley CL. General surgery applicants report the impact of virtual interviews on their rank list and match. Global Surg Educ. 2022;1(1):65. https://doi.org/10.1007/s44186-022-00071-8.
18. Finney N, Stopenski S, Smith BR. Applicant perspectives of virtual general surgery residency interviews. Am Surg. 2022;88(10):2556–60. https://doi.org/10.1177/00031348221103658.

19. Beesley H, Pernar L, Kettoola Y, Hess D. The association between virtual interviewing and geographical distribution of matched residency programs for general surgery applicants. J Surg Educ. 2023;80(2):194–9. https://doi.org/10.1016/j.jsurg.2022.09.018.
20. Zarate Rodriguez JG, Caldwell KE, Donald CM, Wise PE, Awad MM. General surgery virtual residency recruitment in 2021 and 2022: lessons learned. Global Surg Educ. 2023;2(1):82. https://doi.org/10.1007/s44186-023-00160-2.
21. Lamberton T, Tung C, Kaji AH, Neville AL, Singer GA, Simms ER, Lona Y, Virgilio CD. Faculty scoring of general surgery residency interviewees: a comparison of in-person and virtual interview formats. J Surg Educ. 2022;79(6):e69–75. https://doi.org/10.1016/j.jsurg.2022.09.003.
22. Wames WM, Welter M, Folkert K, Elian A, Timmons J, Sawyer R, Shebrain S. Applicants performance in interview for a general surgery residency pre- and during coronavirus disease-19 pandemic. J Surg Res. 2024;293:341–6. https://doi.org/10.1016/j.jss.2023.08.040.
23. Ho JW, Joung RH, Krueger M, Cid C, Holmstrom AL, Schlick CJR, Tatebe LC, Alam HB, Halverson AL, Christopher DA. Understanding general surgery applicant expectations and perceptions in the virtual interview process. J Surg Educ. 2022;79(6):e61–e8. https://doi.org/10.1016/j.jsurg.2022.07.024.
24. Zarate Rodriguez JG, Caldwell KE, Donald CM, Wise PE, Awad MM. Preference signaling for general surgery residency: how should applicants use signaling? J Surg Res. 2024;293:580–6. https://doi.org/10.1016/j.jss.2023.09.023.
25. Pletcher SD, Chang CWD, Thorne MC, Malekzadeh S. The otolaryngology residency program preference signaling experience. Acad Med. 2022;97(5):664–8. https://doi.org/10.1097/acm.0000000000004441. Epub 2021 Oct 5. PubMed PMID: 34618735; PMCID: PMC9028299.
26. Grauer R, Ranti D, Greene K, Gorin MA, Menon M, Zorc S. Characterization of applicant preference signals, invitations for interviews, and inclusion on match lists for residency positions in urology. JAMA Netw Open. 2023;6(1):e2250974. https://doi.org/10.1001/jamanetworkopen.2022.50974. Epub 2023 Jan 3. PubMed PMID: 36662528; PMCID: PMC9860522.
27. Pletcher SD, Chang CWD, Thorne MC, Malekzadeh S, Francis CL, Naemi B, Costa J, Dunleavy D. Interview invitations for otolaryngology residency positions across demographic groups following implementation of preference signaling. JAMA Netw Open. 2023;6(3):e231922. https://doi.org/10.1001/jamanetworkopen.2023.1922. Epub 2023 Mar 1. PubMed PMID: 36881409; PMCID: PMC9993176.
28. Catalanotti JS, Swails JL. Preference signals in residency applications: a potential tool to combat application inflation. J Gen Intern Med. 2023;39:357–8. https://doi.org/10.1007/s11606-023-08451-6.
29. Sorenson JC, Ryan PM, Ward RA, Fornfeist DS. The value of signaling an orthopaedic surgery program: a survey to orthopaedic surgery programs. J Am Acad Orthop Surg Glob Res Rev. 2023;7(6):e23.00050. https://doi.org/10.5435/JAAOSGlobal-D-23-00050. Epub 2023 Jun 2. PubMed PMID: 37276378; PMCID: PMC10241500.
30. Haque WZ, Taub PJ, Hammoud MM. Congestion in the coming residency match: it is time for an interview cap. Acad Med. 2021;96(2):163–4.
31. Farooq S, Mehta A. Modeling the urology residency application and match process: a mathematical argument for application and interview caps. Urology. 2023;173:48–54. https://doi.org/10.1016/j.urology.2022.11.042.
32. Strand EA, Winkel AF, Marzano DA, Morgan HK, Staples H, Hammoud MM. Stakeholder perspectives on limiting residency applications and interviews in obstetrics and gynecology. J Surg Educ. 2022;79(2):362–9. https://doi.org/10.1016/j.jsurg.2021.10.012.
33. Morgan HK, Winkel AF, Standiford T, Muñoz R, Strand EA, Marzano DA, Ogburn T, Major CA, Cox S, Hammoud MM. The case for capping residency interviews. J Surg Educ. 2021;78(3):755–62. https://doi.org/10.1016/j.jsurg.2020.08.033.
34. Carmody JB, Rosman IS, Carlson JC. Application fever: reviewing the causes, costs, and cures for residency application inflation. Cureus. 2021;13(3):e13804. https://doi.org/10.7759/cureus.13804. Epub 2021 Mar 10. PubMed PMID: 33850672; PMCID: PMC8034763.

35. Mitton TJ, Elder R, Hunter JB. A simulation of the effect of interview caps on the national resident matching program match in otolaryngology. Acad Med. 2023;98(4):448–54. https://doi.org/10.1097/acm.0000000000005122. Epub 2022 Dec 12. PubMed PMID: 36515560.
36. Rajesh A, Asaad M. Alternative strategies for evaluating general surgery residency applicants and an interview limit for MATCH 2021: an impending necessity. Ann Surg. 2021;273(1):109–11. https://doi.org/10.1097/sla.0000000000004501. PubMed PMID: 32941286.
37. Association of American Medical Colleges: ERAS 2024 cycle applicant and application data. https://www.aamc.org/data-reports/data/eras-statistics-data. Accessed 2 Mar 2024.
38. Benjamin WJ, Lenze NR, Bohm LA, Thorne MC, Kupfer RA, Sepdham D, Mihalic AP, Abraham R. Evaluating the impact of the novel geographic preferences section on interview rate and residency match outcomes. J Gen Intern Med. 2024;39:–365. https://doi.org/10.1007/s11606-023-08342-w. Epub 2023 Aug 1. PubMed PMID: 37528251.
39. Benjamin WJ, Lenze NR, Bohm LA, Thorne MC, Abraham R, Sepdham D, Mihalic AP, Kupfer RA. Impact of applicants' characteristics and geographic connections to residency programs on preference signaling outcomes in the match. Acad Med. 2024;99(4):437–44. https://doi.org/10.1097/acm.0000000000005551. Epub 2023 Nov 17. PubMed PMID: 37976398.
40. Luu Y, Gao W, Han J, Mihalic A, Vandergriff T. Personal connections and preference signaling: a cross-sectional analysis of the dermatology residency match during COVID-19. J Am Acad Dermatol. 2023;88(6):1381–3.
41. Rajesh A, Asaad M, Chandra A, Rivera M, Stulak JM, Heller SF, Farley DR. What do former residents say about their nondesignated preliminary year? A survey of prelims' experiences in a general surgery residency program. J Surg Educ. 2020;77(2):281–90. https://doi.org/10.1016/j.jsurg.2019.10.003. Epub 2019 Oct 31. PubMed PMID: 31677981.
42. Montero P, Powell R, Travis CM, Nehler MR. Selection, mentorship, and subsequent placement of preliminary residents without a designated categorical position in an academic general surgery residency program. J Surg Educ. 2012;69(6):785–91. Epub 2012 May 30. PubMed PMID: 23111047. https://doi.org/10.1016/j.jsurg.2012.04.009.
43. Pezzi CM, Leibrandt TJ, Augustine RT, Nakao S, Borman KR, Dent TL, Kukora JS. Nondesignated preliminary residents in general surgery: 25-year outcomes. Am J Surg. 2011;202(2):233–6. https://doi.org/10.1016/j.amjsurg.2010.06.033. PubMed PMID: 21810503.
44. Sullivan MC, Yeo H, Roman SA, Jones AT, Bell RH Jr, Sosa JA. Discrepancies in training satisfaction and program completion among 2662 categorical and preliminary general surgery residents. Ann Surg. 2013;257(6):1174–80. https://doi.org/10.1097/SLA.0b013e3182718ef1. PubMed PMID: 23059505.
45. Gates RS, Moreci R, Marcotte K, Paget C, Krumm AE, Yee CC, George BC. Operative experiences of preliminary versus categorical general surgery residents. Global Surg Educ. 2023;2(1):114. https://doi.org/10.1007/s44186-023-00196-4.
46. Ritter KA, Anand RJ, Beard K, Edelman DA, Huth L, Namm J, Hope W, Allen S, Joshi A, Hildreth A, Tu C, Seavey CN, Vilchez V, Lipman J. Impact of surgery program characteristics on fate of non-designated preliminary surgery interns. J Surg Educ. 2020;77(6):e11–9. https://doi.org/10.1016/j.jsurg.2020.06.001.
47. Kearse LE, Stewart S, Williams K, Cornwell EE 3rd, Wilson LL, Williams M. An analysis of preliminary general surgery residents' matriculation into categorical positions. J Surg Educ. 2022;79(6):e25–9. https://doi.org/10.1016/j.jsurg.2022.06.012. Epub 20220728. PubMed PMID: 35907698.
48. Rawlings A, Doty J, Frevert A, Quick J. Finding them a spot: a successful preliminary match curriculum. J Surg Educ. 2018;75(6):e78–84. https://doi.org/10.1016/j.jsurg.2018.09.011.
49. Ha GQ, Go JT, Murayama KM, Steinemann S. Identifying sources of stress across years of general surgery residency. Hawaii J Health Soc Welf. 2020;79(3):75–81. PubMed PMID: 32190839; PMCID: PMC7061032.

50. Kinslow K, Sutherland M, McKenney M, Elkbuli A. Reported burnout among U.S. general surgery residents: a survey of the association of program directors in surgery members. Ann Med Surg (Lond). 2020;60:14–9. https://doi.org/10.1016/j.amsu.2020.10.012. Epub 2020 Oct 14. PubMed PMID: 33072313; PMCID: PMC7556262.
51. Yeo H, Bucholz E, Ann Sosa J, Curry L, Lewis FR Jr, Jones AT, Viola K, Lin Z, Bell RH Jr. A national study of attrition in general surgery training: which residents leave and where do they go? Ann Surg. 2010;252(3):529–34. https://doi.org/10.1097/SLA.0b013e3181f2789c; discussion 34–6. PubMed PMID: 20739854.
52. Ellis RJ, Nicolas JD, Cheung E, Zhang L, Ma M, Turner P, Nussbaum MS, Are C, Smink DS, Etkin C, Bilimoria KY, Hu YY. Comprehensive characterization of the general surgery residency learning environment and the association with resident burnout. Ann Surg. 2021;274(1):6–11. https://doi.org/10.1097/sla.0000000000004796. PubMed PMID: 33605580.
53. Ratanawongsa N, Wright SM, Carrese JA. Well-being in residency: effects on relationships with patients, interactions with colleagues, performance, and motivation. Patient Educ Couns. 2008;72(2):194–200. https://doi.org/10.1016/j.pec.2008.04.010.
54. Salles A, Wright RC, Milam L, Panni RZ, Liebert CA, Lau JN, Lin DT, Mueller CM. Social belonging as a predictor of surgical resident well-being and attrition. J Surg Educ. 2019;76(2):370–7. https://doi.org/10.1016/j.jsurg.2018.08.022.
55. Torres-Landa S, Moreno K, Brasel KJ, Rogers DA. Identification of leadership behaviors that impact general surgery junior residents' well-being: a needs assessment in a single academic center. J Surg Educ. 2022;79(1):86–93. https://doi.org/10.1016/j.jsurg.2021.07.017.
56. Sullivan MC, Bucholz EM, Yeo H, Roman SA, Bell RH, Sosa JA. "Join the club": effect of resident and attending social interactions on overall satisfaction among 4390 general surgery residents. Arch Surg. 2012;147(5):408–14. https://doi.org/10.1001/archsurg.2012.27. PubMed PMID: 22785631.
57. Kamali D, Illing J. How can positive and negative trainer feedback in the operating theatre impact a surgical trainee's confidence and well-being: a qualitative study in the north of England. BMJ Open. 2018;8(2):e017935. https://doi.org/10.1136/bmjopen-2017-017935. Epub 2018 Feb 12. PubMed PMID: 29440141; PMCID: PMC5829657.
58. Lee J, Lin RP, Haney V, Abell BM, Lin PP. Individual, cultural, and systems factors affect surgical residents' experience with medical errors and learning from mistakes. Global Surg Educ. 2023;2(1):55. https://doi.org/10.1007/s44186-023-00133-5.
59. Appelbaum NP, Lee N, Amendola M, Dodson K, Kaplan B. Surgical resident burnout and job satisfaction: the role of workplace climate and perceived support. J Surg Res. 2019;234:20–5. https://doi.org/10.1016/j.jss.2018.08.035.
60. Foote DC, Evans J, Engler T, Gutterman S, Lussiez A, Amortegui D, Bilimoria KY, Johnson JK, Hu Y-Y, Sandhu G. How program directors understand general surgery resident wellness. J Surg Educ. 2022;79(6):e48–60. https://doi.org/10.1016/j.jsurg.2022.07.022.
61. Joung RH, Amortegui D, Silver CM, Mackiewicz NI, Eng JS, Rosenkranz KM, Johnson J, Bilimoria KY, Hu YY. A national mixed-methods evaluation of general surgery residency program responsiveness and the association with resident wellness. J Surg Educ. 2022;79(6):e1–e11. https://doi.org/10.1016/j.jsurg.2022.05.004. Epub 2022 Jun 2. PubMed PMID: 35660306.
62. Bongiovanni T, Yeo H, Sosa JA, Yoo PS, Long T, Rosenthal M, Berg D, Curry L, Nunez-Smith M. Attrition from surgical residency training: perspectives from those who left. Am J Surg. 2015;210(4):648–54. https://doi.org/10.1016/j.amjsurg.2015.05.014.
63. Friedell ML, VanderMeer TJ, Cheatham ML, Fuhrman GM, Schenarts PJ, Mellinger JD, Morris JB. Perceptions of graduating general surgery chief residents: are they confident in their training? J Am Coll Surg. 2014;218(4):695–703. https://doi.org/10.1016/j.jamcollsurg.2013.12.022. Epub 2013 Dec 24. PubMed PMID: 24529805.
64. Gates RS, Bidwell SS, Chen X, Thelen AE, George BC, Krumm AE, Kim GJ. Resident operative autonomy: do community-based programs offer more than university-based programs? Global Surg Educ. 2022;1(1):26.

65. Yeo HL, Abelson JS, Symer MM, Mao J, Michelassi F, Bell R, Sedrakyan A, Sosa JA. Association of time to attrition in surgical residency with individual resident and programmatic factors. JAMA Surg. 2018;153(6):511–7. https://doi.org/10.1001/jamasurg.2017.6202. PubMed PMID: 29466536; PMCID: PMC5875388.
66. Fonseca AL, Reddy V, Longo WE, Gusberg RJ. Graduating general surgery resident operative confidence: perspective from a national survey. J Surg Res. 2014;190(2):419–28. https://doi.org/10.1016/j.jss.2014.05.014. Epub 2014 May 10. PubMed PMID: 24908164.
67. Bucholz EM, Sue GR, Yeo H, Roman SA, Bell RH Jr, Sosa JA. Our trainees' confidence: results from a national survey of 4136 US general surgery residents. Arch Surg. 2011;146(8):907–14. https://doi.org/10.1001/archsurg.2011.178. PubMed PMID: 21844434.
68. Klingensmith ME, Cogbill TH, Luchette F, Biester T, Samonte K, Jones A, Lewis FR, Malangoni MA. Factors influencing the decision of surgery residency graduates to pursue general surgery practice versus fellowship. Ann Surg. 2015;262(3):449–55; discussion 54–5. PubMed PMID: 26258313. https://doi.org/10.1097/sla.0000000000001435.
69. Vick LR, Borman KR. Instability of fellowship intentions during general surgery residencies. J Surg Educ. 2008;65(6):445–52. https://doi.org/10.1016/j.jsurg.2008.07.003. PubMed PMID: 19059176.
70. Hanks JB, Ashley SW, Mahvi DM, Meredith WJ, Stain SC, Biester TW, Borman KR. Feast or famine? The variable impact of coexisting fellowships on general surgery resident operative volumes. Ann Surg. 2011;254(3):476–83; discussion 83–5. PubMed PMID: 21869743. https://doi.org/10.1097/SLA.0b013e31822aa4d5.
71. Hallowell PT, Dahman MI, Stokes JB, LaPar DJ, Schirmer BD. Minimally invasive surgery fellowship does not adversely affect general surgery resident case volume: a decade of experience. Am J Surg. 2013;205(3):307–11; discussion 11. PubMed PMID: 23414954. https://doi.org/10.1016/j.amjsurg.2013.01.005.
72. Dinan KA, Davis JW, Wolfe MM, Sue LP, Cagle KM. An acute care surgery fellowship benefits a general surgical residency. J Trauma Acute Care Surg. 2014;77(2):209–12. https://doi.org/10.1097/ta.0000000000000293. PubMed PMID: 25058243.
73. Woeste MR, Salyer CE, Hammaker AC, Dodwad SJ, Foote DC, Nahmias JT, Callahan ZM, Quillin RC 3rd, Cortez AR. Do general surgery residents begin specializing before fellowship? A multi-institutional study from the US ROPE Consortium. J Am Coll Surg. 2022;235(5):799–808. https://doi.org/10.1097/xcs.0000000000000311. Epub 2022 Oct 17. PubMed PMID: 36102575.
74. Brochu A, Aggarwal R. Research during general surgery residency: a web-based review of opportunities, structure and outputs. J Surg Res. 2018;223:149–54. https://doi.org/10.1016/j.jss.2017.10.024. Epub 2017 Nov 24. PubMed PMID: 29433867.
75. Sue GR, Bucholz EM, Yeo H, Roman SA, Jones A, Bell RH Jr, Sosa JA. The vulnerable stage of dedicated research years of general surgery residency: results of a national survey. Arch Surg. 2011;146(6):653–8. https://doi.org/10.1001/archsurg.2011.12. Epub 2011 Feb 21. PubMed PMID: 21339415.
76. Robertson CM, Klingensmith ME, Coopersmith CM. Prevalence and cost of full-time research fellowships during general surgery residency: a national survey. Ann Surg. 2009;249(1):155–61. https://doi.org/10.1097/SLA.0b013e3181929216. PubMed PMID: 19106692; PMCID: PMC2678555.
77. Robertson CM, Klingensmith ME, Coopersmith CM. Long-term outcomes of performing a postdoctoral research fellowship during general surgery residency. Ann Surg. 2007;245(4):516–23. https://doi.org/10.1097/01.sla.0000245468.98852.42. PubMed PMID: 17414597; PMCID: PMC1877044.
78. Isom CA, Bisgaard EK, Campbell KM, Courtney C, Erickson C, Faber DA, Gauger PG, Greenberg JA, Kassam AF, Mullen JT, Phares A, Quillin RC 3rd, Salcedo ES, Schaffer AJ, Scaria D, Stahl CC, Wise PE, Kauffmann RM, Chen X, Smith JJ, Terhune KP. Does intentional support of degree programs in general surgery residency affect research productivity

or pursuit of academic surgery? A multi-institutional study. J Surg Educ. 2020;77(6):e34–8. https://doi.org/10.1016/j.jsurg.2020.07.008. Epub 2020 Aug 22. PubMed PMID: 32843316.
79. Huffman EM, Anderson TN, Choi JN, Smith BK. Why the lab? What is really motivating general surgery residents to take time for dedicated research. J Surg Educ. 2020;77(6):e39–46. https://doi.org/10.1016/j.jsurg.2020.07.034.
80. Rajesh A, Asaad M, AlJamal YN, Enger TM, Farley DR. Value of research years for international medical graduates applying to general surgery residency. J Surg Educ. 2020;77(6):1350–6. https://doi.org/10.1016/j.jsurg.2020.04.008. Epub 2020 July 31. PubMed PMID: 32741694.
81. DeWane MP, Thomas DC, Longo WE, Yoo PS. Paying the price: understanding the opportunity cost of dedicated research time during surgical training. Am Surg. 2018;84(11):1723–6. PubMed PMID: 30747623.
82. Nickel BL, Roof J, Dolejs S, Choi JN, Torbeck L. Identifying managerial roles of general surgery coordinators: making the case for utilization of a standardized job description framework. J Surg Educ. 2018;75(6):e38–46. https://doi.org/10.1016/j.jsurg.2018.07.003.
83. Locke M, Davis SW. Residency coordinators' social support of residents in family medicine residency programs. Fam Med. 2011;43(8):551–5.
84. Clark CJ, Hildreth A, Migaly J, Sieren L, Carter J, Stewart JHt. Supervisor, colleague, or assistant: general surgery resident perceptions of advanced practitioners. Am Surg. 2018;84(2):294–9. PubMed PMID: 29580361.
85. Eaton B, Hessler L, O'Meara L, Herrera A, Tesoriero R, Diaz J, Bruns B. The impact of advanced practice providers on the surgical resident experience: agree to disagree? Am J Surg. 2019;217(6):1107–11. https://doi.org/10.1016/j.amjsurg.2018.10.014.
86. Kang R, Columbo JA, Kunkel ST, Stucke RS, Sabatino MJ, Tang A, Goodney PP, Rosenkranz KM. Residents' impressions of the impact of advanced practice providers on surgical training. J Am Coll Surg. 2018;226(6):1036–43. https://doi.org/10.1016/j.jamcollsurg.2017.11.019.
87. Kahn SA, Davis SA, Banes CT, Dennis BM, May AK, Gunter OD. Impact of advanced practice providers (nurse practitioners and physician assistants) on surgical residents' critical care experience. J Surg Res. 2015;199(1):7–12. https://doi.org/10.1016/j.jss.2015.05.036.
88. Rosenblatt A, Ballard HA, Amortegui D, Yuce T, Bilimoria KY, Johnson JK, Hu Y-Y. Invisible work: advanced practice providers' role in the education of surgeons. J Surg Educ. 2022;79(6):1353–62. https://doi.org/10.1016/j.jsurg.2022.06.015.
89. Yuce TK, Khorfan R, Jo Rita Schlick C, Joseph Ellis R, Cheung EO, Andrew Greenberg J, Bilimoria KY, Hu Y-Y. Impact of clinical support staff on general surgery residents' education and wellness. J Am Coll Surg. 2020;231(4, Supplement 1):S99. https://doi.org/10.1016/j.jamcollsurg.2020.07.187.
90. Zhao B, Lam J, Hollandsworth HM, Lee AM, Lopez NE, Abbadessa B, Eisenstein S, Cosman BC, Ramamoorthy SL, Parry LA. General surgery training in the era of robotic surgery: a qualitative analysis of perceptions from resident and attending surgeons. Surg Endosc. 2020;34(4):1712–21. https://doi.org/10.1007/s00464-019-06954-0.
91. Tom CM, Maciel JD, Korn A, Ozao-Choy JJ, Hari DM, Neville AL, de Virgilio C, Dauphine C. A survey of robotic surgery training curricula in general surgery residency programs: how close are we to a standardized curriculum? Am J Surg. 2019;217(2):256–60. https://doi.org/10.1016/j.amjsurg.2018.11.006. Epub 2018 Nov 22. PubMed PMID: 30518480.
92. George LC, O'Neill R, Merchant AM. Residency training in robotic general surgery: a survey of program directors. Minim Invasive Surg. 2018;2018:8464298. https://doi.org/10.1155/2018/8464298. Epub 2018 May 8. PubMed PMID: 29854454; PMCID: PMC5964613.
93. Porras Rodriguez P, Kapadia S, Moazzez A, Singer G, Neville A, Yetasook A, Dauphine C. Should robotic surgery training become a general surgery residency requirement? A national survey of program directors in surgery. J Surg Educ. 2022;79(6):e242–7. https://doi.org/10.1016/j.jsurg.2022.06.010. Epub 2022 July 10. PubMed PMID: 35831236.

94. Sheetz KH, Claflin J, Dimick JB. Trends in the adoption of robotic surgery for common surgical procedures. JAMA Netw Open. 2020;3(1):e1918911. https://doi.org/10.1001/jamanetworkopen.2019.18911. Epub 2020 Jan 3. PubMed PMID: 31922557; PMCID: PMC6991252.
95. Caldwell KE, Clanahan JM, Klingensmith ME, Wise PE, Awad MM, Dickinson KJ. National ABSITE preparation practices: a survey of general surgery residency program directors. J Surg Educ. 2024;81(1):56–63. https://doi.org/10.1016/j.jsurg.2023.10.004. Epub 2023 Nov 30. PubMed PMID: 38036385.
96. Smeds MR, Thrush CR, McDaniel FK, Gill R, Kimbrough MK, Shames BD, Sussman JJ, Galante JM, Wittgen CM, Ansari P, Allen SR, Nussbaum MS, Hess DT, Knight DC, Bentley FR. Relationships between study habits, burnout, and general surgery resident performance on the American Board of Surgery In-Training Examination. J Surg Res. 2017;217:217–25. https://doi.org/10.1016/j.jss.2017.05.034. Epub 2017 May 12. PubMed PMID: 28595817.
97. Sobral FA, Bowder AN, Smith L, Ravipati A, Suh MK, Are C. Current status of international experiences in general surgery residency programs in the United States. Springerplus. 2016;5:586. https://doi.org/10.1186/s40064-016-2270-x. Epub 2016 May 11. PubMed PMID: 27247883; PMCID: PMC4864783.
98. Abraham PJ, Abraham MN, Corey BL, Lindeman B, Chen H. Cross-sectional analysis of global surgery opportunities among general surgery residency programs. J Surg Educ. 2020;77(5):1179–85. https://doi.org/10.1016/j.jsurg.2020.03.017. Epub 2020 July 21. PubMed PMID: 32709570.
99. Malhotra NR, Smith JD, Jacobs AC, Johnson CE, Khan US, Ellison HB, Brintz BJ, Millar MM, Cloud WG, Nahmias J, Hendershot KM, Smith BK. High value care education in general surgery residency programs: a multi-institutional needs assessment. Am J Surg. 2021;221(2):291–7. https://doi.org/10.1016/j.amjsurg.2020.09.032. Epub 2020 Sep 28. PubMed PMID: 33039148.
100. Cogbill TH, Klingensmith ME, Jones AT, Biester TW, Malangoni MA. Resident preparation for careers in general surgery: a survey of program directors. J Surg Educ. 2015;72(6):e251–7. https://doi.org/10.1016/j.jsurg.2015.05.001. PubMed PMID: 26073717.
101. Stanley MD, Davenport DL, Procter LD, Perry JE, Kearney PA, Bernard AC. An acute care surgery rotation contributes significant general surgical operative volume to residency training compared with other rotations. J Trauma. 2011;70(3):590–4. https://doi.org/10.1097/TA.0b013e318203386a. PubMed PMID: 21610347.
102. Jarman BT, O'Heron CT, Kallies KJ, Cogbill TH. Enhancing confidence in graduating general surgery residents: establishing a chief surgery resident service at an Independent Academic Medical Center. J Surg Educ. 2018;75(4):888–94. https://doi.org/10.1016/j.jsurg.2017.12.012. Epub 2018 Feb 3. PubMed PMID: 29398631.
103. Zhu Y, Goldstone AB, Woo YJ. Integrated thoracic surgery residency: current status and future evolution. Semin Thorac Cardiovasc Surg. 2019;31(3):345–9. https://doi.org/10.1053/j.semtcvs.2019.04.002.
104. Smith BK, Finlayson SRG, Perler BA, Presson AP, Allen CM, Brooke BS. Comparison of patient outcomes among integrated residency versus fellowship-trained vascular surgeons. Ann Surg. 2022;276(6):e1044–51. https://doi.org/10.1097/sla.0000000000004706. Epub 2020 Dec 18. PubMed PMID: 33351460; PMCID: PMC8875290.
105. Vaysburg DM, Cortez AR, Hanseman DJ, Delman AM, Morris C, Kassam AF, Kutz D, Lewis J, Van Haren RM, Quillin RC 3rd. An analysis of applicant competitiveness to general surgery, surgical subspecialties, and integrated programs. Surgery. 2021;170(4):1087–92. https://doi.org/10.1016/j.surg.2021.03.035. Epub 2021 Apr 18. PubMed PMID: 33879334.
106. Treffalls JA, Treffalls RN, Yan Q, Davies MG. Integrated vascular surgery versus general surgery residency programs: a ten-year comparison using a normalized competitive index. Ann Vasc Surg. 2022;79:409–10. https://doi.org/10.1016/j.avsg.2021.12.065.
107. Tchantchaleishvili V, Barrus B, Knight PA, Jones CE, Watson TJ, Hicks GL. Six-year integrated cardiothoracic surgery residency applicants: characteristics, expectations, and concerns. J Thorac Cardiovasc Surg. 2013;146(4):753–8. https://doi.org/10.1016/j.jtcvs.2013.05.023.

108. Meza JM, Rectenwald JE, Reddy RM. The bias against integrated thoracic surgery residency applicants during general surgery interviews. Ann Thorac Surg. 2015;99(4):1206–12. https://doi.org/10.1016/j.athoracsur.2014.11.053.
109. Tchantchaleishvili V, LaPar DJ, Stephens EH, Berfield KS, Odell DD, DeNino WF. Current integrated cardiothoracic surgery residents: a thoracic surgery residents association survey. Ann Thorac Surg. 2015;99(3):1040–7. https://doi.org/10.1016/j.athoracsur.2014.10.063.
110. Nehemiah A, Roberts SE, Song Y, Kelz RR, Butler PD, Morris JB, Aarons CB. Looking beyond the numbers: increasing diversity and inclusion through holistic review in general surgery recruitment. J Surg Educ. 2021;78(3):763–9. https://doi.org/10.1016/j.jsurg.2020.08.048. Epub 2020 Sep 17. PubMed PMID: 32950431.
111. Meneses E, McKenney M, Elkbuli A. Diversity and inclusion among US general surgery residency programs: translating initiatives into action. Am Surg. 2021;87(1):166–7. https://doi.org/10.1177/0003134820948887. Epub 2020 Oct 20. PubMed PMID: 33081488.
112. Choinski K, Lipsitz E, Indes J, Phair J, Gao Q, Denesopolis J, Koleilat I. Trends in sex and racial/ethnic diversity in applicants to surgery residency and fellowship programs. JAMA Surg. 2020;155(8):778–81. https://doi.org/10.1001/jamasurg.2020.1018. PubMed PMID: 32459323; PMCID: PMC7254440.
113. Wong RL, Sullivan MC, Yeo HL, Roman SA, Bell RH Jr, Sosa JA. Race and surgical residency: results from a national survey of 4339 US general surgery residents. Ann Surg. 2013;257(4):782–7. https://doi.org/10.1097/SLA.0b013e318269d2d0. PubMed PMID: 23001076.
114. Keshinro A, Frangos S, Berman RS, DiMaggio C, Klein MJ, Bukur M, Welcome AU, Pachter HL, Berry C. Underrepresented minorities in surgical residencies: where are they? A call to action to increase the pipeline. Ann Surg. 2020;272(3):512–20. https://doi.org/10.1097/sla.0000000000004209. PubMed PMID: 33074873.
115. Heiderscheit EA, Schlick CJR, Ellis RJ, Cheung EO, Irizarry D, Amortegui D, Eng J, Sosa JA, Hoyt DB, Buyske J, Nasca TJ, Bilimoria KY, Hu YY. Experiences of LGBTQ+ residents in US general surgery training programs. JAMA Surg. 2022;157(1):23–32. https://doi.org/10.1001/jamasurg.2021.5246. PubMed PMID: 34668969; PMCID: PMC8529519.
116. Sandler BJ, Tackett JJ, Longo WE, Yoo PS. Pregnancy and parenthood among surgery residents: results of the first nationwide survey of general surgery residency program directors. J Am Coll Surg. 2016;222(6):1090–6. https://doi.org/10.1016/j.jamcollsurg.2015.12.004. Epub 2015 Dec 18. PubMed PMID: 26776357.
117. Castillo-Angeles M, Smink DS, Rangel EL. Perspectives of US general surgery program directors on cultural and fiscal barriers to maternity leave and postpartum support during surgical training. JAMA Surg. 2021;156(7):647–53. https://doi.org/10.1001/jamasurg.2021.1807.
118. Rangel EL, Castillo-Angeles M, Marincola Smith P, Terhune KP. Parental support policies and benefits: a surgical training program report card of transparency. Ann Surg. 2023;277(6):938–43. https://doi.org/10.1097/sla.0000000000005566. Epub 2022 July 15. PubMed PMID: 35837953.
119. Yehia BR, Cronholm PF, Wilson N, Palmer SC, Sisson SD, Guilliames CE, Poll-Hunter NI, Sánchez J-P. Mentorship and pursuit of academic medicine careers: a mixed methods study of residents from diverse backgrounds. BMC Med Educ. 2014;14(1):26. https://doi.org/10.1186/1472-6920-14-26.
120. Roberts SE, Shea JA, Sellers M, Butler PD, Kelz RR. Pursing a career in academic surgery among African American medical students. Am J Surg. 2020;219(4):598–603. https://doi.org/10.1016/j.amjsurg.2019.08.009.
121. Feeley AA, Feeley IH, Sheehan E, Carroll C, Queally J. Impact of mentoring for underrepresented groups in undergraduate medical education: a systematic review. J Surg Educ. 2023;81:353–66. https://doi.org/10.1016/j.jsurg.2023.11.015.
122. Haque S. 634 future women in surgery and the role of mentorship. Br J Surg. 2022;109(Supplement_6):znac269.229. https://doi.org/10.1093/bjs/znac269.229.

123. Faucett EA, McCrary HC, Milinic T, Hassanzadeh T, Roward SG, Neumayer LA. The role of same-sex mentorship and organizational support in encouraging women to pursue surgery. Am J Surg. 2017;214(4):640–4. https://doi.org/10.1016/j.amjsurg.2017.07.005. Epub 2017 July 12. PubMed PMID: 28716310.
124. Beanlands RA, Robinson LJ, Venance SL. An LGBTQ+ mentorship program enriched the experience of medical students and physician mentors. Can Med Educ J. 2020;11(6):e159–62. https://doi.org/10.36834/cmej.69936. Epub 2020 Dec 7. PubMed PMID: 33349768; PMCID: PMC7749670.

Part III
Excelling in Surgical Training

Chapter 14
Developing Clinical and Technical Skills

Rebecca Moreci, Gabrielle Moore, and Tania K. Arora

Abstract Clinical and technical skill sets are necessary for the successful completion of a surgical residency training program. Each clinical encounter is an opportunity to expand clinical knowledge and practice decision making. Applying fundamentals of history-taking, physical exam technique, and test interpretation is key to skill development. Technical skills involve practice in the clinical and operative settings, but must also be practiced outside the patient care setting to allow for adequate repetition, comfort, and safety. Many of these skills will be taught, but the development and honing of these skill sets will require self-motivation, feedback, and deliberate practice. For both clinical and technical skill development, there are resources and simulation tools to foster competency and graduated autonomy. Additionally, models of micro-assessments provide potential for greater entrustability. While progressing through training, it is crucial to take an active role in utilizing peer and faculty mentors to identify opportunities for professional growth. This chapter will discuss the foundational principles of surgical training, identify core clinical and technical skills, and describe how the development of these various skills will allow for optimal patient care.

The foundation and preparation for a career in surgery begins in medical school and extends into the training years of residency, fellowship, and beyond. This preparation includes both surgical and critical care rotations, acting internships, or elective (medicine, radiology, pathology) rotations that may be useful for developing clinical and technical skills. A feeling of preparation during surgical residency is associated with lower rates of burnout and attrition [1], so any priming is beneficial. Both clinical and technical skill sets take time to develop, but it is important to consider any opportunities that may accelerate and enhance this process. Formal and structured programs for incoming interns designed to improve clinical and technical

R. Moreci
Department of Surgery, Louisiana State University, New Orleans, LA, USA
e-mail: morecir@med.umich.edu

G. Moore · T. K. Arora (✉)
Department of Surgery, Medical College of Georgia, Augusta, GA, USA
e-mail: GABMOORE@augusta.edu; tarora@augusta.edu

A. Gillis, C. B. Aarons (eds.), *A How To Guide For Medical Students*, Success in Academic Surgery, https://doi.org/10.1007/978-3-031-66011-5_14

skills exist both at the institutional [2–8] and national [9, 10] levels. Be aware and attend any surgery boot camps and preparation for residency courses that your medical school or future residency program offers.

Over the last 2 decades, surgical training and education has evolved [11]. There have been reforms in duty hours [12, 13], reductions in trainee autonomy [14], advancements in laparoscopic and robotic training [15–18], increases in trainee diversity [19], transitions to workplace-based knowledge, and development of tools for competency-based skill and judgment assessments. An overarching theme in these changes is the improvement of delivery in patient care and outcomes, better delivery methods of information, and more effective means of assessment.

In this chapter, we will discuss the foundational principles of surgical training, identify processes to develop clinical and technical skills, and highlight unique aspects of the operative experience (Table 14.1). These concepts are ubiquitous to a career in surgery. Basic aptitude begins during the clerkship and these continue maturing throughout the professional journey.

Table 14.1 Types of skills required for surgical residency and examples of how to develop and improve these skills

Skill type	Skill	Example(s) of how to develop this skill
Clinical	Comprehensive history and physical exams	Case-based learning, textbooks, self-assessment question banks
	Diagnosis and workup of surgical patients	Case-based learning, textbooks, self-assessment question banks, morbidity and mortality conference, mock oral exams
	Interpretation of labs and imaging	Case-based learning, textbooks, self-assessment question banks
	Identifying and managing postoperative complications	Case-based learning, textbooks, self-assessment question banks, morbidity and mortality conference, mock oral exams
Technical	Knot tying, suturing	Boot camps, simulation centers, operative experience, deliberate practice
	Skin preparation	Boot camps, operative experience
	Instrument handling	Boot camps, operative experience, deliberate practice
	Procedural skills	Simulation centers, operative experience
	Advanced techniques	Simulation centers, robotics training courses
Non clinical, non technical	Professionalism	Learn from role models and mentors, self-reflection, ask for feedback, attend local and national conferences
	Teamwork	
	Communication	
	Leadership	
	Multidisciplinary collaboration	
	Trust	

14.1 Foundational Principles of Surgical Training

Surgical training consists of skill sets that may be acquired and built upon. These include: clinical skills (history and physical exam, judgment, knowledge of pathophysiology, anatomy, operative steps, medical/surgical decision making, etc.) and technical skills (instrument handling, tying, suturing, respect for tissue, use of minimally-invasive technology etc.). Just as critical are non-clinical/non-technical skills including team based training, multidisciplinary collaboration, professionalism, situational awareness, stress-management, level of organization and efficiency, and ethical decision-making. While the focus of this chapter will be clinical and technical skills, developing proficiency in these "soft" skills will contribute to not only personal and professional growth of the individual trainee but can also create a positive and inclusive work environment for teams.

Teamwork is critical for safe and effective patient care [20]. As a surgical resident, there will be many opportunities for multidisciplinary collaboration both in and out of the operating room (OR). For example, following rounds it is common practice to place orders and call consults. An intern or resident may be tasked with calling a pharmacist to correctly choose a type and dose of antibiotics for a patient, speaking with a social worker to assist with the home or transportation needs, or calling a cardiology consult for a new abnormal rhythm. In the OR, there will be many people with a variety of roles (surgeons, anesthesiologists, trainees, nurses, scrub techs, etc.) working together to ensure optimal patient outcomes. Effective communication within the surgical team and to individuals with varied specialties and levels of training is one primary skill that will enable your success as a surgical resident.

Similarly, professionalism, which can be defined as adherence to ethical standards, accountability and respect to patients, staff and team members, is evaluated in residency as one of the core competencies described in the Accreditation Council for Graduate Medical Education (ACGME) milestones [21]. In spite of its importance in training, many residency programs do not have a standard curriculum for improving and promoting professional practices [22, 23]. Practicing to change behavior is important, though like any skill, without insight and self-reflection this skill is difficult to improve. Patient-centered care and safety is a top priority for any new clinician with ever-growing responsibilities.

Other non-clinical/non-technical skills include leadership, teaching, organization, and trust. While foundational for the success of functional teams, these skills are not formally taught. Instead they are often learned from role models and mentors. While the importance of developing clinical and technical skills is not debated, the interplay and synergy with additional skills is essential to achieving mastery.

For successful development of both types of skills, it is incumbent upon every learner to acknowledge the need for supervision and to ask for help. Asking for help is a skill that requires humility and a recognition of limitations. Honesty and self-awareness will likely to lead to greater entrustment from staff, peers, and faculty [24] and result in a more cohesive team [25, 26].

14.2 Clinical Decision-Making and Critical Thinking

Developing clinical skills involves utilizing medical knowledge to think critically and make evidence-based decisions for patients [27]. There is a continuum of learning that spans from the early years in medical school through the years in independent surgical practice. In transitioning from medical student to intern, any documentation of patient care is part of the medical record, which can carry important legal ramifications, and have real implications in the care of patients. Therefore, detail and accuracy are paramount. This must be balanced with the urgency of the patient's presentation (e.g. stability or instability of vitals), the clinical environment (e.g. clinic, inpatient floor, emergency room or trauma bay), and the competing demands on most residents (e.g. orders, notes, cases etc.). Taking an accurate history involves active listening and query on the patient's complaints, presenting symptoms, past episodes, previous medical problems, surgeries/procedures, medications, allergies, smoking, alcohol and drug use, family diseases and conditions, and a general review of systems. Even a "complete" physical exam can be tailored but should include the vital signs, a general assessment (is the patient cooperative, combative?), a neurologic assessment (is the patient alert and oriented, able to transfer from chair to bed independently?), examination of the chest (listening to heart and lungs to serve as a baseline), abdominal examination (including inspection, auscultation, light and deep palpation), and evaluating the extremities for warmth, edema, and pulses. Specific complaints will require a more detailed exam. The recent objective data (labs, imaging) should be reviewed, documented and interpreted. With practice and volume, these steps will improve and become more efficient. Equally important is the acknowledgment that everyone has limitations and will be at different stages of competency at different times. It is critical to develop a lifelong habit of asking for help and feedback, observing senior residents and faculty perform histories and physicals, and asking for demonstration of important physical findings that you might have missed. Furthermore, you will be expected to begin developing an understanding of the various diagnostic tools, including a multitude of imaging techniques (e.g. CT, MRI, X-ray), measurements (e.g. ankle brachial index, MELD score, FeNA) and when to use them. The next and most important part of a patient's clinical workup is the assessment and plan. This involves interpretation of the history, physical, test results, and a list of action items that address any problems or abnormalities noted. In the field of surgery, plans must differentiate if there are indications to operate. This daunting task will come with time, experience, and practice. Remain calm and continue practicing and asking for feedback. This progression of clinical judgment and decision making processes develop throughout training, beginning with abstract knowledge and transitioning to more concrete knowledge in preparation for independent practice [28].

Just as simulation can improve surgical-technical skills, case-based learning is one of the most common ways both medical students and surgery residents can test medical knowledge and practice decision making. This type of learning, whether at the bedside or in the hallways, allows learners to understand the direct relevance of the disease process and practice analyzing real-world surgical cases. This method allows the learner to connect the patient they just saw with the disease, increasing the likelihood that they will remember it [29]. Case-based learning is also seen in morbidity and mortality (M&M) conferences and mock-oral exam practice, where learners are actively involved. Residents in M&M traditionally present their own patient cases (but may present cases where they were not directly involved) and common complications that may have occurred, reflecting on what occurred during a patient's hospital course or operation that led to a negative outcome. These sessions promote interactive teaching over a wide range of surgical diseases at regular intervals as well as focusing on strategies to improve patient outcomes [30, 31]. Additionally, M&M provides an opportunity for discussion of evidence-based practices and how the literature may support the clinical decisions that are made on a day-to-day basis. This principle of retrospective contemplation, admission of mistakes and seeking data-supported ways to improve is important for the individual, the department, and the hospital system. Mock-oral exam practice places residents in different clinical environments (the inpatient ward, clinic, operating room, and emergency department) and tests the residents' understanding of a patient presentation, physical finding, test results, operative steps and post-operative challenges. The exercise assesses the synthesis of knowledge and application and is a prime opportunity to seek feedback on knowledge gaps, communication style, and confidence with practice with each subsequent exam and real clinical encounter.

There are many resources available for resident learning and self-assessment. For example, these resources can include traditional textbooks [32, 33], journal articles, multiple choice question banks [34–36], review courses, and surgical podcasts [37]. While the examples listed are commonly used by many surgical residents, this is by no means comprehensive. Prior to starting residency, ask residents and faculty for their recommendations of ideal learning tools, what resources your future program uses currently, and what their perceived strengths and weaknesses are. Think critically about the type of learner you are and be honest and realistic about the amount of time you will be able to dedicate to studying outside of the hospital. Whenever possible, track time spent with a calendar for accountability and revising plans, success on multiple choice questions and areas that need more attention, and schedule sessions with a coach/mentor for objective review.

14.3 Technical Proficiency

Surgical and procedural-based specialties require practice and mastery of both clinical knowledge *and* a technical skill set. Therefore, the training can be challenging when compared to counterpart residencies. In order to attain operative mastery, technical proficiency and knowledge of surgical anatomy and physiology is needed. In medical school, a single anatomy course tends to occur in the preclinical years, leaving students to rely on clinical rotations for hands-on experiences to demonstrate understanding and knowledge of anatomy. These experiences can be highly variable based on the rotation, team, and patient. A more formal anatomy curricula for those students pursuing a surgical specialty, including full body dissections with fresh frozen cadavers, mannequins, or animal models has been suggested, though it is difficult to implement one standard program across the country [38, 39]. Watching surgical videos, reviewing anatomy or operative atlases or anatomy mobile applications, and reviewing previous operative dictations are useful adjuncts for students learning anatomy and operative skills [40]. However, beware that publicly accessible videos may vary in quality and usefulness [41]. Some programs employ the American College of Surgeons Entering Resident Readiness Assessment (ACS ERRA) as a needs assessment to understand each new intern's baseline knowledge [10]. Surgical boot camps, occurring either in fourth year of medical school or the beginning of surgical residency, can improve knowledge and confidence in anatomy and basic surgical skills [42]. Asynchronous curricula developed by the Association of Surgical Education, Association of Program Directors in Surgery, and the American College of Surgeons Resident Prep Curriculum is designed for fourth year medical students and can be purchased via an individual subscription or through a program [43].

Technical skills, like most, require practice to achieve mastery. Deliberate practice is defined as focused and repeated tasks utilizing coaching and/or feedback to improve performance on a skill (Fig. 14.1) [44]. The goal is to improve upon existing skills and recognize that everyone starts at a different level. Working on technical skills requires preparation in advance, clear intentions, and desired results shared with a mentor or coach. While repetition is important to hone a skill, deliberate practice can provide more cognitive learning opportunities including the chance to recognize and describe thought processes involved in performing a specific skill [45]. Basic surgical skills can be described as the cornerstone of a strong foundation. Like a house built on solid material, the bricks, wood, and stones that follow

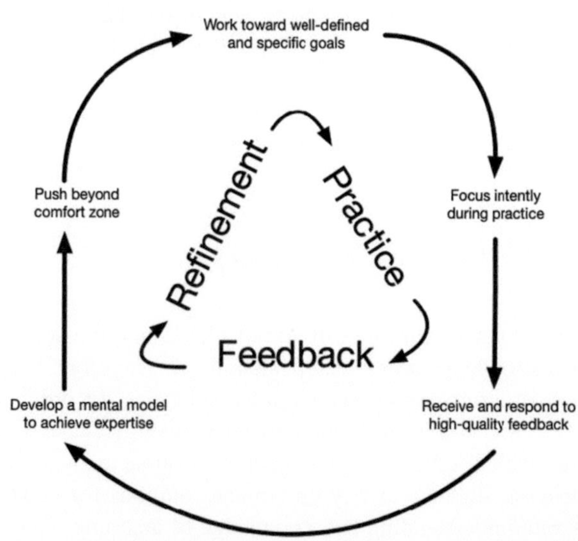

Fig. 14.1 Deliberate practice flow diagram adapted from [75, 76]

will weather a storm. These skills include knot tying, suturing, instrument handling, skin preparation, positioning and draping, and gowning and gloving. It is important to take advantage of any skills preparation courses that your medical school or residency program offers. However, most residency programs understand that their incoming interns will arrive with various levels of experience and comfort. These intern boot camps may help equalize varying levels of skills, but practice outside of any structured program is necessary. Knot tying can be practiced during less busy times at work and at home. Obtain expired or extra suture and ties, discarded operative instruments or basic hemostats and forceps from the OR, wound care closet, or simulation lab. Tying and suturing outside the OR on silicone molds or even on a towel can promote muscle memory and allow for a low-stakes environment to correct mistakes. With greater emphasis of healthcare systems on patient outcomes and operative time, it is imperative to practice skills outside the OR. While there is no replacement for hands-on learning in the OR, this must be balanced with these competing priorities. In the OR, active listening to names of instruments and sutures that are utilized, learning where and why techniques may vary from the textbooks, understanding how patients are appropriately positioned and why, and asking for specific feedback on performance during a case is essential to improve and enhance care for the patient.

As training progresses, residents are exposed to more complex cases, and are expected to employ more advanced surgical techniques, greater efficiency of movement and reflexes to adapt to an emergent change in the case or the patient's status. For all of these skills, there is no replacement for exposure, practice, and feedback. Advanced techniques include laparoscopic and robotic skills as well as the incorporation of the most up-to-date technological instruments and materials. These skills and instruments may even be new for some faculty surgeons. Additionally, residency training incorporates exposure to a variety of surgical specialties. These specialties may differ based on instruments commonly used, organ systems operated on, or open vs. minimally invasive approaches utilized. There will be nuances to each specialty, including the use of loupes or other specialized tools. Loupes allow for magnification of small anatomic structures and fine suturing. While not all residency programs will purchase loupes, try to obtain loupes from a vendor before needed in the OR. Surgical simulation and practice with loupes is recommended to adapt to the magnification and to practice on graft material with 4–0, 5–0 and 6–0 sutures. Some specialties will require the use of more advanced surgical techniques, which is why more senior residents might be expected to scrub these cases. Take advantage of being the first assist in these complex cases and observe the steps and how challenges are managed. These patients will have more complicated post-operative care and understanding the course of the surgery will translate into being able to communicate and care for the patient with greater command of the clinical picture. It is important to emphasize that many technical skills build on each other, therefore focus should be placed on developing accuracy and precision of the fundamental skills. Seek out feedback from senior residents and faculty. Although you may be subject to differing feedback at times, this is the most likely way to ensure accuracy and precision as skills develop. (For more on laparoscopic and robotic practice, see the chapter on simulation).

14.4 Surgical Simulation and Training

Over the last 30 years, the literature has demonstrated the importance of simulation in surgical training as a means of both honing skills in a safe environment and decreasing operative errors [46]. For new learners, there is often a fear of inadvertently harming a patient while intending to practice the principle of nonmaleficence ("first do no harm"). Within surgical fields, there is a balance between protecting patient safety and ensuring trainees' skill development through graduated autonomy and entrustment. While surgical trainees cannot learn how to operate from the sidelines, they can develop fundamental skills and study procedures through simulation-based learning. Given the high variability of student experience on surgical rotations as well as decreasing time spent on the operative blocks, simulation is particularly impactful in early training [47]. When started in medical school, formal surgical simulation courses improve clinical knowledge, technical skills, and confidence for graduating medical students [4, 48]. Okusanya et al. reported that interns who participated in surgical boot camps maintained higher levels of confidence in performing procedures (i.e., thoracostomy tubes and cricothyroidotomies) 6 months into residency as compared to their counterparts [49].

Although this will vary, most surgical training programs will include some form of a simulation curriculum given the significant impact it has on the development of surgical skills. Surgical simulation offers residents high-fidelity training, equipping residents with technical skills directly applicable in the operating room and resulting in superior operative skills compared to those without such specialized training [50]. These simulation activities can include basic knot tying, suturing, central line placement, laparoscopic and robotic techniques while simulation tools can include box trainers, 3-D printed or animal organs, and cadavers. Trainees enrolled in simulation courses achieve higher procedural proficiency than their counterparts and experience fewer operative complications [51]. Moreover, the efficacy of simulation-based learning has been comprehensively demonstrated particularly when prioritizing spaced simulation—a method proven to enhance skill retention over time [52, 53]. This concept finds support in the "consolidation of learning" which occurs as individuals engage in practice during learning sessions and utilize the time in between practice for mental rehearsal [54].

Simulation has been further augmented with the advent of virtual reality (VR). VR has the potential to improve accessibility to surgical simulation while having measurable benefits to trainees. The integration of VR into surgical learning improves residents' surgical efficiency and tissue handling while minimizing operative errors [55, 56]. VR can also be utilized to enhance manual dexterity and performance speed when used as a pre-operative warmup modality [57]. Despite being in its early stages, VR shows promise to become a widespread surgical education tool.

14.5 Operative Experience and Graduated Responsibility

A critical component of resident development is earning graduated responsibility. This involves progressive autonomy within the operating room and in the clinical management of patients. Work hour restrictions (i.e., the 80-h work week limit), the litigious nature of surgery, and the requirement of attending supervision, are some of the barriers residents encounter in gaining operative independence. While these barriers are mechanisms for patient safety as there is an association of resident scrubbed cases with longer operative times and minor complications (i.e., wound infections), it is crucial to emphasize the overall safety of resident participation in surgeries [15, 58]. In order to reconcile patient safety and resident education, surgical curricula have been implemented within training programs to ensure early, level appropriate milestones for residents while assessing progression. Considering this, the American Board of Surgery (ABS) developed training requirements to secure early operative exposure to young trainees including completion of a minimum of 250 cases in the first 2 years of training indicated as first assistant or operating surgeon [59]. Additionally, the ABS developed Entrustable Professional Activities (EPAs) which have been implemented to assess general surgery trainees on core competencies and to evaluate resident advancement and entrustment [60]. This assessment tool aids clinical educators in determining the appropriate level of autonomy given to residents informed by their clinical and operative proficiency (Fig. 14.2) [61]. To facilitate the distribution of EPAs into training programs nationally, the Society for Improving Medical Professions (SIMPL) collaborative developed an easily accessible, cost-free, mobile-based platform designed for collecting the data on learner entrustment [62, 63]. Although EPAs were recently launched in July 2023, they offer a promising approach to standardize graduated autonomy nationally.

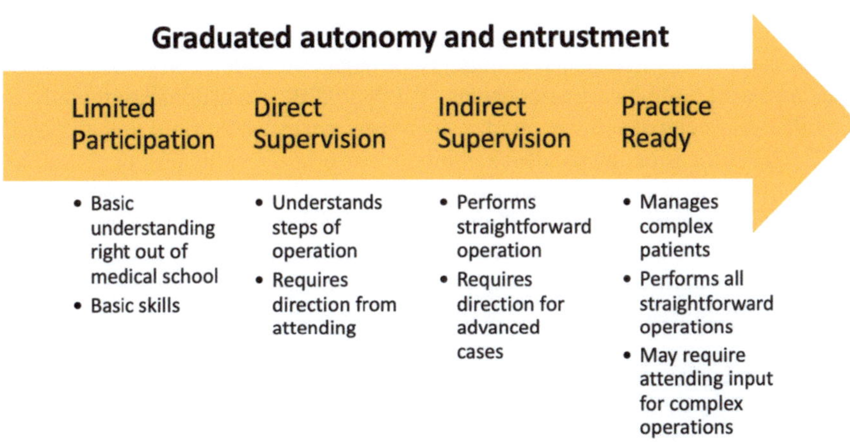

Fig. 14.2 Conceptual framework of grading scale for Entrustable Professional Activities [61]

On an individual level, surgical residents can take an active role in earning operative autonomy early on in their training. This autonomy is largely influenced by non-operative experiences including patient knowledge and ownership, professionalism, positive interpersonal relationships, medical knowledge, and asking for help when clinically necessary [64, 65]. Intraoperative behaviors that are highly associated with greater surgical entrustment include surgical planning, leadership, and problem solving [66]. The importance of building a robust foundation of clinical knowledge and fostering interpersonal skills should not be overlooked.

General surgery trainees establish a foundation of surgical knowledge when rotating through diverse surgical specialties including Acute Care Surgery/Surgical Critical Care, Colorectal, Cardiothoracic, Pediatric, Transplant, Vascular, and Surgical Oncology. Each subspeciality has a unique set of disease processes and cases allowing for trainees to develop mastery of a wide range of surgical techniques. Regardless of one's ultimate career path, each surgical rotation offers unique skills for a surgeon's armamentarium. For example, while on Vascular Surgery rotations, residents learn essential general surgery foundations including gaining proximal and distal control of vessels, formation of vascular anastomoses, and safely operating around major vascular structures [67]. Moreover, a study by Schwartz et al. reported that while the minority of surveyed residents planned to pursue a career in transplant surgery, the majority of these residents felt that the skills acquired on their transplant rotation would prove beneficial to their future career [68]. Recognizing the value in each surgical rotation is paramount to a surgeon's technical success as these key technical principles are applicable across all surgical specialties.

14.6 Continuous Assessment and Feedback

Surgical training, like the mastery of any discipline, requires frequent opportunities to receive feedback and improve skills. Constructive feedback is shared by both faculty and peers, verbally and commonly through end-of-rotation (EOR) evaluations and workplace-based assessments (WBAs). EOR evaluations are thought to provide a more global assessment of resident performance compared to their peers, while WBAs focus on the resident's ability to perform a specific task or procedure [69]. Entrustable Professional Activities (EPAs), as mentioned in the above section, have recently been implemented in all general surgery programs across the country. These frequent, time-efficient WBAs allow residents to be assessed in real-time and be assigned an entrustment score for a variety of core clinical activities.

Residency programs may also employ validated assessment tools, such as the Objective Structured Assessment of Technical Skills (OSATS) [70, 71] or the Zwisch scale [72] to assess surgical performance or autonomy levels, respectively, in the operating room. Additionally, formal semi-annual evaluations are performed by faculty based-Clinical Competency Committees (CCC) [73]. Program faculty will review all resident evaluations as well as their Accreditation Council for

Graduate Medical Education (ACGME) Milestones [21] and then discuss the resident's progress and any concerns that may exist. These meetings, mandated by the ACGME, allow residents another opportunity for feedback and improvement as they continue through training. Finally, informal verbal feedback may be provided regularly though it is easy to miss and impossible to track. Feedback doesn't have to be structured in a formal manner, or even labeled as feedback for it to be highly educational or useful for skill progression. Prepare yourself to receive feedback. When a learner is not ready, this can result in a feeling of shame, shutting down, and resistance to future feedback.

Though there may be multiple avenues for feedback to be provided, it is important to be open and receptive to receiving this feedback. Not all feedback is created equally; individual faculty surgeons vary in the delivery and quality of feedback provided [74]. Many programs employ faculty development programs to empower their faculty to deliver more effective feedback and to try to tailor this to the learner. In order to take an active role in learning and improving, ask for feedback frequently and take note of who provides the most high quality, useful critiques. Be specific when asking for feedback—if you can identify a particular area of improvement, faculty will be more likely to help develop an action plan and less likely to provide generic and unhelpful advice.

14.7 Conclusion

Surgical training requires both clinical knowledge and technical skills to succeed. It is important to start learning the basics in medical school, and continue to practice and sharpen these skills as you advance in residency training. Many of these skills will build upon each other, therefore it is crucial to ensure your techniques are both accurate and precise. Furthermore, there are many non clinical and non technical skills that contribute to your development as an ethical, professional, and team-driven surgeon. All of these skills are important and necessary in providing optimal patient care.

References

1. Engelhardt KE, Bilimoria KY, Johnson JK, Hewitt DB, Ellis RJ, Hu YY, et al. A national mixed-methods evaluation of preparedness for general surgery residency and the association with resident burnout. JAMA Surg. 2020;155(9):851–9.
2. Antonoff MB, Swanson JA, Green CA, Mann BD, Maddaus MA, D'Cunha J. The significant impact of a competency-based preparatory course for senior medical students entering surgical residency. Acad Med. 2012;87(3):308.
3. Brunt LM, Halpin VJ, Klingensmith ME, Tiemann D, Matthews BD, Spitler JA, et al. Accelerated skills preparation and assessment for senior medical students entering surgical internship. J Am Coll Surg. 2008;206(5):897–904.

4. Esterl RM, Henzi DL, Cohn SM. Senior medical student "boot camp": can result in increased self-confidence before starting surgery internships. Curr Surg. 2006;63(4):264–8.
5. Schoolfield CS, Samra N, Kim RH, Shi R, Zhang WW, Tan TW. Evaluating the effectiveness of the general surgery intern boot camp. Am Surg. 2016;82(3):243–50.
6. Neylan CJ, Nelson EF, Dumon KR, Morris JB, Williams NN, Dempsey DT, et al. Medical school surgical boot camps: a systematic review. J Surg Educ. 2017;74(3):384–9.
7. Miller S, Shipper E, Hasty B, Bereknyei MS, Lee EW, Lin D, et al. Introductory surgical skills course: technical training and preparation for the surgical environment. MedEdPORTAL. 2018;14:10775.
8. Bauman B, Kernahan P, Weinhaus A, Walker MJ, Irwin E, Sundin A, et al. An interprofessional senior medical student preparation course: improvement in knowledge and self-confidence before entering surgical training. Adv Med Educ Pract. 2021;12:441–51.
9. ACS [Internet]. [cited 2023 Dec 11]. ACS Fundamentals of Surgery Curriculum. https://www.facs.org/for-medical-professionals/education/programs/acs-fundamentals-of-surgery-curriculum/
10. ACS [Internet]. [cited 2023 Dec 11]. ACS Entering Resident Readiness Assessment (ACS ERRA). https://www.facs.org/for-medical-professionals/education/programs/acs-entering-resident-readiness-assessment/
11. Evolving Educational Techniques in Surgical Training—ClinicalKey [Internet]. [cited 2023 Dec 12]. https://www-clinicalkey-com.proxy.lib.umich.edu/#!/content/playContent/1-s2.0-S0039610915001619?returnurl=null&referrer=null
12. Baldwin K, Namdari S, Donegan D, Kamath AF, Mehta S. Early effects of resident work-hour restrictions on patient safety: a systematic review and plea for improved studies. JBJS. 2011;93(2):e5.
13. Bilimoria KY, Chung JW, Hedges LV, Dahlke AR, Love R, Cohen ME, et al. National cluster-randomized trial of duty-hour flexibility in surgical training. N Engl J Med. 2016;374(8):713–27.
14. Meyerson SL, Teitelbaum EN, George BC, Schuller MC, DaRosa DA, Fryer JP. Defining the autonomy gap: when expectations do not meet reality in the operating room. J Surg Educ. 2014;71(6):e64–72.
15. Torricelli FCM, Barbosa JABA, Marchini GS. Impact of laparoscopic surgery training laboratory on surgeon's performance. World J Gastrointest Surg. 2016;8(11):735–43.
16. Williamson T, Song SE. Robotic surgery techniques to improve traditional laparoscopy. JSLS J Soc Laparosc Robot Surg. 2022;26(2):e2022.00002.
17. Khan MTA, Patnaik R, Lee CS, Willson CM, Demario VK, Krell RW, et al. Systematic review of academic robotic surgery curricula. J Robot Surg. 2023;17(3):719–43.
18. Panait L, Shetty S, Shewokis PA, Sanchez JA. Do laparoscopic skills transfer to robotic surgery? J Surg Res. 2014;187(1):53–8.
19. Davis EC, Risucci DA, Blair PG, Sachdeva AK. Women in surgery residency programs: evolving trends from a national perspective. J Am Coll Surg. 2011;212(3):320–6.
20. Teamwork and Surgical Team–Based Training—ClinicalKey [Internet]. [cited 2023 Dec 29]. https://www-clinicalkey-com.proxy.lib.umich.edu/#!/content/playContent/1-s2.0-S0039610920301134?returnurl=null&referrer=null
21. ACGME Surgery Milestones. Accreditation Council for Graduate Medical Education (ACGME); 2019.
22. Deptula P, Chun MBJ. A literature review of professionalism in surgical education: suggested components for development of a curriculum. J Surg Educ. 2013;70(3):408–22.
23. Keune JD, Kodner IJ. The importance of an ethics curriculum in surgical education. World J Surg. 2014;38(7):1581–6.
24. Sterkenburg A, Barach P, Kalkman C, Gielen M, ten Cate O. When do supervising physicians decide to entrust residents with unsupervised tasks? Acad Med. 2010;85(9):1408.
25. Nemani VM, Park C, Nawabi DH. What makes a "great resident": the resident perspective. Curr Rev Musculoskelet Med. 2014;7(2):164–7.

26. Kennedy TJT, Regehr G, Baker GR, Lingard L. Preserving professional credibility: grounded theory study of medical trainees' requests for clinical support. BMJ. 2009;338:b128.
27. Hale JF, Terrien JM, Quirk M, Sullivan K, Cahan M. The impact of deliberate reflection with WISE-MD™ modules on surgical clerkship students' critical thinking: a prospective, randomized controlled pilot study. Adv Med Educ Pract. 2018;9:757–66.
28. Woelfel IA, Smith BQ, Salani R, Harzman AE, Cochran AL, Chen PX. The long game: Evolution of clinical decision making throughout residency and fellowship. Am J Surg. 2022;223(2):266–72.
29. Irby DM. Three exemplary models of case-based teaching. Acad Med. 1994;69(12):947.
30. Veldenz HC, Dovgan PS, Schinco MS, Tepas JJ. Morbidity and mortality conference: Enhancing delivery of surgery residency curricula. Curr Surg. 2001;58(6):580–2.
31. Slater N, Sekhon P, Bradley N, Shariff F, Bedford J, Wong H, et al. Morbidity and mortality conferences in general surgery: a narrative systematic review. Can J Surg. 2020;63(3):E211–22.
32. US Elsevier Health [Internet]. [cited 2024 Jan 10]. Current Surgical Therapy—9780323796835. https://www.us.elsevierhealth.com/current-surgical-therapy-9780323796835.html
33. Schwartz's Principles of Surgery, 11e | AccessMedicine | McGraw Hill Medical [Internet]. [cited 2024 Jan 10]. https://accessmedicine.mhmedical.com/book.aspx?bookID=2576
34. SCORE | General Surgery Resident Curriculum Portal [Internet]. [cited 2024 Jan 10]. https://www.surgicalcore.org/
35. TrueLearn: SmartBanks for Medical and Licensure Exam Prep [Internet]. [cited 2024 Jan 10]. https://truelearn.com/?utm_source=google&utm_medium=cpc&utm_campaign=pmax&utm_term=%7Bkeyword%7D&utm_content=pmax&gad_source=1&gclid=Cj0KCQiAnfmsBhDfARIsAM7MKi2R1jaBS4LE0JWbl_fqMETqDrRBjTvQJenHqSmUsYF7vtySUtfjwtQaAjsoEALw_wcB
36. ABSITE Quest [Internet]. [cited 2024 Jan 10]. ABSITE Quest | Surgical Question Bank + Exam Prep! https://absitequest.com
37. Behind The Knife: The Premier Surgery Podcast | Surgical Education [Internet]. [cited 2024 Jan 10]. https://behindtheknife.org/
38. Estai M, Bunt S. Best teaching practices in anatomy education: a critical review. Ann Anat Anat Anz Off Organ Anat Ges. 2016;208:151–7.
39. Ocel JJ, Natt N, Tiegs RD, Arora AS. Formal procedural skills training using a fresh frozen cadaver model: a pilot study. Clin Anat N Y N. 2006;19(2):142–6.
40. Selten JW, Nazari T, Andriessen EH, Konings S, Wiggers T, de Jonge J. Standardized videos in addition to the surgical curriculum in Medical Education for surgical clerkships: a cohort study. BMC Med Educ. 2022;22(1):384.
41. Karic B, Moino V, Nolin A, Andrews A, Brisson P. Evaluation of surgical educational videos available for third year medical students. Med Educ Online. 2020;25(1):1714197.
42. Zhang J, Zilundu PLM, Zhang W, Yu G, Li S, Zhou L, et al. The use of a surgical boot camp combining anatomical education and surgical simulation for internship preparedness among senior medical students. BMC Med Educ. 2022;22(1):459.
43. ACS [Internet]. [cited 2024 Feb 13]. ACS/APDS/ASE Resident Prep Curriculum. https://www.facs.org/for-medical-professionals/education/programs/acsapdsase-resident-prep-curriculum/
44. Dearani JA, Gold M, Leibovich BC, Ericsson KA, Khabbaz KR, Foley TA, et al. The role of imaging, deliberate practice, structure, and improvisation in approaching surgical perfection. J Thorac Cardiovasc Surg. 2017;154(4):1329–36.
45. Higgins M, Madan CR, Patel R. Deliberate practice in simulation-based surgical skills training: a scoping review. J Surg Educ. 2021;78(4):1328–39.
46. Zevin B, Aggarwal R, Grantcharov TP. Surgical simulation in 2013: why is it still not the standard in surgical training? J Am Coll Surg. 2014;218(2):294–301.
47. Lind DS, Deladisma AM, Cue JI, Thomas AM, MacFadyen BV, Nesbit RR. Survey of student education in surgery. J Am Coll Surg. 2007;204(5):969–74; discussion 975-976

48. Singh P, Aggarwal R, Pucher PH, Hashimoto DA, Beyer-Berjot L, Bharathan R, et al. An immersive "simulation week" enhances clinical performance of incoming surgical interns improved performance persists at 6 months follow-up. Surgery. 2015;157(3):432–43.
49. Okusanya OT, Kornfield ZN, Reinke CE, Morris JB, Sarani B, Williams NN, et al. The effect and durability of a pregraduation boot cAMP on the confidence of senior medical student entering surgical residencies. J Surg Educ. 2012;69(4):536–43.
50. Sturm LP, Windsor JA, Cosman PH, Cregan P, Hewett PJ, Maddern GJ. A systematic review of skills transfer after surgical simulation training. Ann Surg. 2008;248(2):166–79.
51. Aydın A, Ahmed K, Abe T, Raison N, Van Hemelrijck M, Garmo H, et al. Effect of simulation-based training on surgical proficiency and patient outcomes: a randomised controlled clinical and educational trial. Eur Urol. 2022;81(4):385–93.
52. Moulton CAE, Dubrowski A, Macrae H, Graham B, Grober E, Reznick R. Teaching surgical skills: what kind of practice makes perfect? A randomized, controlled trial. Ann Surg. 2006;244(3):400–9.
53. Luft AR, Buitrago MM. Stages of motor skill learning. Mol Neurobiol. 2005;32(3):205–16.
54. Hall JC. Imagery practice and the development of surgical skills. Am J Surg. 2002;184(5):465–70.
55. Seymour NE, Gallagher AG, Roman SA, O'Brien MK, Bansal VK, Andersen DK, et al. Virtual reality training improves operating room performance. Ann Surg. 2002;236(4):458–64.
56. Portelli M, Bianco SF, Bezzina T, Abela JE. Virtual reality training compared with apprenticeship training in laparoscopic surgery: a meta-analysis. Ann R Coll Surg Engl. 2020;102(9):672–84.
57. da Cruz JAS, Dos Reis ST, Cunha Frati RM, Duarte RJ, Nguyen H, Srougi M, et al. Does warm-up training in a virtual reality simulator improve surgical performance? A prospective randomized analysis. J Surg Educ. 2016;73(6):974–8.
58. Davis SS, Husain FA, Lin E, Nandipati KC, Perez S, Sweeney JF. Resident participation in index laparoscopic general surgical cases: impact of the learning environment on surgical outcomes. J Am Coll Surg. 2013;216(1):96–104.
59. Training Requirements | American Board of Surgery [Internet]. [cited 2024 Jan 7]. https://www.absurgery.org/default.jsp?certgsqe_training
60. Entrustable Professional Activities | American Board of Surgery [Internet]. [cited 2024 Jan 7]. https://www.absurgery.org/default.jsp?epahome
61. General Surgery Entrustable Professional Activities [Internet]. American Board of Surgery; https://www.absurgery.org/wp-content/uploads/2023/08/gsepas_all.pdf
62. George BC, Bohnen JD, Schuller MC, Fryer JP. Using smartphones for trainee performance assessment: A SIMPL case study. Surgery. 2020;167(6):903–6.
63. Bohnen JD, George BC, Williams RG, Schuller MC, DaRosa DA, Torbeck L, et al. The feasibility of real-time intraoperative performance assessment with SIMPL (system for improving and measuring procedural learning): early experience from a multi-institutional trial. J Surg Educ. 2016;73(6):e118–30.
64. Miles VP, Schroll RW, Beaty JS. Empowering the resident learner. J Surg Educ. 2022;79(4):909–17.
65. Chen XP, Sullivan AM, Alseidi A, Kwakye G, Smink DS. Assessing residents' readiness for OR autonomy: a qualitative descriptive study of expert surgical teachers' best practices. J Surg Educ. 2017;74(6):e15–21.
66. Nguyen C, Thompson-Burdine J, Kemp MT, Williams AM, Rivard S, Sandhu G. High vs. low entrustment behaviors in the operating room. Am J Surg. 2021;221(5):973–9.
67. Grabo DJ, DiMuzio PJ, Kairys JC, McIlhenny SE, Crawford AG, Yeo CJ. Have endovascular procedures negatively impacted general surgery training? Ann Surg. 2007;246(3):472–7; discussion 477-480
68. Schwartz JJ, Thiesset HF, Bohn JA, Sloat B, Carricaburu M, Hatch J, et al. Perceived benefits of a transplant surgery experience to general surgery residency training. J Surg Educ. 2012;69(3):371–84.

69. Ahle SL, Schuller M, Clark MJ, Williams RG, Wnuk G, Fryer JP, et al. Do end-of-rotation evaluations adequately assess readiness to operate? Acad Med. 2019;94(12):1946.
70. Niitsu H, Hirabayashi N, Yoshimitsu M, Mimura T, Taomoto J, Sugiyama Y, et al. Using the objective structured assessment of technical skills (OSATS) global rating scale to evaluate the skills of surgical trainees in the operating room. Surg Today. 2013;43(3):271–5.
71. Martin JA, Regehr G, Reznick R, Macrae H, Murnaghan J, Hutchison C, et al. Objective structured assessment of technical skill (OSATS) for surgical residents. Br J Surg. 1997;84(2):273–8.
72. George BC, Teitelbaum EN, Meyerson SL, Schuller MC, DaRosa DA, Petrusa ER, et al. Reliability, validity, and feasibility of the zwisch scale for the assessment of intraoperative performance. J Surg Educ. 2014;71(6):90–6.
73. French JC, Dannefer EF, Colbert CY. A systematic approach toward building a fully operational clinical competency committee. J Surg Educ. 2014;71(6):e22–7.
74. Marcotte KM, Ötleş E, Thelen AE, Gates R, George BC, Krumm AE. Using natural language processing to determine factors associated with high-quality feedback. Glob Surg Educ J Assoc Surg Educ. 2022;1(1):58.
75. Petrosoniak A, Lu M, Gray S, Hicks C, Sherbino J, McGowan M, et al. Perfecting practice: a protocol for assessing simulation-based mastery learning and deliberate practice versus self-guided practice for bougie-assisted cricothyroidotomy performance. BMC Med Educ. 2019;19(1):100.
76. Dkane47. Deliberate Practice: Mental Models [Internet]. Five Twelve Thirteen. 2017 [cited 2024 Feb 19]. https://fivetwelvethirteen.wordpress.com/2017/01/05/deliberate-practice-mental-models/

Chapter 15
Utilizing Technology and Simulation-Based Training

Sophie E. Mayeux and Catherine McManus

Abstract Simulation is a crucial tool for the development of surgical skills. Many important skills can be taught outside of the operating room in a low-risk environment, allowing for detailed feedback and assessment. With new technologies, such as virtual reality or augmented reality, simulation based training resembles more realistic scenarios with imbedded feedback and haptics. Robot assisted surgery also requires the use of simulation to develop competency. Technology and simulation are both critical for a surgeon in training.

15.1 Introduction

Simulation in medicine is defined as replicating aspects of real situations, often immersive, for a guided experience in an interactive manner [1, 2]. It has become a key tool in medical training, quality of care and the maintenance of patient safety [1]. In surgery, simulation allows surgeons and trainees to acquire and practice new skills and knowledge prior to involving patients. Learners are able to prepare for critical situations and improve their skills in a secure, risk-free environment.

In the 1980s–1990s, Reznick et al. at the University of Toronto developed a method to assess and validate resident technical skills [3]. They created models aimed at specific tasks such as suturing, chest tube insertion, and skin closure. Surgeons used a checklist to observe and score students called the Objective Structured Assessment of Technical Skills (OSATS). All residents participated, and the results showed that with each level of training, there was significant improvement in global rating scores. They concluded that technical skills could effectively be measured using simulation [3].

With the advancement of surgical technologies in the 1990s, such as laparoscopy, simulation gained attention as surgeons needed to master this new skill set in

S. E. Mayeux · C. McManus (✉)
Department of Surgery, Columbia University Irving Medical Center, New York, NY, USA
e-mail: sm3104@cumc.columbia.edu; cm3304@cumc.columbia.edu

A. Gillis, C. B. Aarons (eds.), *A How To Guide For Medical Students*, Success in Academic Surgery, https://doi.org/10.1007/978-3-031-66011-5_15

a controlled, low stakes environment while maintaining patient safety [4, 5] Although the initial box-trainer systems were relatively simple, with exercises like suturing foam or dropping beans into an elevated cup, studies demonstrated that practice with the first laparoscopic simulators improved laparoscopic dexterity as measured in the simulated environment [4, 5]. Korn Doffer et al. built a set of laparoscopic exercises to develop basic laparoscopic skills known as the "Southwestern" video trainer stations. In their multi-institutional study, they found that task and performance scores in the training environment correlated with laparoscopic experience. They also found that residents who received just 5 h of simulator training scored significantly better on a scale of operative performance compared to controls [6].

15.1.1 Simulation for Surgeons in Training

Often the first exposure that students have to simulation is in medical school with a cadaver dissection during their anatomy course. For students interested in a procedural based specialty, the ASE and ACS created a simulation-based surgical curriculum for medical students to develop surgical examination and procedural skills [7, 8].

Effective and efficient training of surgical residents became crucial with the introduction of the 80-h work week in 2003. Traditionally, surgical trainees learned and mastered their craft by being present in the hospital and getting hands on experience. However, surgical educators had to shift away from this model and adapt novel methods to train safe and competent surgeons within a limited timeframe. Surgical simulation utilizes concepts of adult learning theory such as cognitive pretraining and deliberate practice to allow trainees to build a foundation of knowledge and skills so they can be more prepared for and get more out of patient care experiences [9].

The American Board of Surgery (ABS), the American College of Surgeons (ACS), the American Surgical Association (ASA), the Association of Program Directors in Surgery (APDS), the Association for Surgical Education (ASE), and the Residency Review Committee for Surgery of the Accreditation Council on Graduate Medical Education (RRC-S), all major stakeholders in surgical education, have endorsed use of simulation in surgical education [4, 10]. For example, simulation-based sessions, also referred to as surgical "bootcamps," to prepare students for surgical residency are quite common. They include technical skills, interpersonal skills, communication, and systems-based practice [8, 11]. During residency, simulation is used continuously for skill development and refinement including suturing, knot-trying, laparoscopy, central line placement, and robotic surgery [8].

Importantly, simulation is not just for development of technical skills. Nontechnical skills, such as communication, situational awareness, and decision-making under pressure have been linked to adverse events [12]. Simulations have been developed to assess and improve resident communication and interpersonal skills in the operating room [13]. Another example of communication is "VitalTalk," an evidence-based communication skills teaching model focused on difficult conversations [14].

15.1.2 Simulation Beyond Residency

Simulation is a critical teaching tool used throughout a surgeon's career. As surgical techniques continue to evolve, experts need to find a safe way to be introduced to new technology and practice new skills. Practicing surgeons may use simulation not only to improve their technical skills, but also to enhance their teaching skills. For example, Stefanidis et al. successfully created a coaching curriculum for surgeons using simulation to improve and give feedback on technical and non-technical skill sets [15]. Simulation is also used to equip educators with the skills required to be an efficient educator and to standardize instructional methods [8, 16]. For instance, MacKenzie et al. successfully created a national laparoscopic train-the-trainer curriculum in which they focused on teaching skills such as performance-enhancing feedback and trainer intervention [8]. Their simulation-based curriculum showed improvement in long and short-team trainee performances.

15.2 Types of Simulation

15.2.1 Animal and Cadaver Labs

There are several ways to achieve surgical simulation, both with organic models, such as live animals or cadavers, as well as inorganic models, such as simulators or synthetic models [2]. Animal labs are effective because they share many of the same features as humans, including the need for anesthesia and adequate hemostatic control. Trainees can therefore practice every element of an operation from technical skills to avoiding to managing complications when they arise [17]. However, prohibitive factors exist for animate labs including the cost, limited availability, as well as ethical and legal concerns [2].

Cadaver labs also provide a unique opportunity to understand details of human anatomy [18]. Commonly reserved for advanced specialty instructional courses, cadaver labs can simulate surgical procedures (both open and laparoscopic) and endoscopy (upper endoscopy, colonoscopy) [2]. Several disadvantages associated with cadaver labs include difficult acquisition, high maintenance costs, and the absence of psychological considerations that are associated with patient care [2].

15.2.2 Virtual Reality

Virtual reality (VR) simulations were first used for medical training in the 1990s. These computer-based systems provide a safe and ethical way to repeatedly practice surgical techniques in a realistic virtual environment, allowing trainees to become accustomed to surgical procedures at their own pace [19, 20]. VR simulations have been shown to shorten the learning curve and avoid risks associated with entering new environments, both of which are important to the learner and to experienced personnel [20]. Surgical VR simulators are particularly effective at developing the user's technical psychomotor skills because they can be used repeatedly and require very little time and resources to set up [21]. A key feature is the ability for VR to provide real-time haptic feedback as well as performance metrics such as time to complete a task, number of errors made, and economy of movement [22]. This unique and automatic feedback from the simulator allows trainees to not only practice repeatedly but to also improve their skills without the need for constant supervision [23].

VR simulation can provide training across a wide range of skills, both technical and nontechnical. For example, VR systems can teach basic tasks such as laparoscopic suturing and knot-tying, in addition to more complex technical tasks including microdissection and tumor aspiration [24, 25]. In a meta-analysis, Mao et al. showed VR was a cost-effect method for improving surgical skill acquisition and efficiency for residents and medical students [26]. Lohre et al. conducted a randomized control trial of 18 senior orthopedic surgery residents to assess if VR could improve operative knowledge and complex procedural skills. One group watched a surgical training video of a reverse total shoulder replacement while the other group used a VR platform for learning key steps, and both groups then completed the operation on a cadaver. Residents in the VR group completed the cadaver exercise faster than the control group. They always had a significantly higher mean technical score including implant position. They concluded that VR training demonstrated learning efficiency and can be a helpful tool for both training and assessment [27].

Patient-specific VR simulations have also been used as a method to practice a procedure preoperatively. These simulations are anatomically accurate, help surgeons reduce errors, and allow for a discussion of the surgical plan with the operating team and the patient [28]. In 2015, Makiyama et al. created a patient-specific simulator for laparoscopic renal surgery which allowed surgeons to practice procedures with various anatomical variations including ureters and renal vessels [29].

Regarding non-technical skills, Cohen et al. used VR to simulate trauma and emergency responses. They assessed participants on skills such as appropriate triage, timing, communication, team orientation, adaptability, and situational awareness [30]. Another study incorporated VR into a neurosurgical course for medical students and found that VR training may improve confidence which can contribute to improved self-efficacy and participation during surgical rotations [31].

As VR technology advances, these technical features, such as improved technical feedback and realism, will improve. Consequently, widespread, standardized use of these simulators has been suggested in surgical training [17].

15.2.3 Augmented and Mixed Reality

Augmented reality (AR) and mixed reality (overlay of digital information in physical world) were initially developed to assist with telementoring in remote areas but have also been shown to have positive effects on performance for surgical trainees [32]. For example, Rojas-Munoz et al. used an augmented reality headset to project instructions directly into the wearer's field of view to teach trauma situations such as fasciotomies and cricothyroidotomies. In this study, medical students and residents were taught to perform leg fasciotomies either using telementoring with their AR headset or by independently reviewing the procedure. They found that students who used the AR headset achieved greater technical skills scores and made fewer errors. They concluded that AR telementoring can help surgical knowledge and skill [33].

15.2.4 Robotic Assisted Surgical Training

With the rise of robotic-assisted surgery over the last decade, simulation training has been recognized as a crucial step in developing the necessary skills that are unique to operating with the da Vinci system. More specifically, robotic training includes bedside and console training. The bedside training consists of learning about procedure-specific port placements, robot docking, and understanding robotic arm ergonomics [34]. While there are no published metrics to measure technical performance of the bedside assistant, they are an important part of the operation [35].

The da Vinci system has specific simulators to train on the console. Surgeons can practice in a virtual environment looking through the same viewer as during an operation which promotes a smooth transition from simulation to surgery [36]. Virtual exercises range from simple tasks like tissue manipulation and knot-tying, to more advanced high-fidelity simulation such as cholecystectomy. Similar to VR simulators, robot simulators can provide specific feedback including completion time, number of errors, and a motion analysis [36]. Validity studies have shown that the use of robotic simulators accelerates initial console training [36, 37]. Basic skills such as camera movement and finger control can be learned on robotic simulators. More advanced skills such as suturing or diathermy can be learned via simulator or, more frequently, during wet labs such as with a live animal or cadaveric models [34].

For future directions of robotic training, there is a need for a universal curriculum with objective and subjective measures of proficiency, access to simulations for all learners, and a digital platform to guide learners through their training [38].

15.2.5 3D Printing

Other recent innovations in surgical simulation include patient-specific prototyping, such as 3D printing. 3D models can be used from patient imaging, such as CT or MRI, to build synthetic models of patient-specific organs or vasculature [34]. 3D printed models can help with surgical planning and operative feasibility [39]. It has been used for operations such as kidney and liver transplants, complex pancreatic resections, tracheal stenosis repairs, and biliary tree procedures [40].

15.2.6 Artificial Intelligence and Machine Learning

Artificial intelligence (AI) is the capability of a machine to execute cognitive processes similar to the human brain. It allows computer systems to reason, perform mental tasks and problem-solve [41]. Machine learning (ML) is a subset of AI technology that allows computer systems to learn and make predictions based on data and pattern recognition [41]. In medicine, AI can be used for learning and teaching. For example, it has been used to create case-based learning systems to evaluate student responses and improve clinical thinking [42]. Within surgical training, AI has become an increasingly popular tool to enhance surgical training and to enhance the capabilities and accuracy of surgical simulators [43]. Although surgical simulators can offer trainees an opportunity to practice skills, they do not provide feedback at the level of a skilled surgeon. However, using historical data, AI technology can enhance the effectiveness of simulators to generate algorithms and models capable of predicating accuracy [43, 44]. For example, Fazlollahi et al. developed an AI-enhanced curriculum to teach neurosurgical techniques to medical students. The curriculum objectives were chosen by an algorithm that analyzed metrics and selected 4 that were significantly associated with expertise. Feedback on these metrics were delivered by the Virtual Operative Assistant (VOA), an intelligent tutoring system that evaluates the competency level of the learning. The cohort exposed to the VOA was compared to a control cohort and performance outcomes were assessed. Participants in the AI—enhanced curriculum group showed significant improvement in safety metrics and bimanual control of the operative field when compared to the control group [45].

AI can also be used to improve surgical quality and patient outcomes. For example, Korndorffer et al. used AI to annotate over 100 laparoscopic cholecystectomy videos for disease severity, fulfillment of the critical view of safety criteria, surgical phases, and intraoperative events. Surgeons then reviewed these videos and recorded whether AI annotations were correct. Surgeons agreed with 75% of critical view of safety components and 99% of the AI-annotated intra-operative events. As shown in this study, AI can impact surgical education, skill development, and even quality and safety [46].

15.3 Conclusion

Surgical training has evolved from the "see one, do one, teach one" model to one that includes simulation for standardization, assessment and feedback. The secure, risk-free environment allows trainees to gain technical experience and self-confidence. The evolution of technology in surgical simulation has allowed for improved collaboration, realistic experiences, and customization [19]. Surgical simulation has an innovative future as we develop more personalized, immersive systems to prioritize skill and patient safety.

References

1. Agha RA, Fowler AJ. The role and validity of surgical simulations. Int Surg. 2015;100:350–7.
2. Cardoso SA, Suyambu J, Iqbal J, et al. Exploring the role of simulation training in improving surgical skills among residents: a narrative review. Cureus. 2023;15:e44654.
3. Reznick R, Regehr G, MacRae H, Martin J, McCulloch W. Testing technical skill via an innovative "bench station" examination. Am J Surg. 1997;173:226–30.
4. Scott DJ, Cendan JC, Pugh CM, Minter RM, Dunnington GL, Kozar RA. The changing face of surgical education: simulation as the new paradigm. J Surg Res. 2008;147:189–93.
5. Moore MJ, Bennett CL. The learning curve for laparoscopic cholecystectomy. The southern surgeons club. Am J Surg. 1995;170:55–9.
6. Korndorffer JR, Clayton JL, Tesfay ST, Brunner WC, Sierra R, Dunne JB, Jones DB, Rege RV, Touchard CL, Scott DJ. Multicenter construct validity for southwestern laparoscopic videotrainer stations. J Surg Res. 2005;128:114–9.
7. American College of Surgeons. ACS/ASE Medical Student Simulation-Based Surgical Skills Curriculum. 2013. https://www.facs.org/for-medical-professionals/education/programs/acsase-medical-student-simulation-based-surgicalskills-curriculum/. Accessed 7 Jan 2024
8. Perone J, Anton NE, Gardner AK. The various roles of simulation throughout the surgeon lifecycle. Resources in Surgical Education; 2018.
9. McManus C, Lee JA. A review of innovations in surgical education: melding metacognition and technology. Laparosc Surg. 2022;6:27.
10. Bell RH. Surgical council on resident education: a new organization devoted to graduate surgical education. J Am Coll Surg. 2007;204:341–6.
11. American College of Surgeons. ACS/ASE/APDS Resident Prep Curriculum. 2014. https://www.facs.org/education/program/resident-prep. Accessed 7 Jan 2024.
12. Robertson ER, Hadi M, Morgan LJ, Pickering SP, Collins G, New S, Griffin D, McCulloch P, Catchpole KC. Oxford NOTECHS II: a modified theatre team nontechnical skills scoring system. PLoS One. 2014;9:e90320.
13. Fleetwood VA, Veenstra B, Wojtowicz A, Kerchberger J, Velasco J. Communication through simulation: developing a curriculum to teach interpersonal skills. Surgery. 2018;164:802–9.

14. Nakagawa S, Fischkoff K, Berlin A, Arnell TD, Blinderman CD. Communication skills training for general surgery residents. J Surg Educ. 2019;76:1223–30.
15. Stefanidis D, Anderson-Montoya B, Higgins RV, Pimentel ME, Rowland P, Scarborough MO, Higgins D. Developing a coaching mechanism for practicing surgeons. Surgery. 2016;160:536–45.
16. Mackenzie H, Cuming T, Miskovic D, et al. Design, delivery, and validation of a trainer curriculum for the national laparoscopic colorectal training program in England. Ann Surg. 2015;261:149–56.
17. Tan SSY, Sarker SK. Simulation in surgery: a review. Scott Med J. 2011;56:104–9.
18. Sturm LP, Windsor JA, Cosman PH, Cregan P, Hewett PJ, Maddern GJ. A systematic review of skills transfer after surgical simulation training. Ann Surg. 2008;248:166–79.
19. Badash I, Burtt K, Solorzano CA, Carey JN. Innovations in surgery simulation: a review of past, current and future techniques. Ann Transl Med. 2016;4:453.
20. Rizzetto F, Bernareggi A, Rantas S, Vanzulli A, Vertemati M. Immersive virtual reality in surgery and medical education: diving into the future. Am J Surg. 2020;220:856–7.
21. Blackburn SC, Griffin SJ. Role of simulation in training the next generation of endoscopists. World J Gastrointest Endosc. 2014;6:234–9.
22. Satava RM. Historical review of surgical simulation—a personal perspective. World J Surg. 2008;32:141–8.
23. Seymour NE, Gallagher AG, Roman SA, O'Brien MK, Bansal VK, Andersen DK, Satava RM. Virtual reality training improves operating room performance: results of a randomized, double-blinded study. Ann Surg. 2002;236:458–63; discussion 463
24. Delorme S, Laroche D, DiRaddo R, Del Maestro RF. NeuroTouch: a physicsbased virtual simulator for cranial microneurosurgery training. Neurosurgery. 2012;71:32–42.
25. Gallagher AG, McClure N, McGuigan J, Crothers I, Browning J. Virtual reality training in laparoscopic surgery: a preliminary assessment of minimally invasive surgical trainer virtual reality (MIST VR). Endoscopy. 1999;31:310–3.
26. Mao RQ, Lan L, Kay J, Lohre R, Ayeni OR, Goel DP, de Sa D. Immersive virtual reality for surgical training: a systematic review. J Surg Res. 2021;268:40–58.
27. Lohre R, Bois AJ, Pollock JW, Lapner P, McIlquham K, Athwal GS, Goel DP. Effectiveness of immersive virtual reality on orthopedic surgical skills and knowledge acquisition among senior surgical residents: a randomized clinical trial. JAMA Netw Open. 2020;3:e2031217.
28. Endo K, Sata N, Ishiguro Y, Miki A, Sasanuma H, Sakuma Y, Shimizu A, Hyodo M, Lefor A, Yasuda Y. A patient-specific surgical simulator using preoperative imaging data: an interactive simulator using a three-dimensional tactile mouse. J Comput Surg. 2014;1:10.
29. Makiyama K, Yamanaka H, Ueno D, Ohsaka K, Sano F, Nakaigawa N, Yao M, Kubota Y. Validation of a patient-specific simulator for laparoscopic renal surgery. Int J Urol. 2015;22:572–6.
30. Cohen D, Sevdalis N, Patel V, Taylor M, Lee H, Vokes M, Heys M, Taylor D, Batrick N, Darzi A. Tactical and operational response to major incidents: feasibility and reliability of skills assessment using novel virtual environments. Resuscitation. 2013;84:992–8.
31. Atli K, Selman W, Ray A. A comprehensive multicomponent neurosurgical course with use of virtual reality: modernizing the medical classroom. J Surg Educ. 2021;78:1350–6.
32. Suresh D, Aydin A, James S, Ahmed K, Dasgupta P. The role of augmented reality in surgical training: a systematic review. Surg Innov. 2023;30:366–82.
33. Rojas-Muñoz E, Cabrera ME, Lin C, Andersen D, Popescu V, Anderson K, Zarzaur BL, Mullis B, Wachs JP. The system for telementoring with augmented reality (STAR): a head-mounted display to improve surgical coaching and confidence in remote areas. Surgery. 2020;167:724–31.
34. Sridhar AN, Briggs TP, Kelly JD, Nathan S. Training in robotic surgery-an overview. Curr Urol Rep. 2017;18:58.
35. Hazen JK, Scott DJ, Holcomb CN. The effect of bedside assistant technical performance on outcomes in robotic surgery. J Robot Surg. 2023;17:711–8.

36. Liu M, Curet M. A review of training research and virtual reality simulators for the da Vinci surgical system. Teach Learn Med. 2015;27:12–26.
37. Hung AJ, Jayaratna IS, Teruya K, Desai MM, Gill IS, Goh AC (2013) Comparative assessment of three standardized robotic surgery training methods. BJU Int 112:864–871
38. Porterfield JR, Podolsky D, Ballecer C, Coker AM, Kudsi OY, Duffy AJ, Meara MP, Novitsky YW. structured resident training in robotic surgery: recommendations of the robotic surgery education working group. J Surg Educ. 2024;81:9–16.
39. Chandak P, Byrne N, Coleman A, Karunanithy N, Carmichael J, Marks SD, Stojanovic J, Kessaris N, Mamode N. Patient-specific 3D printing: a novel technique for complex pediatric renal transplantation. Ann Surg. 2019;269:e18–23.
40. Meyer-Szary J, Luis MS, Mikulski S, et al. The role of 3D printing in planning complex medical procedures and training of medical professionals-cross-sectional multispecialty review. Int J Environ Res Public Health. 2022;19(6):3331. https://doi.org/10.3390/ijerph19063331.
41. Amin A, Cardoso SA, Suyambu J, et al. Future of artificial intelligence in surgery: a narrative review. Cureus. 2024;16(1):e51631. https://doi.org/10.7759/cureus.51631.
42. Wang M, Sun Z, Jia M, Wang Y, Wang H, Zhu X, Chen L, Ji H. Intelligent virtual case learning system based on real medical records and natural language processing. BMC Med Inform Decis Mak. 2022;22:60.
43. Park JJ, Tiefenbach J, Demetriades AK. The role of artificial intelligence in surgical simulation. Front Med Technol. 2022;4:1076755.
44. Rubalcava NS, Guetter CR, Kapani N, Martinez Quinones P. How artificial intelligence is expected to transform surgical training. In: American College of Surgeons. 2023. https://www.facs.org/for-medical-professionals/news-publications/news-andarticles/bulletin/2023/august-2023-volume-108-issue-8/how-artificial-intelligence-isexpected-to-transform-surgical-training/. Accessed 28 Jan 2024.
45. Fazlollahi AM, Yilmaz R, Winkler-Schwartz A, Mirchi N, Ledwos N, Bakhaidar M, Alsayegh A, Del Maestro RF. AI in surgical curriculum design and unintended outcomes for technical competencies in simulation training. JAMA Netw Open. 2023;6:e2334658.
46. Korndorffer JR, Hawn MT, Spain DA, Knowlton LM, Azagury DE, Nassar AK, Lau JN, Arnow KD, Trickey AW, Pugh CM. Situating artificial intelligence in surgery: a focus on disease severity. Ann Surg. 2020;272:523–8.

Chapter 16
Strategies for Succeeding During Intern Year: Perspectives from Recent Surgical Interns

Courtney Rentas and Chukwuma Eruchalu

Abstract The intern year of surgical residency is both a challenging and rewarding period marked by significant personal and clinical development. Advancement of technical skills, establishment of mentorship relationships, and expansion of clinical knowledge and acumen are paramount to success during the intern year. The chapter that follows outlines core attributes of successful surgical interns and the methods used to develop these qualities.

16.1 Core Attributes of a Successful Surgical Intern

There is considerable variability in the breadth and depth of opportunities for academic and clinical preparation for graduate medical training across US Medical Schools. Additionally, mechanisms of assessment as well as educational objectives for medical students vary, introducing heterogeneity in the competencies and qualities that students develop. Consequently, surgical educators, in conjunction with other leaders in the Graduate Medical Education community, expressed concerns regarding the preparedness of some graduating medical students for surgical residency training. In order to address this issue, the Association of Program Directors in Surgery (APDS) convened at the 2015 APDS Spring Meeting and published a consensus list of core Entrustable Professional Activities (EPAs) that residents could be expected to perform on their first day of residency [1]. Some examples of these initial EPAs include the ability to "gather a history and perform a physical examination," "recommend and interpret common diagnostic and screening tests,"

Courtney Rentas and Chukwuma Eruchalu contributed equally with all other contributors.

C. Rentas · C. Eruchalu (✉)
Department of Surgery, University of Michigan, Ann Arbor, MI, USA

Department of Surgery, Massachusetts General Hospital, Boston, MA, USA
e-mail: corentas@med.umich.edu; ceruchalu@mgh.harvard.edu

A. Gillis, C. B. Aarons (eds.), *A How To Guide For Medical Students*, Success in Academic Surgery, https://doi.org/10.1007/978-3-031-66011-5_16

"document a clinical encounter in the patient record," "provide an oral presentation of a clinical encounter," "form clinical questions and retrieve evidence to advance patient care," "collaborate as a member of an interprofessional team," and "contribute to a culture of safety and improvement," along with an assortment of basic procedural skills [1]. Interestingly, when studied, students' ratings of their competencies were higher than those of their program directors for nearly every EPA domain, suggesting potential misalignment of perception versus reality regarding students' level of preparedness across these key competencies for early residents [1].

The 2015 APDS survey that described core EPAs has now been integrated into the fabric of surgical education [1, 2]. Furthermore, review of the EPA framework allows for identification of common themes across competencies, which enables the definition of several core attributes of successful surgical residents in the first year and beyond. Indeed, follow-up studies at the multi-institutional level have emphasized key preparatory domains for entering interns, including practice-based learning, interpersonal communication, professionalism, and systems-based practice, as well as the importance of incorporating experiential learning at the senior medical student level to inculcate these qualities [3, 4]. A non-exhaustive list of foundational competencies of successful residents includes (1) clinical knowledge and the ability to appropriately research information to fill knowledge gaps (2) effective interpersonal communication in both oral and written form (3) organization and task prioritization (4) honesty and integrity (5) receptiveness to feedback and (6) capacity for self-introspection and commitment to self-improvement.

16.1.1 Clinical Knowledge and Information Gathering

The overarching mission of graduate surgical educators is to develop clinically and technically excellent surgeons. Therefore, clinical and anatomic knowledge are key to the success of surgical residents. Interns enter residency with varying levels of clinical knowledge, largely owing to differences in didactic- and hospital-based experiences at the medical student level. Therefore, successful interns are able to leverage academic resources to fill in their own knowledge gaps. At this stage, entering interns have likely already identified their ideal learning styles and academic adjuncts. Commonly utilized educational resources include online clinical databases such as UpToDate, surgical textbooks, anatomical atlases, and video-based didactic content. Senior residents and faculty surgeons are also important informational resources. Irrespective of the medium, interns should be able to efficiently query the resource to identify the relevant information to address the clinical question at hand. Specific clinical challenges commonly faced by interns include:

- Medication dosing and common side effects,
- The interpretation of abnormal laboratory values and imaging tests,
- Treatment of pain and nausea,
- Evaluation of postoperative fever,

- Management of surgical drains, and
- The initial diagnostic assessment and therapeutic management of an unstable or decompensating patient (e.g. a postoperative patient who develops hypotension, oliguria, delirium, or atrial fibrillation).

Interns should expect to be frequently confronted by unfamiliar clinical scenarios and face new challenges on a regular basis, regardless of the extent of their clinical experiences at the undergraduate medical level. In this way, clinical knowledge foundation at the start of residency is less important than the ability to effectively and efficiently acquire new knowledge and integrate this knowledge into existing clinical frameworks.

16.1.2 Effective Interpersonal Communication

Strong interprofessional and patient-centered communication skills are vital for all interns; nevertheless, validated communication curricula are not widely implemented across programs [5]. The surgical intern will regularly serve as the "responding clinician," the first point of contact regarding the care of an inpatient. As such, the intern is typically the first to be notified of any change in the patient's clinical status and will serve as the liaison between the surgical team and the nursing as well as consulting teams. Therefore, it is critically important that interns cultivate effective communication skills, both in oral and written form. Nursing teams rely on accurate written documentation of daily plans for patient care as well as clear verbal communication regarding any updates or changes. When paged about a concern, successful interns will collaborate with nurses in a timely fashion, ideally in-person, to arrive at a mutually agreeable solution. Additionally, interns must be able to communicate clinical questions accurately and succinctly to consulting services to allow for efficient advancement of patient care. When unsure of the best course of action, successful interns will expeditiously communicate with their supervising residents or faculty surgeons to clarify the optimal plan. They will not "worry alone."

Moreover, the surgical intern serves as the liaison between the surgical team and the surgical patient, as they are typically the provider who spends the most time in the patient room throughout the day. Thus, the intern must cultivate patient-centered communication skills, which allow for translation of medical information into accessible language as well as the incorporation of shared decision-making [5]. Relatedly, the surgical intern is often tasked with explaining invasive procedures to patients and obtaining informed consent. Nevertheless, strategies for framing effective informed consent discussions are not regularly included in medical curricula. Interns with exceptional communication skills are able to shift the focus of these interactions from technical jargon describing a surgical problem to an accessible and collaborative discussion regarding therapeutic options, treatment alternatives, and desired quality of life outcomes [6]. For example, the "Best Case/Worst Case" communication framework has emerged as a strategy for promoting shared decision-making in challenging or high-stakes clinical scenarios [6]. This framework is particularly beneficial for junior residents as it shifts focus away from the technical details of a given surgical intervention and places emphasis instead on humanistic attributes such as empathetic listening and values alignment. Importantly, with deliberate practice in both simulated environments and real-life clinical scenarios, interpersonal communication skills improve over time [7].

16.1.3 Organization and Task Prioritization

Surgical interns will frequently be confronted with competing demands and the perceived need to attend to multiple responsibilities simultaneously. While attempting to complete one task, an intern may be paged with several additional requests. Therefore, strong organizational skills are necessary for managing the extensive cognitive load of information and daily tasks with which interns are inundated on a regular basis. First-year residents must cultivate a system that ensures that tasks are not inadvertently neglected. Furthermore, when faced with a list of competing demands, effective interns must prioritize tasks to ensure that care is advanced for all patients on the service as smoothly as possible. In general, consults should be called, diagnostic tests ordered (and the appropriate scheduling personnel contacted), medications updated, patient-facing tasks completed, and plans communicated verbally to nurses prior to turning attention to writing daily progress notes or completing other tasks that do not require the assistance of other hospital personnel. Patients who are proceeding to the operating room and those who are ready for hospital discharge are prioritized, as are patients who are more clinically complex or sick. Furthermore, successful interns will be adaptable, recognizing that unpredictable circumstances often necessitate rearrangement of task priorities throughout the day.

16.1.4 Integrity

Personal integrity is perhaps the most valuable core attribute of a successful intern. Supervising residents and faculty often spend much of the day off the surgical floor in the operating room or in the clinic. Therefore, as the team member primarily entrusted with completion of patient care tasks, surgical interns must be trustworthy and dependable. Although interns will often have assistance from Advanced Practice Providers, senior residents and faculty will expect interns to take ownership of the patients on the service, and they must be able to trust that interns will do what they say that they will do. This personal integrity should be intentionally cultivated from the very first interactions of residency. Interns must be honest, especially in situations during which disclosing the truth means discussing a potential error (e.g. when forgetting to complete a task or perform a specific physical exam maneuver).

Notably, senior surgical residents, faculty, and program leadership must cultivate an environment of psychological safety, in which mistakes can be discussed openly and leveraged as opportunities for growth.

16.1.5 Receptiveness to Feedback

Surgical interns will receive performance-related feedback, both explicit and implicit, on a regular basis. Feedback is often delivered informally by senior residents and surgical faculty, and this feedback occurs in various settings, including the operating room, inpatient floor, and surgical clinic. Given the breadth of skills and competencies that must be developed during surgical residency, direct constructive feedback regarding areas for improvement will be a regular occurrence, particularly during the intern year. Therefore, interns must approach these interactions with an open mind and with a focus on identifying tangible mechanisms for future growth. Effective feedback discussions will center on actionable and objective areas for improvement rather than subjective assessments of personal characteristics. For many residents, feedback on clinical and technical performance is ideally delivered through direct mechanisms and in close temporal proximity to the event [8]. Nevertheless, there is a continued need to formalize structured interventions for delivering high-quality feedback in perioperative settings as well as utilizing debriefing practices after challenging clinical encounters in order to more systematically reflect on training experiences and cultivate growth [9, 10].

16.1.6 Capacity for Self-Introspection and Commitment to Self-Improvement

Finally, successful surgical residents will possess the capacity to reflect inwardly on their strengths, weaknesses, and opportunities for improvement. Although residents will receive frequent performance-related feedback from external sources, which can inform these deliberations, effective interns will create space for intentional personal reflection on clinical experiences in order to identify areas for growth. The capacity for self-introspection and recognition of existing personal limits are important manifestations of emotional maturity that allow adult learners to take ownership of their personal development and optimize the potential for growth. Successful surgical interns will adopt a growth-focused mindset that is centered on consistent self-improvement across educational competencies.

16.2 Deliberate Practice and Technical Skills Training

Competency-based surgical education is gaining momentum as the medical field aims to ensure that surgical residents achieve the technical skills required to provide safe patient care [11–15]. The ability to develop and refine the basic surgical skills necessary to demonstrate competency, without compromising patient safety, is accomplished at the trainee level largely through simulation training, which has become the standard of training in most graduate medical education programs [15]. In addition to providing a safe environment for learners to acquire technical skills, simulated environments demonstrate transferability of skills in the operating room (OR) [16, 17]. While participating in simulation training as a junior resident can result in technical competency, mastery of such skills requires deliberate practice [18].

According to psychologist Anders Ericsson, achieving competency in a new skill typically requires only 50 hours of effort, after which the action can be practiced and repeated without active engagement [19]. Ericsson suggests that while working to perfect a new skill, a learner cannot expect to progress by simply repeating tasks he or she has grown comfortable with. Instead, repetition must be applied to challenging tasks aimed at addressing the learner's weaknesses. If this meaningful repetition is followed by assessment and feedback, Ericsson states that performance improvement can be achieved; he coined this learning style "deliberate practice" [19, 20]. Deliberate practice is therefore incumbent on intense, meaningful training and preparation. Because it requires significant time and repetition, it is most commonly employed in the setting of simulation training during surgical residency.

Much like elite athletes, if future surgeons desire to perform at the highest level, they must continuously strive to grow their skillset. Surgical residents cannot achieve or maintain mastery of technical skills without consistent deliberate practice outside of the operating room [20]. Simulation labs provide a safe, readily-accessible environment for learners to engage in deliberate practice and junior residents should therefore incorporate time in these settings into their weekly routines. An important and often-overlooked component of deliberate practice is obtaining feedback. It is therefore imperative that junior residents seek feedback on their technical skill development intraoperatively from senior residents, fellows, and attending surgeons. Surgical residents are expected to achieve excellent technical skills to provide safe care to patients; the development and refinement of these skills begins during the intern year.

16.3 Developing a Mentorship Network

Meaningful mentorship is critical in surgical training and requires ongoing support throughout residency [21]. Strong mentorship can improve the resident experience and protect against burnout and attrition rates [22–24]. Junior residents should seek a variety of mentorship relationships as they navigate their training environment.

For example, near-peer mentors who are a single step ahead of a mentee (PGY2, PGY3 residents) have comparatively small differences in knowledge level and training; these relationships are extremely advantageous to interns learning to navigate their new roles and responsibilities. Alternatively, junior residents often find mentors in faculty members who provide long-term research and career guidance. Whatever the style, effective mentoring should be a dynamic relationship that evolves as the learner progresses in their own training [21]. Strong mentors are defined by many traits which should be considered by junior residents seeking to invest in a mentorship relationship; a non-exhaustive list of essential traits of a good mentor includes the following: commitment, empathy, versatility, model of excellence, and communicates optimism [21, 25].

16.3.1 Commitment to Mentoring

Not all mentors are created equally; good mentors possess a firm belief that they are capable of making a difference in the lives of others. They are understanding that mentorship requires a significant investment of time and energy, and yet they persist in pursuing these relationships. Mentors should be invested in the development of their mentees without the promise of personal gains. While finding a mentor during surgical residency who possesses the time and energy it takes to fully invest in this relationship can be challenging and may take several attempts, the benefits can be substantial and are worth the effort.

16.3.2 Empathy

The best mentors are empathetic to the challenges junior residents face daily; while often not facing the same challenges at their stage of training, they are able to reflect on their own experience during surgical residency to offer guidance and support. Much like good doctors listen to and accept the concerns of their patients without judgment, good mentors must be willing to listen and accept the concerns of their mentees to support them. When mentees do not feel their distresses are heard and appreciated, the mentee/mentor relationship becomes stagnant, and the trust required to move the relationship forward comes to a halt as well. Finding a mentor, whether a near-peer or a senior faculty member, who can empathize with the difficulties the mentee is facing personally, professionally, or both, is paramount to building a strong, lasting mentorship.

16.3.3 *Versatility*

Mentors should be able to adapt to meet the needs of their mentees. The mentorship needs of a surgical intern are different from that of a surgical chief resident, and a good mentor understands that and can adjust to provide what is required by each. To make such adjustments, good mentors must possess a deep understanding of what they have to offer and an innate ability to anticipate the needs of their mentees.

16.3.4 *Model of Excellence*

Good mentors model admirable behaviors for surgical residents. They attend and participate in educational conferences. They conduct research that advances the field forward. They are prepared for their clinical and operative responsibilities. They attend workshops to enhance their surgical skills. They serve in leadership positions within their departments. Most importantly, they share what they have learned from these endeavors with their mentees and subsequently challenge them and support them to achieve similar pursuits.

16.3.5 *Communicates Optimism*

One of the most important traits of a good mentor is the ability to communicate a genuine belief that their mentees can overcome the challenges they are presently faced with and achieve success in the future. Strong mentors capitalize on opportunities to uplift their mentees and reaffirm their potential in both public and private settings. Crucially, they give mentees the self-confidence necessary to grow in the challenging field of surgery.

16.4 Conclusion

Intern year can be challenging for all surgical trainees. This should be a transformative year that will set residents up for success as lifelong learners and health care professionals. Therefore, adopting a growth mindset, utilizing helpful resources, deliberate practice, and cultivation of mentorship are fundamental tools for success.

References

1. Lindeman BM, Sacks BC, Lipsett PA. Graduating students' and surgery program directors' views of the association of American medical colleges core entrustable professional activities for entering residency: where are the gaps? J Surg Educ. 2015;72(6):e184–92.
2. Brasel KJ, Lindeman B, Jones A, Sarosi GA, Minter R, Klingensmith ME, et al. Implementation of entrustable professional activities in general surgery: results of a national pilot study. Ann Surg. 2023;278(4):578–86.
3. Minter RM, Amos KD, Bentz ML, Blair PG, Brandt C, D'Cunha J, et al. Transition to surgical residency: a multi-institutional study of perceived intern preparedness and the effect of a formal residency preparatory course in the fourth year of medical school. Acad Med. 2015;90(8):1116–24.
4. LaFemina J, Ahuja V, Alseidi A, Balters M, Brasel K, Clark C, et al. APDS consensus statement: ideal senior medical student experiences for preparedness for general surgery internship. J Surg Educ. 2021;78(1):69–75.
5. Kapadia MR, Lee E, Healy H, Dort JM, Rosenbaum ME, Newcomb AB. Training surgical residents to communicate with their patients: a scoping review of the literature. J Surg Educ. 2021;78(2):440–9.
6. Taylor LJ, Nabozny MJ, Steffens NM, Tucholka JL, Brasel KJ, Johnson SK, et al. A framework to improve surgeon communication in high-stakes surgical decisions: best case/worst case. JAMA Surg. 2017;152(6):531–8.
7. Newcomb AB, Liu C, Trickey AW, Lita E, Dort J. Patient perspectives of surgical residents' communication: do skills improve over time with a communication curriculum? J Surg Educ. 2018;75(6):e142–9.
8. Pascarella L, Marulanda K, Duchesneau ED, Sanchez-Casalongue M, Kapadia M, Farrell TM. Preferred feedback styles among different groups in an academic medical center. J Surg Res. 2023;288:215–24.
9. McKendy KM, Watanabe Y, Lee L, Bilgic E, Enani G, Feldman LS, et al. Perioperative feedback in surgical training: a systematic review. Am J Surg. 2017;214(1):117–26.
10. Evans TR, Burns C, Essex R, Finnerty G, Hatton E, Clements AJ, et al. A systematic scoping review on the evidence behind debriefing practices for the wellbeing/emotional outcomes of healthcare workers. Front Psychiatry. 2023;14:1078797.
11. Sonnadara RR, Mui C, McQueen S, Mironova P, Nousiainen M, Safir O, et al. Reflections on competency-based education and training for surgical residents. J Surg Educ. 2014;71(1):151–8.
12. Alman BA, Ferguson P, Kraemer W, Nousiainen MT, Reznick RK. Competency-based education: a new model for teaching orthopaedics. Instr Course Lect. 2013;62:565–9.
13. Competence by design: the rationale for change [Internet]. Royal College of Physicians and Surgeons of Canada. [cited 2024 Jan 19]. http://www.royalcollege.ca/rcsite/cbd/rationale-why-cbd-e
14. Overview [Internet]. www.acgme.org. [cited 2024 Jan 31]. http://www.acgme.org/acgmeweb/tabid/430/ProgramandInstitutionalAccreditation/NextAccreditationSystem/Milestones.aspx
15. de Montbrun S, Louridas M, Grantcharov T. Passing a technical skills examination in the first year of surgical residency can predict future performance. J Grad Med Educ. 2017;9(3):324–9.
16. Vanderbilt AA, Grover AC, Pastis NJ, Feldman M, Granados DD, Murithi LK, et al. Randomized controlled trials: a systematic review of laparoscopic surgery and simulation-based training. Glob J Health Sci. 2014;7(2):310–27.
17. Zendejas B, Brydges R, Hamstra SJ, Cook DA. State of the evidence on simulation-based training for laparoscopic surgery: a systematic review. Ann Surg. 2013;257(4):586–93.
18. Higgins M, Madan CR, Patel R. Deliberate practice in simulation-based surgical skills training: a scoping review. J Surg Educ. 2021;78(4):1328–39.
19. Ericsson KA. Deliberate practice and acquisition of expert performance: a general overview. Acad Emerg Med. 2008;15(11):988–94.

20. Wollstein Y, Jabbour N. Building surgical expertise through deliberate practice. Ear Nose Throat J. 2022;101(9_suppl):47S–51S.
21. Steelman K, Fleifel D, Waheed M, Vaidya R. Mentorship in a surgical residency: a comprehensive review of the literature. Cureus. 2023;15(8):e43422.
22. Bingmer K, Wojnarski CM, Brady JT, Stein SL, Ho VP, Steinhagen E. A model for a formal mentorship program in surgical residency. J Surg Res. 2019;243:64–70.
23. Foote DC, Donkersloot JN, Sandhu G, Ziegler K, Lau J. Identifying institutional factors in general surgery resident wellness and burnout. Am J Surg. 2022;223(1):53–7.
24. Shen MR, Zhuo L, Madison K, Bredbeck BC, Kemp MT, Santos-Parker JR, et al. How we do it: an innovative general surgery mentoring program. J Surg Educ. 2022;79(5):1088–92.
25. Rowley JB. The good mentor. Educational Leadership. 1999;56(8):20–2. https://eric.ed.gov/?id=EJ585660

Chapter 17
Strategies for Succeeding in Residency Programs: A Program Director's Perspective

Jennifer Yu and Paul E. Wise

Abstract As the classic adage states, residency training in any specialty is a marathon, not a sprint; but what may be a more accurate analogy is that residency training is akin to the physical and psychological preparation *before* the race even occurs. For any young surgeon, this is arguably the most critical period in their career, since everything subsequent to residency is built upon the foundation of what a trainee ingrains during this initial time spent learning to care for patients both inside and outside of an operating room. The running of the marathon, just like sitting for the Boards and entering the first year of practice, becomes the test of all of the prior days, months, and years of technical practice, cross-training, and mental roadmapping. In this chapter, we seek to describe strategies for success as residents embark on this journey toward becoming independent clinicians and surgeons.

17.1 Getting Started

17.1.1 Knowledge Base

As a general surgery resident, having a solid base of medical knowledge is crucial. Understanding the distinctions between normal anatomy and surgical anatomy gives perspective on how physiologic processes will be impacted by surgery, and it is always helpful to participate in the operating room (OR) even as an observer to then appreciate how intra-operative management may change a patient's

J. Yu
Abdominal Transplant Surgery, Washington University School of Medicine in St. Louis, St. Louis, MO, USA
e-mail: j.yu@wustl.edu

P. E. Wise (✉)
Department of Surgery, Washington University School of Medicine in St. Louis, St. Louis, MO, USA
e-mail: wisepe@wustl.edu

A. Gillis, C. B. Aarons (eds.), *A How To Guide For Medical Students*, Success in Academic Surgery, https://doi.org/10.1007/978-3-031-66011-5_17

postoperative course (including potential complications). The range of general surgery is such that it is vital to appreciate how the anatomy and pathophysiology over multiple organ systems are interrelated. Learning the fundamentals of surgical techniques and perioperative care are priorities in the early years of residency, as these, along with medical knowledge, are the building blocks which will more effectively bolster a resident's ability to assess and manage patients with increasing levels of complexity. Utilization of textbooks, journals, and online resources as routine aids while preparing for cases or clinics can be a useful habit to develop, not only in being able to discuss issues in-depth with both patients and faculty, but also in maintaining an awareness of clinical advances and changes in practice patterns in different subspecialties over time. Educational conferences may vary between institutions, but this traditional format will help to expand a resident's knowledge base as well through didactic lectures and academic peer interaction. Finally, a strong knowledge base will help with the annual in-service training exam and ultimately Board certification and licensure (see "Sect. 17.7" below).

17.1.2 Skill Development

In addition to gaining medical knowledge, surgical skill development is essential for success towards advancing through the years of residency. Seeking opportunities to observe and to assist in cases is the most time-honored tradition in training, and through repetition of action, hands-on experience, and attention to detail, residents gradually progress through developing basic skills of suturing, instrument handling, and knot-tying. These foundational skills then lead to appreciating and performing more challenging techniques of dissection and reconstruction. All of these skills become critical to competency-based education, the modern basis for feedback and skills assessment in surgical training. Simulation labs and skill workshops are becoming increasingly required in surgical training programs, being common as tools within the surgical education armamentarium. These are extremely useful adjuncts for practicing skills in a low-stakes setting where residents can become more comfortable with a variety of procedures prior to performing them in an operating room. Some programs will expect a certain level of skills performance in the lab before skills may be attempted in the OR.

It is also absolutely imperative to realize that technical proficiency is irrelevant without its counterpart of appropriate clinical judgment. The ability to recognize "sick" versus "not sick" (and to know what to do about it) is just as critical as knowing how to perform any operation to fix the problem. Furthermore, non-technical skills have been increasingly acknowledged as domains in which trainees must reach a level of competency, and this extends to communication, teamwork, situational awareness, leadership, and decision-making [1]. Skill development in these areas in turn impacts operative performance and patient outcomes.

17.2 Building Your Network

17.2.1 Peers

Creating a network with fellow trainees, both senior and junior, enhances not only learning opportunities throughout residency but also promotes professional growth and collaboration as well as lays the groundwork for relationships in practice. The significance of one's peers in training cannot be understated, and this interaction provides the basis for the development of both academic relationships as well as long-lasting friendships and personal bonds. Shared experiences and collaborative learning can offer valuable insights and perspectives that enhance the overall educational process, and the sense of community and camaraderie that organically develops amongst trainees is unequivocally necessary in mitigating the intensity of the experience of surgical training. By reviewing clinical cases, patient scenarios, and management strategies with their peers, residents can broaden their knowledge base and refine clinical skills. Furthermore, by discussing challenging experiences, residents are able to offer emotional support, share coping strategies, and create an environment that allows for open discourse. Fostering a culture of mutual respect and teamwork should be a priority for all residents, as this can help to combat burnout, to promote overall well-being, and to provide encouragement in a demanding work environment. Senior residents and fellows can be excellent role models and teachers for junior residents in refining leadership skills, while junior residents are in turn learning communication styles and teamwork.

17.2.2 Faculty

Equally important to peers are connections that residents build with faculty members. These are essential for mentorship, professional development, and career guidance. Every surgeon can recall at least one pivotal faculty mentor in their training who made an impact on the path of their surgical career. In the clinical domain, Surgery remains at its heart an apprenticeship-style vocation in which faculty are the "masters" to the trainee "apprentices." Trainees learn through clinical interactions and graduated autonomy under the watchful eye of the attending staff. This in turn shapes the very nature with which an individual surgeon may approach different clinical problems, patient management strategies, and operative techniques. Beyond the OR, faculty mentors are key in opening doors to educational resources, networking, and research and professional collaborations. Cultivating relationships with faculty in different subspecialties, either through research collaborations or clinical experiences, allows residents to explore potential areas of interest and expertise in a supportive setting.

17.3 Day-to-Day

17.3.1 Maintaining Motivation

Surgical residency can be exceptionally demanding, requiring resilience and motivation to succeed. This is what ultimately drives residents to excel in their training, to work continuously to improve their skills, and to provide quality patient care despite long hours and stressful situations. The transition from medical school to intern year involves an indescribably enormous paradigm shift in adapting the knowledge gained through years of study and building even more on top of that foundation while donning the mantle of a physician's responsibilities for the first time. The challenging and complex nature of medicine and healthcare can be overwhelming and difficult to understand, especially early in residency, so maintaining a sense of equilibrium and purpose can be a constantly shifting objective. Each resident must find intrinsic motivation through their own passion for surgery and in developing their abilities as physicians to care for patients in this unique way. Self-reflection and setting realistic short- and long-term goals can help to reframe the residency training period, which is finite and objective-oriented. For every individual, it is important to recall even in the smallest of moments the impact that one can make in patients' lives and to celebrate the milestones that one achieves along the way [2].

17.3.2 Professionalism

Maintaining professionalism is paramount in surgery, encompassing integrity, ethics, communication, and interpersonal skills. This is, first and foremost, the principal creed to which residents must adhere in their training, which is what will ultimately shape them as future independent surgeons. Ethical standards must be upheld without question, as the well-being and lives of patients depends upon this, and professional standards of conduct should be at the forefront of every interaction and decision made in the care of patients. Demonstrating professionalism involves communicating effectively with peers and colleagues, collaborating in interdisciplinary settings, and being accountable for one's decisions. Respect and empathy are of the utmost importance, both in working with other physicians as well as with patients, and this commitment to lifelong learning and self-improvement is an essential quality to develop throughout surgical training. Program Directors will expect professionalism above all other characteristics in a trainee.

17.3.3 *Teamwork*

Surgery is inherently a team-based specialty that requires collaboration and cooperation among multidisciplinary teams. Developing strategies for effective communication (especially closed-loop communications), inclusivity, and teamwork is imperative, as collaborating with nurses, hospital and clinic staff, anesthesiology faculty and trainees, advanced care providers, and other healthcare professionals forms the backbone of any surgeon's work. By fostering a culture of safety, residents are able to effect far more efficient and effective care for patients and create a much more pleasant working environment for themselves and others.

17.4 Year-to-Year

17.4.1 *Personal Growth*

Residency is not just about clinical training but also about significant maturation, personal growth and development, and increasing responsibility. Setting realistic expectations for one's own progress can aid in developing a feasible overall training plan, and having external guideposts such as regular performance review with mentors and faculty regarding evaluations and competency metrics is helpful in providing objective goals. These are required per the ACGME, and known as "milestones"—available online as expected metrics to be achieved before training can be completed [3]. The competency-based "entrustable professional activities" ("EPAs") as required by the American Board of Surgery (ABS) have added an additional layer for feedback and assessing progress in training [4]. It is important to take time to reflect on strengths and weaknesses, as well as areas for improvement, as these will all fluctuate with different training experiences. Seeking feedback from mentors, supervisors, and peers creates a platform for discussion and allows for a deeper understanding of one's performance and progress.

17.4.2 *Leadership*

Developing leadership skills is an integral part of personal and professional growth during residency, and this maturity as a clinician comes with experience and often through emulating more senior trainees and faculty. Every phase of training presents different challenges and roles, each requiring adaptation of previously learned behavior patterns and growth in taking on more responsibilities, such as teaching more junior trainees and managing patient care. Formal leadership roles within residency programs, such as serving on committees, organizing educational events, or leading quality improvement projects, are also excellent opportunities to build leadership skills, to network, and to provide perspective on possible future jobs. Residency is a crucial time to cultivate a leadership style and to learn how to take initiative, as these become dynamic components of independent practice. Some residency programs offer formal leadership education, and/or formal leadership training can be available for residents from national organizations, such as the American College of Surgeons [5].

17.4.3 Developing a Support System

Surgical residency is perhaps the most emotionally and physically demanding (and rewarding!) experience of every surgeon's life, so having a strong support system in place secures a vital source of encouragement and emotional support over the years of training. Communication is important, as friends, family, and significant others can be bastions of normalcy apart from what can be a chaotic work life, while fellow residents and colleagues who understand the professional challenges of training can empathize and provide camaraderie. Seeking mentors for advice on professional and personal life can be rewarding and key to training success. Senior residents, faculty members, and training program alumni, above and beyond mentors, are also valuable resources who can offer guidance and perspective based on their own experiences within training.

17.5 Career/Specialty

17.5.1 General Surgery

The breadth and depth of general surgery remain key components of its appeal, as it not only provides a solid training foundation in the fundamentals of surgical management of disease and critical care, but also offers pathways into a multitude of subspecialties through additional fellowship training. Residency ensures that trainees have a well-grounded clinical knowledge base and technical skillset through interaction with a wide variety of patient populations and surgical procedures. Rotations on subspecialties within general surgery, such as trauma, surgical oncology, transplant, and pediatric surgery, can offer additional insight into career trajectories. Individual programs may be structured differently in terms of rotations and roles within each residency year, but the requirements and expectations set forth by the ABS for graduating residents helps level the playing field by confirming sufficient exposure to different case types and experiences.

17.5.2 Surgical Subspecialties

In addition to general surgery, residents can consider pursuing fellowship training in a surgical subspecialty to further refine technical skills and build expertise. Diverse career paths in academic medicine, private practice, research, and global health are all highly tenable tracks arising from general surgery residency or from a diverse array of subspecialties, which can include cardiothoracic surgery, transplant surgery, or surgical critical care, amongst others. Mentorship from senior surgeons, collaboration in research initiatives, and/or additional elective rotations can help trainees explore subspecialties or to springboard into more specialized areas of interest and find their niche as they progress into the early stages of their career.

17.6 Research/Electives

17.6.1 Internal Vs. External Opportunities

Though each program varies in structure, residency training may offer formal or informal opportunities for research experiences and elective rotations (research opportunities should be included as part of clinical training, even if additional segregated research time or professional development time is not desired by the trainee). Even if dedicated research or elective time is not built into the residency curriculum, residents should still seek to take advantage of clinical work-adjacent opportunities, such as participating in clinical trials, retrospective studies, or quality improvement projects (these are part of the "milestones", of note). External research support such as fellowships, societal or federal grants, or inter-institutional projects may also provide resources for residents to explore an array of clinical research or elective interests. Presentations at local, regional, or national conferences can further allow for networking with colleagues, knowledge sharing, and career advancement.

17.6.2 Beyond Basic Science

Cultivating a sense of intellectual curiosity along with a drive to continually improve patient care is pivotal in expanding our understanding of the impact of surgery through clinical, translational, and health services research. By addressing clinically relevant research questions, surgeons are able to improve patient safety and care outcomes in often immediately applicable ways and to advance the field in developing new surgical techniques, devices, care pathways, and/or healthcare delivery models. Multidisciplinary research teams which reflect clinical care structures can help to ameliorate biases, to address disparities in care, and to improve interprofessional communication. An increasing focus on surgical education research, curriculum development, and performance analysis also represents a growing discipline in which surgeons continue to change and enrich the training archetype.

17.7 Standardized Exams

17.7.1 ABSITE

The ABS In-Training Examination (ABSITE) is a low-stakes, standardized, multiple choice, online written exam administered annually to assess the knowledge and progress of general surgery residents [6]. Performance on the exam has clear implications on future qualifying Board exam performance (see "Board Exams" below) [7, 8]. Developing a study plan to prepare for the ABSITE, including review of core surgical textbooks, practice questions, and online resources should be a priority for residents each year. Study groups, review courses, and mock exams can also help gauge readiness and identify areas for improvement. Studying high-yield topics and surgical principles relevant to the ABSITE format and content in relation to daily patient care can solidify knowledge elements and understanding. While the exam is considered low-stakes, it can have fellowship or residency promotion implications, so each trainee should have an appreciation for the import of their ABSITE performance in the context of their program and their future.

17.7.2 Board Exams

The ABS qualifying exam (QE) and certifying exam (CE) are the final steps in becoming a Board-certified general surgeon after successfully completing residency training. The QE is a multiple-choice online written exam designed to test a candidate's fundamental medical knowledge in surgery and related topics, and passage of the QE is required to then sit for the oral CE (currently offered in a virtual format). ABSITE performance is a useful indicator of the likelihood of passing the QE as noted above, while mock oral exams have been found to correlate with performance on the CE [8]. Residents should begin preparing for the ABS exam early in residency by incorporating board review materials into a general study routine. Similar to ABSITE preparation, using resources such as review books, question banks, and online courses can help to review core surgical principles and clinical concepts. Board review courses and workshops may also be useful adjuncts to reinforce knowledge and practice test-taking strategies, especially for those who struggle with ABSITE and/or mock orals performance.

17.8 Life/Work Integration

Residency is an extraordinary experience in every surgeon's career, and trainees are tested to their full capacity in managing the physical and psychological demands of their jobs. Long hours and intense workloads weigh heavily on personal lives and well-being, and the recognition of means to reduce stressors and to optimize the working environment within surgical training continues to evolve. Duty-hour restrictions and the ongoing integration of competency assessments (e.g., EPAs) will provide additional clarity in the coming years in tailoring training duration and content for individual residents. Managing time and setting boundaries should be a high priority for every resident, and sustaining well-being by appreciating the importance of exercise, nutrition, sleep, and stress management is critical. Each individual resident should seek an equilibrium that allows them to maintain their passion for their work and to pursue their growth as surgeons yet find fulfillment in their relationships with others and lives outside of surgical training. Residency programs and institutional graduate medical education systems will offer a variety of resources to support resident well-being and work-life integration, so residents should query their program leadership about what is available to them and how they can best access these resources.

References

1. McCulloch P, et al. The effects of aviation-style non-technical skills training on technical performance and outcome in the operating theatre. BMJ Qual Safety. 2009;18(2):109–15.
2. L'Huillier JC, et al. Thriving as a surgical intern: three tips from the collaboration of surgical education fellows (CoSEF). Ann Surg Open. 2023;4(3):e306.
3. The Accreditation Council for Graduate Medical Education. Surgery Milestones. https://www.acgme.org/specialties/surgery/milestones/
4. The American Board of Surgery. Entrustable Professional Activities (EPAs). https://www.absurgery.org/get-certified/epas/
5. The American College of Surgeons. ACS Residents as Teachers and Leaders. https://www.facs.org/for-medical-professionals/education/programs/acs-residents-as-teachers-and-leaders/
6. The American Board of Surgery. In-Training Examinations. https://www.absurgery.org/get-certified/for-programs/in-training-exams/
7. The American Board of Surgery. Relationship Between ABSITE Scores and the Probability of Passing the QE. https://absurgerydata.shinyapps.io/relationqeabsite/
8. Nguyen J, et al. Predictive factors of first time pass rate on the American Board of Surgery certification in general surgery exams: a systematic review. J Surg Educ. 2021;78(5):1676–91.

Part IV
Building a Career in Academic Surgery

Chapter 18
Balancing Clinical, Research, and Teaching Responsibilities

Deanna L. Palenzuela Rothman and Roy Phitayakorn

Abstract There are several steps medical students can start to embark on an academic surgery career. Academic surgeons are traditionally involved in patient care, research, and teaching, and are often affiliated with universities. Aspiring academic surgeons should clarify their professional objectives, seek out mentorship, and gain research experience. Mentorship, a pivotal factor for academic success, should come from individuals who have a successful track record and can offer genuine guidance. Engaging in research helps develop practical skills and sets the stage for a competitive residency application. Joining surgical societies can offer insights into surgical advancements and networking opportunities. During residency, aligning clinical focus with research interests facilitates a synergistic approach to academic surgery, where clinical practice informs research, and vice versa. There is no single path to becoming an academic surgeon, but early preparation, mentorship, and a clear alignment of clinical and research interests are key strategies for success.

18.1 Introduction: What Is Academic Surgery?

Before we discuss building a career in academic surgery, we must first define what it means to be an academic surgeon. Traditionally, an academic surgeon is engaged in the three pillars of teaching hospitals and excelled at patient care, scientific research, and medical student/resident physician teaching endeavors [1–4]. To have access to each of those areas of expertise, academic surgeons are typically affiliated with a university-based medical school. In this way, academic surgery is distinguished from community-based or private practice programs, where the surgeon is privately employed and not affiliated with a hospital and/or university [5, 6]. In these other settings, while research and teaching are still a possibility, the primary role of the surgeon is clinical practice.

D. L. Palenzuela Rothman (✉) · R. Phitayakorn
Massachusetts General Hospital, Boston, MA, USA
e-mail: DPALENZUELA@mgh.harvard.edu; RPHITAYAKORN@mgh.harvard.edu

A. Gillis, C. B. Aarons (eds.), *A How To Guide For Medical Students*, Success in Academic Surgery, https://doi.org/10.1007/978-3-031-66011-5_18

At this point in your medical training, the best way to begin a path towards academic surgery is to define your professional vision and goals. Clearly defining your goals now can help you identify the best training pathway to meet these goals, define career development activities, and seek appropriate mentors to help you on your journey [7]. The aim of this chapter is to provide guidelines for academic activities in medical school, residency, and beyond to assist with shaping your personal vision and setting goals for a future in academic surgery.

18.2 Where to Begin as a Medical Student

There are several steps you can begin taking as a medical student to start defining your vision/goals and shaping your future career in academic surgery.

18.2.1 Seeking Mentors

Mentorship is critical in all stages of training and is often cited as the most important factor to academic success [2, 7–9]. Mentors can provide advocacy, role-modeling, sponsorship, teaching, and advice for students as they develop their academic interests [7, 10]. When identifying a mentor, there are several factors that should be considered [10]. The first factor is their professional and personal history. Ideal mentors should be successful within their respective fields to best serve as a role model for your own pathway. Additionally, mentors who are known to have fostered mentoring relationships in the past will likely have more experience guiding mentees. Next, a strong mentor should be generous with their time and expertise. They should be willing and able to meet with you and have honest, meaningful discussions with genuine interest in your success. Lastly, a mentor should be someone you trust, and can interact with on a personal level. The best mentors are those who you feel comfortable turning to and enjoy meeting with on a regular basis.

For medical students, mentorship can be found in many different forms. For example, a mentor can be a more senior medical student giving pointers on how to succeed in the surgery clerkship, a senior resident reviewing your residency application, or an attending surgeon providing insight into their personal path to academic surgery. Ideally, you should have a team of mentors with each mentor complimenting different areas of your future career interests. Often, medical schools will provide academic advisors that may also serve a mentorship role. However, the best surgical mentors will likely be found during your surgical clerkship and sub-internships. During your clinical rotations, identify resident physician and attending surgeon mentors that you believe fulfill your ideal mentor characteristics, and begin fostering those relationships.

18.2.2 Gaining Research Experience

Medical school is a great time to begin exploring different areas of research. As previously mentioned, participating in significant research endeavors is one of the hallmarks of an academic surgeon, and productivity is often defined by numbers of publications, citation metrics such as an h-index, and successful procurement of internal/external research funding [11].

You should consider exploring research as a medical student for several reasons. First, there are many different areas of research, and therefore by getting involved in research early, a student can begin identifying which areas best align with their interests. Some examples of different research areas and their definitions are included in Table 18.1. In addition, participating in research projects allows for the acquisition of many practical skills, including but not limited to project management, research design, Institutional Review Board applications, budget management, data collection, hands-on lab techniques, quantitative and/or qualitative analysis, oral presentations, and abstract/manuscript preparation and writing. All these skills will continue to be valuable throughout training and their future career in academic surgery. Lastly, meaningful participation in research projects will help a student stand out during the residency application process. Engaging in research activities suggests dedication to surgical investigation, acquisition of critical skills, and interest in an academic career, all of which will contribute to a competitive residency application.

There are several avenues through which you can identify potential research opportunities. Leveraging mentors' experiences is a great first place to start. Depending on the mentor, they may be involved in research themselves, or may be able to connect you with other colleagues engaged in research. In this way, the mentor can act as an advocate or sponsor for their mentee, integrating them in research activities. Another way is by reaching out to investigators directly. Often medical schools and affiliated hospitals have a research website, which lists principal investigators and their areas of active research. If you know an area of research you are interested in pursuing, exploring your institution's research website or using www.PubMed.gov could help you identify potential research mentors already working in those fields. Additionally, some institutions offer summer research internships, especially for students who are underrepresented in medicine (URiM), which are great opportunities to gain research experience while building relationships with investigators at different institutions.

18.2.3 Surgical Society Involvement

As you consider a career in academic surgery, you should also consider joining an academic surgical society. Surgical societies offer many benefits for medical students including insight into the most up-to-date advances in surgical research and

Table 18.1 List of research areas and their descriptions

Area of research	Description
Basic science	Basic science research is an investigation aimed at expanding scientific knowledge and understanding fundamental principles without any immediate practical application. It often involves lab-based experimentation, observation, and theoretical work to explore the underlying principles governing a particular phenomenon or system
Translational	Translational research refers to the process of applying findings from basic scientific research to develop practical applications that benefit human health or society. It bridges the gap between fundamental scientific discoveries (often made in laboratories) and their implementation in clinical or real-world settings
Clinical	Clinical research refers to scientific investigations conducted with human subjects to study health and disease in order to discover, evaluate, and validate new treatments, medications, procedures, or medical devices. It involves systematically gathering data and evidence through experiments or observations in clinical settings or through human volunteer participation
Education	Education research is a systematic inquiry into various aspects of the educational process, aiming to understand, improve, and enhance teaching, learning, educational policies, and systems. Education research often employs various methodologies, including quantitative and qualitative approaches, surveys, experiments, case studies, and longitudinal studies
Health policy	Health policy research involves the systematic investigation and analysis of various aspects of healthcare systems, policies, and interventions to understand their impact, effectiveness, and implications on public health outcomes. It aims to inform decision-makers, policymakers, healthcare providers, and stakeholders about the development, implementation, and evaluation of health policies
Quality improvement	Quality improvement research focuses on systematically studying and implementing strategies to enhance the quality, safety, efficiency, and effectiveness of healthcare delivery. It involves the continuous evaluation and refinement of processes, practices, and systems within healthcare settings to ensure optimal patient outcomes and satisfaction. Quality improvement research often draws upon methodologies such as Plan-Do-Study-Act (PDSA) cycles, six sigma, lean methodology, and other systematic approaches to drive improvements in healthcare delivery
Diversity, equity, and inclusion/disparities	Diversity, equity, and inclusion (DEI) research or disparities research focuses on investigating and understanding disparities, inequalities, and underrepresentation across various social, economic, and cultural dimensions within different contexts, including healthcare, education, employment, and society at large. The ultimate goal is to generate evidence-based insights and actionable recommendations to address inequalities, promote diversity, advance equity, and create more inclusive environments and societies
Innovation	Innovation research refers to the process of discovering, developing, and applying new ideas, technologies, treatments, or methodologies to improve health care. This area of research encompasses a wide range of activities, including: Drug discovery and development, medical devices and equipment, healthcare technology, and biomedical research

(continued)

Table 18.1 (continued)

Area of research	Description
Global surgery	Global surgery research is an interdisciplinary field focused on addressing disparities in surgical care worldwide, especially in low- and middle-income countries. It encompasses studying access to and quality of surgical services, workforce training, and capacity building. This research also involves analyzing the economic and policy aspects of surgical care, investigating surgical epidemiology, and innovating in surgical techniques for resource-limited settings. The ultimate aim is to ensure that safe, effective, and affordable surgical care is accessible to all, irrespective of geographic or economic barriers

Table 18.2 Academic Surgical Societies with Reduced Membership Fees for Medical Students

Society	2023 Student membership fee	Website
American College of Surgeons (ACS)	$20	https://www.facs.org/for-medical-professionals/membership-community/membership-benefits/medical-student-members/
Association for Academic Surgery (AAS)	$25	https://www.aasurg.org/apply-for-membership/
Association of Women Surgeons (AWS)	$25	https://www.womensurgeons.org/membership-categories
American Medical Association	$20	https://www.ama-assn.org/member-benefits/member-eligibility-dues/ama-membership-dues

education, networking opportunities through committees and conferences, and medical student specific curricula with curated resources. Many societies also offer greatly discounted membership to medical students, so there is no better time to begin getting involved. A list of some example academic societies with free or reduced membership fees for students are included in Table 18.2.

18.3 What to Look for During Residency

Residency is the time to nurture the academic surgery seeds that were planted as a medical student. During residency, you can continue to cultivate your academic growth while refining your clinical and research areas of interest.

18.3.1 Finding the Best Residency Fit

The first step is to identify the surgical residency program that will best fit your developing career goals. While other chapters in this book explore this process in more detail, there is an additional consideration worth mentioning at this point. As previously noted, academic surgeons are traditionally affiliated with academic institutions. Therefore, for a student seriously considering a career in academic surgery, we would recommend applying to surgical residency programs associated with a medical school and/or a university. However, academic opportunities are not exclusively found at academic institutions. Independent academic medical centers, which are sometimes labeled as community programs, can also provide opportunities for scholarship along with meaningful relationships with faculty mentors [5]. Overall, while the decision of where to apply for surgery residency is multifaceted, we would recommend exploring program websites ahead of time to confirm the programs offer opportunities aligned with your career goals and discussing these options with your mentorship team.

18.3.2 Identifying Potential Mentors in Your Field of Interest

In the previous section, we discussed how to identify a good mentor. While these guidelines still hold true in residency, the purpose of a mentor during residency training shifts towards focusing on specific clinical and research interests. To that end, mentors in this stage should be attendings currently practicing in your surgical field of interest, and/or who have experience in your research area of interest. The professional standing of the chosen mentor plays an important role at this point. A mentor who is well-respected by colleagues and recognized as an expert in their field through a record of publications, presentations, and/or grants can serve as an inspiration and role model for a mentee [10]. Additionally, an established mentor can help open doors for their mentee by facilitating networking and connecting them with related opportunities [10].

Finding a potential mentor as a resident can often happen organically when interacting with attendings during clinical rotations. Additionally, some residencies offer dedicated mentorship programs to connect you with attendings in the department that have similar clinical or research interests. Another potential avenue to identify a mentor is by leveraging the experiences of senior residents. Residents who have already matched into your field of interest can provide insight into strong mentors that successfully guided them on their own path.

18.3.3 Preparing for Academic Development Time

General surgery resident physicians at academic surgery programs often have the opportunity to take 1–2 years of academic development time within their surgical training, usually after the second or third clinical year. Overall, a third of all categorical general surgery residents in the United States decide to interrupt their training to pursue at least 1 ear of full-time research [12]. Residency programs that are academic, large, and affiliated with fellowship positions tend to have more research residents than other programs [13]. For resident physicians interested in an academic surgical career, the academic development years offer a great opportunity to focus on building their scholarly repertoire and research expertise. Notably, resident physicians who take advantage of this dedicated research time are more likely to be appointed as academic faculty, successfully obtain NIH funding, and have greater publications per year as attendings [14, 15], reaffirming the correlation between academic development time and future academic success.

Preparing for academic development time requires thorough self-reflection. The research years can help lay a foundation for a career in academic surgery, so it is important to ask yourself what that ideal career would look like. What clinical areas of surgery are you interested in? What kind of research have you enjoyed? Is there an experience you have had so far that you disliked? Where do you see yourself in 5–10 years after finishing residency or fellowship? Taking the time to reflect will help you delineate clear goals for success during your academic development years.

18.4 Aligning you Clinical Focus and Research Interests

In the introduction to this chapter, we discussed how an academic surgeon is the "triple threat," involved in clinical activities, research, and teaching. Although this balance may seem to be difficult to achieve, one strategy is to align your clinical focus and research interests. In doing so, your clinical work can inform your research development, and vice-versa. To illustrate this strategy, we have included a few "Academic Surgeon Phenotypes" as examples:

- A metabolic and bariatric surgeon interested in clinical outcomes research utilizes the Metabolic and Bariatric Surgery Accreditation and Quality Improvement Outcomes (MBSAQIP) database to investigate long term outcome differences between patients who underwent laparoscopic versus robotic sleeve gastrectomy.
- A transplant surgeon whose clinical focus is renal and pancreas transplantation is the principal investigator for a basic science lab focused on trialing pancreatic islet cell transplantation in mice.
- An acute care and trauma surgeon at a busy academic center in the central city is involved in health care policy research investigating gun violence among minors.

In each of the above examples, the surgeon's clinical and research interests build on and augment each other. In this way, rather than having separate academic silos, the surgeons' interests are aligned and interwoven thus demanding less cognitive task switching and dedicated time. Regardless, it is important to note that there is no single way to be an academic surgeon. Each surgeon is unique and therefore develops their own way to balance their academic endeavors. We recommend taking note of the many different career paths and trajectories of the academic surgeons you encounter to help inform your own future goals.

18.5 Conclusion

The essence of pursuing a career in academic surgery revolves around excelling in clinical practice, research, and teaching within a university-affiliated setting. Defining your goals early in your medical training sets the course for achieving these objectives. While there is no one singular pathway to becoming an academic surgeon, taking steps to prepare early in training, seeking academic opportunities, and learning from diverse career trajectories can aid in shaping your own goals for a fulfilling career in academic surgery.

References

1. Staveley-O'Carroll K, et al. Developing the young academic surgeon. J Surg Res. 2004;118(2):109–13.
2. Rosengart TK, et al. The seven attributes of the academic surgeon: critical aspects of the archetype and contributions to the surgical community. Am J Surg. 2017;214(2):165–79.
3. Soybel DI. The education of an academic surgeon. J Surg Res. 2001;97(1):1–8.
4. Balch CM. The academic surgeon as a clinical investigator. J Surg Res. 1986;40(5):413–20.
5. Jones J, Sidwell RA. Residency surgical training at an independent academic medical center. Surg Clin. 2016;96(1):147–53.
6. Goudreau BJ, et al. Academic or community practice? What is driving decision-making and career choices. Surgery. 2018;164(3):571–6.
7. Lin LO, et al. A primer for success as an early career academic plastic surgeon. Plast Reconstr Surg Glob Open. 2022;10(1):e3947.
8. Lee TC, et al. The road to academic surgical leadership: characteristics and experiences of surgical chairpersons. Surgery. 2020;168(4):707–13.
9. Cochran A, et al. Barriers to advancement in academic surgery: views of senior residents and early career faculty. Am J Surg. 2013;206(5):661–6.
10. Scogg Scoggins CR, Pollock RE, Pawlik TM. Surgical mentorship and leadership. Building for Success in Academic Surgery. 2018:2018.
11. Valsangkar NP, et al. Determining the drivers of academic success in surgery: an analysis of 3,850 faculty. PLoS One. 2015;10(7):e0131678.
12. Robertson CM, Klingensmith ME, Coopersmith CM. Prevalence and cost of full-time research fellowships during general surgery residency–a national survey. Ann Surg. 2009;249(1):155–61.
13. Sue GR, et al. The vulnerable stage of dedicated research years of general surgery residency: results of a national survey. Arch Surg. 2011;146(6):653–8.

14. Andriole DA, Klingensmith ME, Fields RC, Jeffe DB. Is dedicated research time during surgery residency associated with surgeons' future career paths? A national study. Ann Surg. 2020;271:590–7.
15. Hsieh H, et al. Formal research training during surgical residency: scaffolding for academic success. Am J Surg. 2014;207(1):141–5.

Chapter 19
Understanding the Intersection of Social Media and Mentorship in Surgery and Medicine

Alison S. Baskin and Julie Ann Sosa

Abstract Mentorship is a key component of success in surgery that benefits both mentors and mentees. It is associated with increased academic productivity, funding, leadership roles, and career advancement. For students and trainees, early mentorship may play a role in specialty or career selection, scholarly output, and residency or fellowship match. Until recently, mentor-mentee dyads have connected through traditional communication channels; however, in an increasingly virtual world, academic communities are adopting new ways to communicate, including over social media platforms. Given its ability to transcend constraints of geography, hierarchy, and time, social media can be used as a communication tool to establish and improve mentoring relationships. Specifically, social media can be used to strengthen preexisting mentoring relationships, identify new mentorship opportunities both locally and remotely, and facilitate modern mentorship models, such as team mentorship and near-peer mentorship. Furthermore, it increases the durability of mentor-mentee relationships and helps to expand and diversify mentorship networks, which may especially benefit female and underrepresented in medicine students and trainees. Despite the many advantages of social media, it is not a replacement for traditional local mentorship and must always be used in an intentional and professional manner. In this chapter, not only do we discuss the benefits of using social media for mentorship, but we also explore some of the challenges of balancing virtual and local mentorship, recognize potential concerns raised by social media use, and provide suggestions on how to leverage social media to optimize your virtual mentorship experience.

A. S. Baskin · J. A. Sosa (✉)
Department of Surgery, University of California, San Francisco, CA, USA
e-mail: alison.baskin@ucsf.edu; julie.sosa@ucsf.edu

A. Gillis, C. B. Aarons (eds.), *A How To Guide For Medical Students*, Success in Academic Surgery, https://doi.org/10.1007/978-3-031-66011-5_19

19.1 Introduction

Mentorship is a key component of success in many professional fields, and surgery is no exception. In a mutually beneficial relationship, mentors pass along knowledge, strategy, and acquired experiences to mentees, ensuring their ongoing achievement and fulfillment [1, 2]. Mentorship influences the arc of professional development across the career continuum, which for some individuals begins as early as grade school. Effective mentorship is associated with increased academic productivity, successful funding, leadership roles, job retention, and advancement of both mentors' and mentees' careers [3, 4]. For students and trainees, early mentorship may play a role in specialty or career selection, scholarly output, and residency or fellowship match [3]. Due to the positive impact mentorship can have, it is never too early for medical students and surgical trainees to seek out mentors within their fields of interest.

Until recently, mentors and mentees have connected through traditional communication channels; however, in a world more virtual than ever before, we have adapted the ways in which we communicate. Integration of social media into the professional environment is a prime example of how communication within the academic workplace has evolved. In a study assessing 650 physicians' use of social media across different surgical and medical specialties, 71% had at least one social media profile [5]. Surgeons, in comparison to medicine physicians, had greater social media activity and more followers [5]. In a short period, academic communities have embraced social media as an emerging communication tool, appreciating its ability to transcend constraints of geographic location, hierarchy, and time [6–8]. We have seen an association between social media and successful patient and public health advocacy efforts, galvanizing movements and campaigns, increased networking opportunities, and the promotion of professional pursuits; yet, we have also realized that social media can increase stress in the workplace [9]. Despite potential concerns of increased use of social media, particularly in professional settings, it has successfully extended and enhanced mentorship opportunities for students and trainees within specialties in medicine and surgery.

Recognizing how communication has evolved in today's virtual world, this chapter explores the intersection of surgical mentorship and social media, including how virtual platforms can enhance and transform traditional mentorship models (Fig. 19.1). We highlight how social media can promote existing mentorships, help students and trainees identify new mentorships, expand and diversify professional and mentorship networks, and provide opportunities for near-peer mentoring [10]. We discuss some of the challenges of balancing virtual and local mentorship, recognize potential concerns raised by social media use, and provide suggestions on how to leverage these platforms to optimize your virtual mentorship experience.

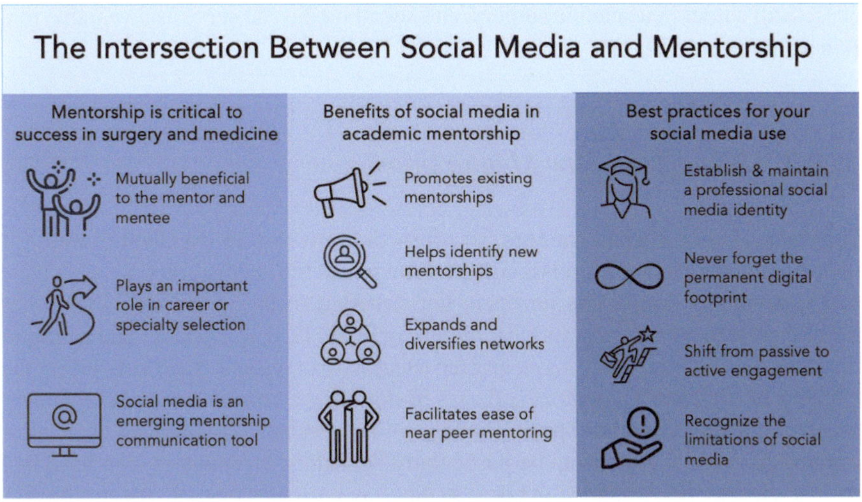

Fig. 19.1 Understanding the intersection between social media and mentorship in surgery and medicine

19.2 Leveraging Social Media for Mentorship

19.2.1 Promoting Existing Mentorships

If you are a current social media user, you already may have noticed how virtual platforms are used to promote existing mentorships. In a few words and a single click, a mentor can amplify the work of a mentee, celebrate their accomplishments, and make introductions to potential colleagues or collaborators [1, 4]. Mentees often reciprocate with words of appreciation for their mentor. Through this mutually beneficial exchange, a mentee's work is disseminated, and their visibility in the academic community increased. At the same time, their success serves as a positive reflection of their mentor [1].

Freed from constraints of geographic location and time, social media enhances existing relationships by facilitating flexible and real-time communication. Nearly a quarter of medical faculty report using social media daily, meaning that for many, social media is already a part of their regular communication practices [11]. Mentor-mentee dyads may find it appealing to utilize social media for content sharing or simple communication touchpoints: for example, sharing an article or scholarship opportunity, or quickly checking-in. Social media can serve as a platform to track a mentee's performance—specifically, if a mentee posts about project updates or shares individual or group achievements. As students and residents advance through their training and careers, social media also can help sustain valuable mentor-mentee relationships from prior career stages through virtual mentorship by allowing both parties to keep each other abreast of new and ongoing professional pursuits. As many successful professionals emphasize, maintaining relationships is key to a successful career in academic surgery, and social media can serve as a valuable tool to help do so.

19.2.2 *Identifying New Mentorships*

For medical students and trainees, social media provides an excellent avenue for identifying new mentoring relationships. It increases the accessibility mentees have to mentorship by imparting an open, flat structure to the traditional, sometimes intimidating, academic and surgical hierarchy [1, 6, 12, 13]. Mentees struggling to find local mentorship may have greater success over virtual platforms given the larger pool of potential mentors and ease of initiating contact via social media avenues. Some mentors may speak publicly about personal experiences from their training or careers, which can be particularly appealing for mentees who have had similar experiences. Mentorship borne in this way promotes mutual vulnerability, as mentees may be more likely to divulge challenges they face, and mentors may have particularly insightful perspectives and offer more targeted advice informed by a shared experience. This may be especially valuable for female and underrepresented in medicine (URiM) students and trainees facing undue challenges in surgical career development and in surgical subspecialties with limited diversity. A recent study evaluating social media's role in cardiothoracic surgery mentorship found that social media not only increased female surgeons' access to female mentors, but when compared to other surgical subspecialties, female cardiothoracic surgeons were more likely to report building a larger network of same-gender mentorship pairings with the help of social media [7].

Through targeted social media groups, affinity group communities, or specific hashtags, you may more effectively identify mentors with similar niche interests or who practice in medical or surgical subspecialty fields that are unfortunately plagued with ongoing gender or racial bias. Social media may improve the durability of mentorships by transforming brief in-person exchanges, such as those at academic meetings or during residency, fellowship, or job interviews, into longer-term relationships [12].

19.2.3 *Expanding and Diversifying Networks*

As more surgeons embrace social media for professional use, mentorship networks expand and diversify. Telementoring promotes equitable access to high-quality mentorship because mentees are not limited by a potential scarcity of local mentors and can connect with mentors located remotely [7]. In recognizing mentorship as a critical component to mitigating gender and racial disparities in surgery, social media, too, becomes a valuable tool for increased equity in the field [2]. URiM mentees who are disproportionately impacted by a lack of available mentorship at their home institutions are likely to benefit most [14]. Virtual mentorship is cost-effective and promotes work-place efficiency by saving the money and time frequently required for in-person meetings, which can increase the feasibility of mentorship for both you and your mentor.

In many ways, we have adapted our communication within academic surgery to suit today's virtual world. Mentorship, too, has evolved to include more than just the traditional mentor-mentee relationship. Given the ease of networking on social media, team-based mentorship, which is becoming increasingly desirable, may be more easily attained [1]. Further, social media allows individuals to both give and receive mentorship through indirect relationships. On social media platforms, mentors can disseminate career or training advice to broad audiences (see, for example, Tweetorials and the Association of Women Surgeons' #DearIntern initiative) [15]. Meanwhile, mentees may solicit advice from open social media forums or affinity group communities where they can receive input from a large audience of peer and senior mentors. While this type of mentorship does not, and should not, replace traditional mentor-mentee relationships, it augments the mentorship experience by enabling you to gain additional perspectives and a greater sense of community engagement and support.

19.2.4 Fostering near Peer Mentoring

As you advance in your medical education and residency training, you will discover new opportunities to not only be a mentee, but also to serve as a mentor to others. Surgery's hierarchical structure means that at nearly all stages of your training and early career, you will have built-in opportunities to mentor fellow students and trainees. Near-peer mentorship is an excellent way for senior students and junior residents to build and practice mentorship skills at an early stage in their careers. It cultivates rising leaders who can recognize their own potential and ongoing transformation into competent and capable physicians, while affording mentees the perspective of someone who recently navigated a similar stage of their training or career [16, 17].

For students and trainees, virtual platforms make peer mentoring convenient and easily accessible, especially for individuals already using social media. Due to the COVID-19 pandemic, which significantly altered the residency application and match process, residency and fellowship interviews have become primarily virtual [18]. Although this shift has resulted in improved efficiency, reduced financial costs, and greater equity, it has limited the connections applicants across institutions form with one another. In times past, applicants on the interview trail would meet at social gatherings and interview days, oftentimes on more than one occasion. This provided an opportunity for medical students across institutions to build relationships with one another, even if they ultimately ended up at different residency institutions. Social media has helped bridge this gap and allowed applicants to get to know each other beyond the brief interactions that occur during a virtual interview day. Over social media channels, students and trainees from different institutions and geographic regions can share resources, exchange stories and advice drawn from their personal experiences, and answer each other's questions.

19.3 Optimizing Social Media for Mentorship

Currently, the most popular social media platforms used for surgical mentorship are X (formerly Twitter) and Facebook; others include Instagram and LinkedIn [7]. Our observations and experiences suggest there is a learning curve to using social media in the academic setting across these platforms and, especially, to learning how to balance virtual and in-person interactions. Best practices of social media in mentorship ensure that it (1) enhances, and does not hurt, preexisting mentorship models across all platforms, and (2) enables you to present your best self. If you are wondering how you can best leverage social media to optimize your virtual mentorship experience, you are not alone. Here, we aim to provide some fundamental principles to guide your professional social media use, recognizing that as social media use evolves, these principles may too (Fig. 19.2).

19.3.1 Establishing Social Media Identity

Whether you already have a social media profile, or are considering creating one, it is important to ensure it presents a positive image of who you are. Your handle and/or username should accurately reflect your personal identity and be professional, aligning with the values and ethics of the medical profession [19, 20]. When writing a descriptive bio for your social media profile, in addition to sharing basic information about yourself (e.g., year of medical school or training, academic or research institution), consider including information on your clinical or research interests or professional highlights. Also be sure to share your participation in conferences, workshops, and medical projects [20]. This can help you identify mutual interests with potential mentors or peers, which may lead to future mentoring relationships or collaborations. While we encourage you to generate a profile representing your authentic self, exploring the profiles of others in the surgical or medical fields can offer inspiration on how to best present yourself. If you are new to using social media for professional networking, it is okay, and even encouraged, to observe how individuals interact over the platform before you engage in greater depth, especially given that different social media platforms cater to different users and serve varying functions [19, 21].

Some individuals will create more than one account on a single social media platform, distinguishing between personal and professional accounts. The American Medical Association recommends considering separating personal and professional content online to maintain appropriate professional boundaries [22]. While this will

Topic	Social Media Best Practices
Establishing a Social Media Identity	▪ Choose a handle or username reflecting your personal identity in a professional manner ▪ Provide a descriptive bio including information about yourself, your clinical or research interests, and professional highlights ▪ Explore the profiles of others in the surgical or medical fields for inspiration on how to use social media as a health care professional
Consideration of Separate Accounts	▪ Consider creating separate personal and professional accounts to maintain boundaries and curate your content ▪ Ensure all content posted to personal accounts is information you would be willing to share publicly
The Permanent Digital Footprint	▪ Maintain awareness of the policies set by your affiliated institutions ▪ Include a disclaimer that the views and opinions posted on your social media account represent your own ▪ Operate under the assumption that posted content will be available to anyone and at anytime
Shifting from passive to active engagement	▪ Follow professional societies and join affinity group communities unique to your personal interests ▪ Participate in live discussion events ▪ Connect online with potential colleagues and mentors you meet at social and professional events to broaden your network
Defining goals and determining needs	▪ Develop a clear vision of your goals and desired achievements ▪ Determine what you hope to gain from a mentor ▪ Reflect on your role and responsibilities as the mentee in a mentoring relationship
Seeking New Mentorship Online	▪ Initiate contact with a potential mentor by showing interest in their work and/or participating in their sponsored live events or webinars ▪ Explore whether a local mentor or colleague knows the potential mentor and is willing to facilitate an introduction ▪ Introduce yourself authentically and include who you are, what you do, and why you want to connect ▪ Respect others' time and bandwidth for providing mentorship
Balancing virtual and in-person mentorship	▪ Aim to discuss confidential or sensitive matters during face-to-face interactions (whether in-person or video conference) ▪ Recognize virtual mentorship is not a replacement for in-person mentorship and should instead be used as an adjunct ▪ Respect your own feelings towards social media and whether you have the capacity for online social engagement

Fig. 19.2 Recommended best practices for professional social media use in mentorship

allow you to curate the content you feature on one account, we recommend exercising great caution in doing so, as there can be an illusion of privacy associated with personal accounts. All content you post online, whether on a personal or a professional account, should be information you would be willing to share publicly. On professional accounts, some encourage sharing personal details about yourself (e.g., hobbies, family, nonwork-related activities) to demonstrate your multifaceted nature [19]. The goal is to selectively share personal experiences and genuinely connect with others over social media, while maintaining a professional demeanor; however, you should never feel obligated to provide personal information you would like to keep private [20].

19.3.2 Social Media's Permanent Footprint

As medical students and soon-to-be physicians, not only do you represent yourself, but you also represent the medical profession [23]. Although social media may provide a contemporary approach to mentorship, be sure to extend traditional standards of professionalism to your interactions with potential and current mentors. Like all forms of digital communication, what you post on social media is permanent and cannot be erased. Given your role as a training medical professional, your online presence is held to a different set of standards. Always maintain an awareness of the policies set by your affiliated institutions and provide a disclaimer explicitly stating that your expressed views are your own and do not necessarily reflect the views of your affiliations [24]. Most educational and medical institutions have social media policies describing best practices and outlining boundaries related to professionalism. One review article published in *Journal of the American College of Surgeons* outlined best practices for surgeons' social media activities based on seven sets of guidelines developed by medical and surgical organizations [13]. Key recommendations included being aware of social media policies set by employers and practices, operating under the assumption that posted content will be available to anyone in perpetuity, and actively maintaining a professional online presence.

19.3.3 Shifting from Passive to Active Engagement

After creating a social media account, the next step to leveraging social media for your mentorship experience is to move from a state of passive to active engagement. To get started, we recommend following professional societies and joining affinity group communities unique to your interests. Search for hashtags relevant to your clinical and research interests and identify high volume contributors to tailor your online experience. Participate in live discussion events, often advertised on society or organization accounts, to learn, network, and explore new ideas or topics [25, 26]. When included in these virtual groups, you are more likely to hear about organized virtual and in-person events for networking; for example, the Society for Vascular Surgery's Mentor Match connects vascular surgeons at all career stages via the online community, SVS*Connect* [27, 28].

When soliciting new mentorship over social media, like communicating through traditional channels, it is important to be respectful, intentional, and engaged. The first step in seeking mentorship is to develop a clear vision of your goals and desired achievements [1, 29]. It will be difficult for any mentor to help you achieve your goals if you do not know what they are yourself. If you have then identified a potential mentor on social media who you think would be well-positioned to provide guidance, initiate contact by engaging with their online presence [29]. This can manifest in many ways, such as showing interest in their work and/or participating in live events or webinars where they are contributors. Once you have established an initial touchpoint, we recommend introducing yourself through a direct message over social media or via email (if their address is publicly available) or by asking a colleague or faculty member at your local institution whether they know the individual and are willing to facilitate an introduction. Provide a brief introduction of who you are, what you do, and why you want to connect with them [29]. Specifically, describe how their work or professional experiences are relevant to your interests or have inspired you. Ask if they would be willing to briefly chat with you. If the potential mentor agrees to talk with you, be sure to follow up and thank them for their time. When chatting, be specific about your goals and expectations [24]. What specific guidance are you seeking? Are you interested in a specialized topic in which they possess expertise? Are you encountering obstacles in your professional endeavors that you think they may be able to assist you with? Always be mindful of their schedule and availability when arranging times to meet. Lastly, recognize not all potential mentors have the bandwidth to provide mentorship, which requires a lot of time and energy. Others may feel they are not well suited to meet your needs. Respect when someone tells you their limitations. Regardless of the outcome, be gracious and appreciative, and know there are a plethora of other opportunities for connection.

19.4 Recognizing the Limitations of Social Media

Although there are many benefits to social media, it is not a replacement for in-person mentorship. To optimize the mentorship experience over social media, we must ensure communication is confidential and secure when necessary. Hybrid mentorship formats, featuring both virtual and in-person components (when feasible), may offer the improved accessibility and efficiency of the virtual experience while also providing opportunities for face-to-face interactions to discuss sensitive or confidential matters. Platforms supporting secure communication between mentor-mentee dyads, widespread dissemination of information and advice, and easy networking are likely to be the most conducive to positive mentorship experiences. We also must recognize that social media can contribute to the potential strains that medical students, trainees, and professionals already experience. Specifically, building a strong social media presence can be demanding, potentially creating yet another task among the long list of responsibilities mentors and mentees bear [30]. Additionally, there are concerns that social media can pose a threat to trainee wellbeing when others' successes (e.g., awards won and research grants received) are shared across these virtual platforms [31]. It may contribute to feelings of inadequacy or competition. Ultimately, the decision to use social media is a personal one, and only you can decide whether it is right for you.

19.5 Conclusion

In today's virtual world, the role of social media in mentorship is evolving. Social media helps strengthen preexisting mentoring relationships, identify new ones, and facilitates modern mentorship models; however, it does not fully replace traditional local mentorship. To optimize the mentorship experience, it is the role of the profession to bring intentionality and creativity to the forefront of the virtual mentorship landscape so that we can learn how to better support medical students and trainees throughout their journey in the medical field. At the same time, students and trainees ought to be flexible, adaptive, and professional when turning to social media for mentorship. As you progress through successive training and career stages, new mentorship needs will arise, and you will find that stage-specific approaches to acquiring the appropriate mentorship will be required—adapt your use of social media accordingly [16]. As you embark on your own professional journey, know that social media can be a valuable tool to help launch preliminary mentoring relationships, even if it does not serve as your final destination, and ultimately the decision to use social media is a personal one. We are hopeful that as both mentors and mentees become more adept at using social media, virtual communication platforms will continue to lessen the demands of quality mentorship, increase the bandwidth of both parties for dedicated participation, and foster meaningful connections to ensure mutual fulfillment.

*This chapter was adapted from the authors' previously published manuscript: Leveraging social media for mentorship in surgery, available in Surgery (*https://doi.org/10.1016/j.surg.2023.04.056*).*

References

1. Chopra V, Vaughn V, Saint S. The mentorship guide: helping mentors and mentees succeed. Michigan Publisher; 2019.
2. Edwards JA. Mentorship of underrepresented minorities and women in surgery. Am J Surg. 2021;221(4):768–9.
3. Raborn LN, Janis JE. Overcoming the impact of COVID-19 on surgical mentorship: a scoping review of long-distance mentorship in surgery. J Surg Educ. 2021;78(6):1948–64.
4. Chung DH. Society of university surgeons mentorship: fostering personal relationships. Surgery. 2012;152(3):304–8.
5. Hameed I, Oakley CT, Ahmed A, Naeem N, Robinson NB, Hameed NUF, et al. Analysis of physician use of social media. JAMA Netw Open. 2021;4(7):e2118213.
6. Corsini EM, Boeck M, Hughes KA, Logghe HJ, Pitt SC, Stamp N, et al. Global impact of social media on women in surgery. Am Surg. 2020;86(2):152–7.
7. Luc JGY, Stamp NL, Antonoff MB. Social media as a means of networking and mentorship: role for women in cardiothoracic surgery. Semin Thorac Cardiovasc Surg. 2018;30(4):487–95.
8. Antonoff MB. Using social media effectively in a surgical practice. J Thorac Cardiovasc Surg. 2016;151(2):322–6.
9. Onyango JM, Bowe SN. Seeing is believing: how social media is challenging physician stereotypes. J Grad Med Educ. 2019;11(5):495–7.

10. Baskin A, Sosa JA. Leveraging social media for mentorship in surgery. Surgery. 2023;174(2):395–7.
11. Pearson D, Bond M, Kegg J, Pillow T, Hopson L, Cooney R, et al. Evaluation of social media use by emergency medicine residents and faculty. West J Emerg Med. 2015;16(5):715–20.
12. McLuckey MN, Gold JA, O'Glasser AY, Hingle S, Spencer A, Fick LB. Harnessing the power of medical twitter for mentorship. J Grad Med Educ. 2020;12(5):535–8.
13. Logghe HJ, Boeck MA, Gusani NJ, Hardaway JC, Hughes KA, Mouawad NJ, et al. Best practices for surgeons' social media use: statement of the resident and associate society of the American college of surgeons. J Am Coll Surg. 2018;226(3):317–27.
14. Roberts SE, Shea JA, Sellers M, Butler PD, Kelz RR. Pursing a career in academic surgery among African American medical students. Am J Surg. 2020;219(4):598–603.
15. Markham MJ, Gentile D, Graham DL. Social media for networking, professional development, and patient engagement. Am Soc Clin Oncol Educ Book. 2017;37:782–7.
16. Ahmadmehrabi S, Farlow JL, Wamkpah NS, Esianor BI, Brenner MJ, Valdez TA, et al. New age mentoring and disruptive innovation—navigating the uncharted with vision, purpose, and equity. JAMA Otolaryngol Neck Surg. 2021;147(4):389–94.
17. Ramin SK, Suresh A. Paying it forward: near peer mentorship in medical school makes an impact. Acad Med J Assoc Am Med Coll. 2024;99(6):e31.
18. Gupta S, Grier Arthur L, Chandler N, Danielson P, Downard C, Ehrlich P, et al. Is the changing landscape of fellowship recruitment during COVID-19 here to stay? J Pediatr Surg. 2022;57(10):445–50.
19. Ponce SB, Barry MM, Dizon DS, Katz MS, Murphy M, Teplinsky E, et al. Netiquette for social media engagement for oncology professionals. Future Oncol. 2022;18(9):1133–41.
20. Prasad N. Staying professional on social media as a medical student [internet]. 2023. https://blog.blueprintprep.com/medical/staying-professional-on-social-media-as-a-medical-student/
21. Gifford ED, Mouawad NJ, Bowser KE, Bush RL, Chandra V, Coleman DM, et al. Society for Vascular Surgery best practice recommendations for use of social media. J Vasc Surg. 2021;74(6):1783–1791.e1.
22. American Medical Association. Professionalism in the use of social media [Internet]. https://code-medical-ethics.ama-assn.org/ethics-opinions/professionalism-use-social-media
23. Social Media Best Practices for Healthcare Students [Internet]. 2022. https://www.joyce.edu/blog/social-media-best-practices-for-healthcare-students/
24. Keating J. Social media guidelines for medical students and physicians [internet]. 2016. https://www.amsa.org/social-media-guidelines-medical-students-physicians-2/
25. Luc JGY, Varghese TK, Antonoff MB. Participating in a TweetChat: practical tips from the thoracic surgery social media network (#TSSMN). Ann Thorac Surg. 2019;107(3):e229–33.
26. Retrouvey M, Keefe B, Kotsenas A, McGinty G, Patel AK. Women in radiology: creating a global mentorship network through social media. J Am Coll Radiol. 2018;15(1):229–32.
27. Society for Vascular Surgery. Mentor Match [Internet]. https://vascular.org/trainees-students/mentoring-groups/mentor-match
28. Society for Vascular Surgery. SVS Connect [Internet]. https://svsconnect.vascular.org/home
29. LinkedIn. How can you find a mentor using social media? [Internet]. 2023. https://www.linkedin.com/advice/1/how-can-you-find-mentor-using-social-media-qzxwf?trk=organization_guest_main-feed-card_feed-article-content
30. Han B. Social media burnout: definition, measurement instrument, and why we care. J Comput Inf Syst. 2018;58(2):122–30.
31. Rosenbaum L. Being well while doing well—distinguishing necessary from unnecessary discomfort in training. Malina D, editor. N Engl J Med. 2024;390(6):568–72.

Part V
Work-Life Integration as an Academic Surgeon

Chapter 20
Fostering Productive Mentor-Mentee Relationships

Julia L. Beilis and James A. Lee

Abstract Medical school is one of the most transformative periods in a doctor's life as they transition from learner to professional, explore the myriad of available opportunities (research, clinical practice, administration, innovation, etc.), and plot the shape of their future career. Creating effective mentorship relationships is critical to navigating this dynamic phase of life and setting up future success. This chapter will discuss the essential elements of fruitful mentor-mentee relationships from choosing the right mentor to structuring and cultivating the relationship.

20.1 Introduction

Medical school is one of the most transformative periods in a doctor's life as they transition from student to professional, explore available opportunities (research, clinical practice, administration, innovation, etc.), and plot the trajectory of their future career. Fruitful mentor-mentee relationships are an essential aspect of your growth as a physician. The best relationships extend beyond mere academic guidance and clinical expertise; rather, they propel your professional development, provide emotional support, and cultivate a sense of community within the medical field. Maintaining a productive bond is an active process that should be driven by the mentee. This chapter will discuss how to choose, structure, and cultivate successful mentor relationships.

J. L. Beilis
Cleveland Clinic Cole Eye Institute, Cleveland, OH, USA

J. A. Lee (✉)
Department of Surgery, Columbia University Medical Center, New York City, NY, USA
e-mail: jal74@cumc.columbia.edu

A. Gillis, C. B. Aarons (eds.), *A How To Guide For Medical Students*, Success in Academic Surgery, https://doi.org/10.1007/978-3-031-66011-5_20

20.2 Choosing the Right Mentor(s)

It is critical to understand that rather than just one mentor, you will need a team of mentors, each of whom offer specialized knowledge bases and varying experiences. For example, you may have a mentor in your clinical area of interest, a senior medical student who can help you understand the nuances of the curriculum, and a research mentor. If you are a member of an underrepresented minority group, consider finding a mentor who shares your background and has navigated the challenges you are likely to face. While mentors are often thought of as more senior faculty members, the most effective relationships can occur with people at several different levels and tracks. It is far more important that the mentor's experiences match your specific needs rather than just seeking out the most prominent person in the field. It is also essential to recognize the difference between mentors and sponsors or advocates. *Mentors* share their knowledge and provide guidance while sponsors use their social and institutional connections to provide opportunities. *Sponsors* open doors to opportunities, while the mentor enables you to to make the most of those chances. While these roles can intersect and diverge at various times throughout the relationship, it is critical to understand the differences and how to interact with them effectively. Additionally, expect the composition of your team to change as your needs change over time. In recognition of this natural evolution, Kram et al. codified the stages of individual mentor relationships as initiation, cultivation, separation, and redefinition where it is assumed that the mentor-mentee relationship may ultimately end or at the very least change significantly [1].

The most important step in choosing a mentor team is a thorough needs assessment in which you identify your personal and professional aspirations ranging from long-term career goals to more practical day-to-day questions. Instead of relying on your mentor to do the work of figuring out how to help you, consider what type of guidance you need and in what areas—do you need practical advice, psychosocial support, career advice, etc.? An honest and thorough appraisal of your needs will help you select appropriate mentors. In addition to how well the mentors align with your needs, also consider whether they would be an engaged and interested participant. Ask yourself if they have other successful mentor-mentee relationships, or are their schedules too dense to have these sorts of relationships. When you are ready to ask someone to be your mentor, determine if you have contacts who would be willing to broker an introduction, attend their office hours, or send a concise message requesting a brief meeting to discuss the possibility. No matter how you make the initial approach, enter the meeting with a clear "ask" and plan for how to structure the relationship.

20.3 Structuring the Relationship

When embarking on a mentor-mentee relationship, it is important to set expectations up-front and communicate clearly. Your job as the mentee is to make the relationship as frictionless as possible. You should:

- **Define mutually agreeable goals for the relationship**:
- It is important to not assume that you are both automatically aligned on objectives. Detail the areas in which you would like their guidance. Defining your goals will allow your mentor to better tailor their advice to you. For example, if you need help navigating how to become active in a research lab, be specific so they do not think you are looking for advice on how to be successful in the residency match. As the relationship progresses, these areas will naturally evolve, and setting clear goals helps the mentor frame their thinking. At the same time, this relationship should be mutually beneficial. Ask your mentor what they hope to gain from the relationship. Are they doing it to "give back," do they need help with their work, etc.
- **Define the logistics**:
- Set up a consistent schedule for meetings. One of the keys to a successful relationship is developing trust and "learning to authentically engage with one another" [2]. This level of comfort only comes with familiarity, which can be facilitated by the structure of regular interactions. Ask your mentor how often they think you should meet and in what format (in-person, phone, video, etc). Ask if it is ok to contact them for advice between meetings, but stress that you will only do so if there is something important and/or time-sensitive. Also ask if it is fine if you send them updates on projects or progress on advice they have given. If they agree, ask how they prefer to be contacted.

20.4 Cultivating the Relationship

- **Ease into the relationship** and get to know one another. As with any relationship, the mentor-mentee bond requires time to fully develop and mature. Start by asking for guidance on items that do not require a lot of work or time to prepare on their part. As you get to know one another, you can ask for more involved or time-intensive help, such as: reviewing your CV, reading over personal statements, etc. Get to know each other personally as well as professionally. Do not be afraid to share your more vulnerable side as it can lead to moments of constructive feedback and deepen your relationship. Furthermore, let your mentor know of any unique challenges, such as if you are part of an underrepresented minority in medicine. These discussions may lead to self-growth on both sides.

- **Respect their time**
  - Show up to all meetings on time.
  - Respond to your mentor's outreach quickly and thoughtfully.
  - Complete agreed upon tasks in a timely fashion.
  - Prepare and send an agenda in advance of each meeting. Think about the specifics of what you want to cover—advice on a situation, support if you are struggling, or sponsorship for a position. On your own, explore the nuances of your questions and research your own solutions. Practice how you will present the issues. After the meeting, send a summary email of what you discussed and action items for you to accomplish.
  - If you do ask for guidance between scheduled meetings, make the "ask" as easy to address as possible. Ideally, formulate it as a yes/no question, so that your mentor can expand on as they see fit. If it is a more involved issue, ask if you can meet to discuss with a rough estimate of how long you think the conversation will take.
- **Be proactive**
  - Act on advice from your mentor in a timely fashion. Few things will sour the relationship more than if the mentor feels like you are not invested in it.
  - Explore the next logical step(s) of your mentor's advice through your own research and initiative. Look for ways to apply lessons learned to other areas of your life.
  - If they are amenable to communicating between scheduled meetings, provide brief interim updates that demonstrate how you are following through and have applied the advice they have given.
- **Cultivate a growth-mindset**
  - Ask for specific feedback and receive it non-defensively. Listen to your mentor's feedback with an open mind and try to extract as much value as possible. You may not always agree with what they say and do not always have to take their advice, but having a growth-mindset will present you with invaluable opportunities to learn and mature.
- **Reciprocate**
  - The best mentor-mentee relationships are mutually beneficial. As you get to know one another, ask your mentor how you can be helpful to them. Do they need help writing a book chapter? Do they have another mentee who could benefit from your experiences and expertise?
- **Be prepared to alter or end the relationship**
  - Some mentor relationships will either reach their logical conclusion or may not be the right fit. If you feel that the relationship is not productive or a good match, your mentor likely feels the same way. Have an honest conversation with your mentor if you feel like the relationship needs to be altered or con-

cluded. Having a frank conversation may alleviate existing issues. When seeking to end a mentor relationship, make sure to thank them for their time and guidance and part on amicable terms.

20.5 Conclusion

Mentor-mentee relationships significantly contribute to the success of medical students as they embark on their journey to becoming compassionate, skilled, and resilient physicians. Creating active and effective mentorship relationships is essential to navigating this dynamic phase of life and setting up future success.

References

1. Kram KE. Mentoring at work: developmental relationships in organizational life. [Internet] Academy of Management Journal; 1985. [cited 2024 16 Jan]. https://doi.org/10.2307/2392687.
2. Byars-Winston A, Dahlberg ML. The science of effective mentorship in STEMM. [Internet] National Academies of Sciences, Engineering, and Medicine; Policy and Global Affairs; Board on Higher Education and Workforce; Committee on Effective Mentorship in STEMM; 2019. [cited 2024 16 Jan]. https://www.ncbi.nlm.nih.gov/books/NBK552775/.

Chapter 21
Achieving Personal and Professional Fulfilment

Lauren Curwick and Brenessa Lindeman

Abstract When passion and work collide, one achieves the ultimate personal and professional fulfillment. In this chapter, we take holistic approach to accomplishing this. We discuss defining your purpose and self-reflection, goal setting and strategic planning, creating an environment of belongingness and mentorship, and setting realistic expectations and promoting self-care.

21.1 Introduction

Feeling fulfilled is essential to maintain purpose, passion, and compassion for the patients we care for on a daily basis. While conversations in medicine are becoming more encouraging with an emphasis on wellness, rates of burnout remain alarmingly high. A metanalysis was conducted evaluating rates of burnout across all surgical specialties, which found an average rate of 47% with rates as high as 77% in some surgical subspecialities. Associated negative factors included poor work-life balance and work-related issues while positive factors included career advancement and good relationships with co-residents [1]. It is more important now than ever to focus on what makes you fulfilled and channeling that in both your personal and professional life. One strategy to achieve such fulfillment is to seek work-life integration, defined as coordinating and blending different aspects of life into a whole where work, family, friends, and self are valued, and time is distributed proportionally [2]. Work-life integration was further described by authors from the University of California Berkeley Haas School of Business as an approach that creates synergies between all areas that define life, including work, family, community, personal well-being, and health [3]. Reaching one's full potential inside and outside of work is key to combating burn out and finding fulfillment. In this chapter, we will focus

L. Curwick (✉) · B. Lindeman
University of Alabama at Birmingham, Birmingham, AL, USA
e-mail: lacurwick@uabmc.edu; blindeman@uabmc.edu

A. Gillis, C. B. Aarons (eds.), *A How To Guide For Medical Students*, Success in Academic Surgery, https://doi.org/10.1007/978-3-031-66011-5_21

on a holistic approach to achieving personal and professional fulfillment in academic surgery with an emphasis on work-life integration.

21.2 Defining Your Purpose

An article from the Journal of Plastic & Reconstructive Surgery entitled "Finding Meaning in Life" attempts to unpack this weighty topic through defining several pillars to achieving this ultimate goal [4]. One of these pillars is purpose, and we agree that having a clear definition of your own purpose is fundamental before establishing your goals.

Self-reflection is essential in defining your purpose and establishing your why. The following are prompts to reflect on:

- What do you feel is your calling in life?
- What excites you?
- What are your skills and strengths?
- What are your values?
- How do you define success, and what does success look like to you?
- Where do you see your career in the next 5, 10, 15 years?

The answers to these questions likely look different for each individual, and the answers to these questions can change over the duration your career. Thus, continuing to engage in self-reflection is important, and intentionally building this in at a regular interval (i.e., every 6 months or every year) or preceding planned times of transition (e.g., applying for residency, taking academic development time, applying for fellowship, etc.) can help ensure that the goals you're pursuing are consistent with your purpose and not simply on auto-pilot based on a prior plan.

The next step is to channel your passions. While considering your passions, determine how you can integrate these into your work. Examples include:

- An interest in leadership leading to pursuit of an MBA with the goal of taking on a leadership position that involves finance.
- A creative side with the goal of becoming involved in medical illustrations for research articles and book chapters.
- A passion for political change and becoming involved in policy change in health care and surgery.
- An interest in research resulting in working toward a PhD with the goal of running a lab.
- A passion for education and becoming involved in medical student and resident education and paving the way to become a medical student clerkship director, residency program direction, or to enhance education nationwide.

Take time to consider the activities and causes that are important to you. Never stop exploring your passions and what fuels them. Finding ways to incorporate them into your daily work leads to the ultimate professional and personal fulfillment.

21.3 Goal Setting and Strategic Planning

Thinking about what you envision for yourself over the course of residency and beyond can be daunting, and it can be difficult to map out how to get where you want to be. However, establishing a well thought-out, organized plan can maximize your productivity and make these life goals feel more manageable to achieve.

First, consider your priorities. As highlighted in the article by Gade and Yeo (2019), they developed a time management grid inspired by the book *The Seven Habits of Highly Effective People* by Stephen Covey, as a way to organize priorities (Table 21.1) [1, 5]. Determine what is most important to you, and ultimately your goals should be influenced by these.

Goal-setting should include both long-term and short-term goals, and should be set for both your professional and personal life (either separately or together depending on your degree of work-life integration). Like developing a strategic plan for a company, it is incredibly valuable to establish specific, actionable objectives for each goal with deadlines for these objectives (Fig. 21.1). A Twelve-step Approach for Academic Development Planning in Academic Surgery was published in *Annals of Surgery Open* in 2022, as a guide toward helping those interested in a surgical career achieve success in developing their own strategic plan [6]. Having a strategic plan of sorts for your career trajectory makes accomplishing the big tasks seem more manageable by breaking them into small tasks. While this document is not meant to be static and will also change over time as you re-evaluate your goals, it creates an actionable plan for moving forward. It is important to be realistic with yourself as you develop your timeline. Throughout training you evolve and with that, your priorities and goals can shift as you hone in on your areas of interest. Set time aside at specific time intervals, to reassess your plan and what areas need to be tweaked.

21.4 Strategic Plan

Strategic Priority/Goal 1: List your specific short- or long-term goal.

Deliverable: List what achieving this goal look like, and how you measure success.

Table 21.1 Grid to map out priorities

	Important	Less Important
Urgent	Action: Do now	Action: Delegate/push Back
Less urgent	Action: Plan/do soon	Action: Avoid/do last

Strategic Priority/Goal 1: List your specific short- or long-term goal.

Deliverable: List what achieving this goal look like, and how you measure success.

Objectives in support of the strategic priority	Timeline	Resources
List actionable objectives here	Complete by _	List references and resources that will guide your progress here
	Complete by _	
	Complete by _	

Fig. 21.1 Strategic plan example

Objectives in support of the strategic priority	Timeline	Resources
List actionable objectives here	Complete by _	List references and resources that will guide your progress here
	Complete by _	
	Complete by _	

Schedules in residency and throughout your future career are unpredictable. However, staying as organized as possible is key to success. Whether it's your phone or a planner, keeping a calendar with deadlines, meetings, and to do lists can help you stay on track. It is important to be realistic with yourself, continuously readjust based on changing circumstances, and give yourself grace for when you make a mistake. As a surgical resident, your top priority is taking care of patients and learning how to be a good surgeon. Take time as a first-year resident to learn how to be efficient, provide compassionate patient care, and learn key skills in the OR. Time at the hospital ebbs and flows, so plan ahead on when you may be able to start to integrate more. For example, schedule meetings on rotations that may be more flexible in the future rather than on a rotation that is busy and unpredictable. When you feel like you can find time to start to integrate more into your academic career, start with taking on one project at a time as to not spread yourself too thin. You know yourself best, continuously reassess where you are and how far you have come.

Ultimately, creating well thought-out plans, staying organized, and continuous self-assessment can lead to feelings of accomplishment and fulfillment.

21.5 Creating a Supportive Environment

Lambert et al. conducted four studies that found a sense of belonging and social support is strongly correlated with perception of meaning of life [7, 8]. There are many ways to find a sense of belonging in surgical residency.

For residency, you are selected by a program who is excited to train you. They are investing in you and your future as a surgeon and want nothing more than to see you succeed. In addition, your co-residents are your teammates and friends. Support each other every step of the way. While in residency, life outside of medicine continues to pass by which can feel isolating. It's important to nurture your relationships with your colleagues, and to be there for each other. If a major life event occurs during your training, be open with your colleagues, listen to each other, and don't be afraid to ask each other for help.

Determine what characteristics you hope to possess as a surgeon. As you rotate on various services throughout your training, find mentors who exhibit these qualities to guide you in the right direction. It can be helpful to discuss goals for your future and set regular meeting times to touch base on these goals. While it can be fulfilling finding mentors, it can be even more fulfilling becoming a mentor. Don't lose sight of what it is like to be a medical student. Pay it forward and serve as a role model and mentor for students. Prior to starting residency, write down the qualities you found most admirable in residents you worked with. Throughout your training, look back at this list as a reminder about your priorities, particularly for times when things feel too busy or overwhelming.

Extend your social circle even broader. Attend national meetings and join surgical societies and committees. While academic surgery is large, it can start to feel like a close-knit community as you start to surround yourself with others sharing similar passions and interests. Creating this supportive, collaborative environment is another step toward not only professional fulfillment, but also personal fulfillment as your sense of belonging grows.

Lastly, the challenges of residency aren't only felt by you, but also by the loved ones in your life. Discuss your short- and long-term goals with family, and ensure they understand that their input is important to you. While time can be unpredictable throughout your career, set time aside each week to devote quality time with your partner or someone that you care about. Involve these individuals in work opportunities outside of the hospital, such as conference meetings away, holiday parties, co-residents' and their children's birthday parties, etc. This allows your outside-work support system and family to become more integrated in your work life and get to know your colleagues who you spend so much time with. Cultivating a supportive, encouraging environment at home further sets you up for success.

21.6 Invest in Yourself

"You can't take care of your patients if you don't take care of yourself." We have all heard variations of this during residency, and it is absolutely true. It can feel nearly impossible to build healthy habits in residency as you are torn between your professional commitments with long hours, personal and family commitments, sleep, and exercise. We would not be transparent if we said we have a perfect balance but find ways to build healthy habits early on in order to be your best self during training and beyond. This can take many forms, including things like downloading an exercise app on your phone for short workouts to fit in a few times a week, having groceries delivered, setting aside time for meditation, or meal prepping on off weekends. Making these tasks as convenient as possible can help you be more successful.

As a student, you have endless opportunities presented to you throughout medical school. From student organizations to research projects, there is often sufficient time to be involved in many various interests. However, as one transitions to residency, your time becomes more limited, and any spare time is that much more valuable. Like medical school, there are many opportunities presented to residents to be involved in—leadership opportunities, committee involvement, research, and the list goes on. It is important to understand your capacity, and to set boundaries. Get comfortable with saying no to allow yourself to give your all to your other commitments, your patients, and your personal life.

Make time for things you care about outside of medicine. There is always the sense that there is more that can be done. However, it is important to set aside time to reset and invest time in your passions outside of medicine. Building time into your schedule to continue to take time to pursue your hobbies, even if it is a couple of times a month, can help you recharge.

Lastly, practice gratitude. You've come so far. Residency can feel like the highest of highs and lowest of lows. Dive in and enjoy every second of it.

References

1. Jesuyajolu D, et al. Burnout among surgeons and surgical trainees: a systematic review and meta-analysis of the prevalence and associated factors. Surgery in Practice and Science. 2022;10:100094. https://doi.org/10.1016/j.sipas.2022.100094.
2. Gade L, Yeo HL. Work-life integration and time management strategies. Clin Colon Rectal Surg. 2019;32(6):442–9. https://doi.org/10.1055/s-0039-1693011.
3. Wei JL, Villwock JA. Balance versus integration: work-life considerations. Otolaryngol Clin N Am. 2021;54(4):823–37. https://doi.org/10.1016/j.otc.2021.05.007.
4. Dwivedi S, Chung K. Finding meaning in life. Plast Reconstr Surg. 2023;152(3):477–81. https://doi.org/10.1097/PRS.0000000000010534.
5. Covey S. The seven habits of highly effective people. New York, NY: Free Press; 2004. p. 151.
6. Selvakumar S, Ang D, Elkbuli A. Twelve-step approach for academic development planning in academic surgery: climbing the academic uphill with strong and steady steps. Ann Surg Open. 2022;3(1):e119. https://doi.org/10.1097/AS9.0000000000000119.
7. Lambert NM, Stillman TF, Hicks JA, Kamble S, Baumeister RF, Fincham FD. To belong is to matter: sense of belonging enhances meaning in life. Personal Soc Psychol Bull. 2013;39(11):1418–27. https://doi.org/10.1177/0146167213499186.
8. MacKinnon NJ, Rosema D, Cyca P. Career and life fulfillment and planning for medical trainees, and physicians. Int J Med Educ. 2022;13:305–6. https://doi.org/10.5116/ijme.6372.17ba.

Part VI
Embracing Diversity and Inclusion in Surgery

Chapter 22
The Resident Perspective—A Part and Apart from the Surgical Workforce

Imani E McElroy

Abstract Surgical training is a complex experience for any trainee. For those from underrepresented backgrounds this experience becomes even more difficult as we navigate spaces structured for our exclusion. There is a significant emotional tax on trainees when tasked to carry the burden of being at the center of DEI efforts for their program or institution. Being cognizant of the sociopolitical turmoil of our current day and the efforts to defund DEI require us to be more forthright in our efforts to bolster and protect DEI principles within our institution and society.

> *I tell my students, 'When you get these jobs that you have been so brilliantly trained for, just remember that your real job is that if you are free, you need to free somebody else. If you have some power, then your job is to empower somebody else. This is not just a grab-bag candy game.—Toni Morrison*

In this chapter, I write a perspective that describes my journey as someone who finds themselves walking the balance of wanting change but also wanting freedom. Freedom to fall in love with surgery and grow within our training paradigm without the weight of imposter syndrome, shifting goal posts, and the minority tax. I do not claim to be an expert in diversity, equity, and inclusion (DEI) nor will I pretend to have a panacea for the system. I simply offer up the lessons I have learned as someone who has fought for diversity, equity, and inclusion in surgery and society. The desire to do this work is founded in a sense of justice that was cultivated by my mother and grandmother who have spent their lives dedicated to working with at-risk youth and under-resourced communities. The mantra of "lift as you rise" is a key tenant of my family ethos and is the underlying motivation for why I continue to invest in these efforts.

Navigating surgical residency is a balancing act involving learning how to diagnose surgical pathology, mastering the technical steps to fix said pathology, and discerning when not to cut. This balance requires focus, discipline, and adaptability in a fast-paced environment that is built to be rigorous and demanding. As surgeons our greatest growth comes from leaning into discomfort and using that discomfort

I. E. McElroy (✉)
Department of Surgery, Massachusetts General Hospital, Boston, MA, USA
e-mail: imcelroy@usc.edu

A. Gillis, C. B. Aarons (eds.), *A How To Guide For Medical Students*, Success in Academic Surgery, https://doi.org/10.1007/978-3-031-66011-5_22

to hone key skills. Within this system, there is an expectation of trust not just between doctors and patients, but between trainees and their attendings. Trainees are trusted with increasing autonomy as they progress through and prove they are ready. However, trainees also inherently must be able to trust their attendings to fulfill their fiducial duty to teach them and guide them. For those that come from underrepresented backgrounds, this same environment can shift from rigorous and demanding to outright hostile and unwelcoming. The ability to trust a system that was constructed to exclude and take advantage of people from underrepresented and under resourced communities can present as a minefield. And when faced with the decision to speak up or stay quiet to protect our careers, many of us find ourselves stuck in an existential debate of how to survive and thrive in an environment built to suffocate us.

For me, staying quiet became an untenable way to live and I found myself speaking up and out more frequently as my training progressed. This was a calculated risk that I felt I had to take due to the emotional toll I found myself living under otherwise. Luckily, I was able to find support within my department and allies that were willing to take up the charge with me and I was able to avoid significant backlash. But I also have ruffled my fair share of feathers and time will tell if that has lasting effects on my career. Speaking up also came with its own stresses as I found myself suddenly on numerous committees and task forces with the aim of being not only the resident representative but also the representative for my various degrees of minoritization. The mental tax I feel from navigating these roles remains at times overwhelming.

There is an inevitable power inequity that trainees face when tasked with sitting on committees and task forces. We must learn to navigate making our superiors, and potential future employers, uncomfortable with the information and perspective we carry when asking for change. It is a fine line to walk between concerned colleague and angry Black woman. Meanwhile, I still have the same responsibilities of my co-residents to learn the ever-growing number of techniques to treat surgical pathology. I still am faced with the emotional rigors of patient care and the stumbles of residency that we all face with inexperience and bad patient outcomes. And I still face the same biases associated with being a queer, Black, women in a conservative field. While I chose to be vocal about my displeasure with the lack of progress within surgery and medicine in addressing DEI, the subsequent spotlight only increased the scrutiny I face as an underrepresented trainee.

As the demographics of medicine and surgery shift to reflect the ever-changing American population, the importance of DEI programs and initiatives has never been more relevant. Unfortunately, DEI and those that invest their time and energy in its development find themselves in the crosshairs of a political firestorm. Multiple states across the United States are currently working to cut DEI program funding or in some cases ban their existence outright. These efforts effectively compound the already existing resistance to efforts to establish DEI as a legitimate entity that should be embraced. As a queer Black trainee, watching these efforts and hearing the forceful rejection of DEI principles and, by extension the individuals supported by them, often feels like a personal attack. Prior to the summer of 2020 when the

United States supposedly had its "Great Awakening", much of the struggle in working with DEI was getting society to understand the system level barriers of systemic racism and white supremacy in addition to this work not being considered academically rigorous. Funding supporting DEI initiatives was scarce, career advancement and academic promotion remained limited, and much of the burden remained on those with the least amount of power to fix the system.

With the commodification of DEI that happened following the riots of the summer of 2020 there were promises to invest in DEI and creation of new academic positions and task forces to address DEI on institutional and systemic levels. However, as we now know, many of those promises failed to be turned into tangible action items and early reports show a familiar trend of women and minorities being funneled into diversity positions with still limited opportunity for career advancement. And now the subsequent political backlash, many of us find ourselves in a battle to maintain basic rights and privileges that many people take for granted.

I cannot predict how academic surgery will move to protect DEI initiatives and those that work relentlessly to create a more equitable and just society. But I can implore those that come to the table of DEI that there is much work to be done and we all will benefit from DEI efforts personally, professionally, and globally. The time is now to act, we cannot afford to wait and see what happens.

Chapter 23
Recognizing Unconscious Bias and Its Impact on Patient Care and Outcomes

Crystal D. Taylor and Lesly A. Dossett

Abstract Unconscious bias refers to social stereotypes, attitudes, or beliefs held about certain groups of people formed outside of our conscious awareness. It is an innate component of human decision-making prone to error and can affect patient outcomes. Unconscious bias should be recognized at all levels of training. Many strategies are available for mitigating unconscious bias, which requires the intentional effort and consideration of the participant. Although increased cognitive resources are needed to prevent bias, doing so is well worth the effort to improve patient care.

23.1 Introduction

In humans, perceptions of reality are based on received information and experiences, which develop into automatic thinking. This allowed decision-making to become more efficient over time [1]. Decision-making involves type 1 and type 2 processes [2]. Type 1 processes are often known as heuristics or mental shortcuts as they are fast, unconscious, intuitive, and require limited cognitive effort, allowing for rapid decision-making. Type 2 processes, on the other hand, are slower, conscious, analytical, and require more mental effort. These two processes combine the dual process theory [2]. Many of our daily activities use type 1 processes through serial associations where one event automatically triggers the following [3]. For example, someone presents to the emergency department with a chief complaint of chest pain to which you order an electrocardiogram and troponin level to look for myocardial infarction. In using heuristics based on lectures you learned in medical school you instinctively equate chest pain to a heart attack, but may overlook additional history that the patient provided such as upper respiratory symptoms, fever, and productive cough making the diagnosis of pneumonia more likely. We are prone

C. D. Taylor · L. A. Dossett (✉)
University of Michigan, Ann Arbor, MI, USA
e-mail: tacrysta@med.umich.edu; ldossett@med.umich.edu

A. Gillis, C. B. Aarons (eds.), *A How To Guide For Medical Students*, Success in Academic Surgery, https://doi.org/10.1007/978-3-031-66011-5_23

to using heuristics, which usually work well but are vulnerable to error. When errors do occur, they are seldom corrected [3]. This can lead to bias, which is an inherent part of human judgment.

Unconscious bias, also commonly known as implicit bias, refers to social stereotypes, attitudes, or beliefs held about certain groups of people formed outside of our conscious awareness. This ultimately affects our interactions and understanding with those around us and can have unintended consequences [4]. The term was introduced by Anthony G. Greenwald and Mahzarin R. Banaji in 1995, at which time they argued that social behavior often operates unconsciously. Consequently, past experiences can influence judgment in an implicit manner, which can impact attitudes, stereotyping, and self-esteem [5]. It is important to note that unconscious bias does not require the individual to subscribe to or allocate attention to its expression. This is in contrast to explicit bias, where the individual is aware of their evaluation of another, believes this evaluation to be valid to some extent, and has the time and motivation to act on it in the current situation [6].

The racial and ethnic makeup within the United States is more diverse than in prior years. This creates a unique opportunity for healthcare professionals to care for individuals from many backgrounds, beliefs, and cultures. It is, therefore, essential to be aware of unconscious bias and its effect on patient care. Preferences for or against particular groups can translate to tangible differences in patient outcomes. This can ultimately contribute to health disparities and can generate patient mistrust of providers or institutions within the healthcare system. This chapter will review common types of unconscious bias in healthcare, the impact of unconscious bias on patient care, how to recognize unconscious bias, and strategies for mitigation.

23.2 Common Types of Unconscious Bias in Healthcare

Medicine is a dynamic profession that allows physicians to observe and treat rare conditions, teach and learn from others, and become an integral part of a patient's life. Medical students are taught the ethical principles of beneficence, maleficence, autonomy, and justice early in their medical education [7]. As physicians, we are expected to make objective recommendations and provide impartial care to all patients. In reality, this is a much more challenging task, given the pervasive nature of bias. Many types of unconscious bias permeate the healthcare setting. The most commonly encountered biases are race, age, gender, education, socioeconomic status, and overweight/obesity.

Racial bias impacts multiple aspects of society. Healthcare is not immune to its effects. In 2003, the Institute of Medicine published the landmark report *Unequal Treatment,* which documented that individuals from minority groups received fewer procedures and poorer quality of care in comparison to their white counterparts. These differences persisted even after adjusting for income, education, disease severity, medical comorbidities, and health insurance [8]. It increased attention to healthcare inequities and noted that healthcare professionals' unconscious bias contributes to deficits in quality care.

Age bias, also called ageism, is an important type of unconscious bias to consider as individuals live longer and access healthcare often. It has previously been shown that one out of five adults over the age of 50 experiences discrimination in the healthcare setting [9]. Further work has demonstrated that many adults ages 50–80 years regularly experience at least one form of everyday ageism, which is associated with poor mental and physical health [10]. Other studies have demonstrated that physicians are less likely to recommend patients for surgery and involve patients in medical decision-making in older adults [11, 12]. As many physicians primarily treat older adults, ageism can potentially influence this population's care negatively.

Gender bias is commonly seen in healthcare in the context of pain presentation and management. A review performed by Samulowitz and colleagues noted that men presenting with pain were seen as stoic, tolerated pain, denied pain, and avoided seeking healthcare for fear of pain as a perceived weakness. In contrast, women presenting with pain were perceived as hysterical, emotional, and malingerers and experienced a longer time for diagnosis and treatment [13]. Discrimination against LGBTQ adults is prevalent in healthcare. In a study performed by Casey et al., one in six LGBTQ adults reported avoiding healthcare due to anticipated discrimination, while 16% reported discrimination during healthcare encounters [14]. This can result in delayed presentation of illness and treatment.

It is well known that higher levels of education are associated with improved health outcomes. Higher educational attainment is linked to more stable jobs, leading to higher income and wealth accruement that can be used to improve health behaviors and overall health. Adults with lower levels of educational attainment report worse general health, more chronic conditions, and increased functional limitations and disability [15]. Intricately connected with educational attainment is socioeconomic status (SES). Individuals with lower SES have lower life expectancy, suffer from more chronic conditions, receive fewer diagnostic tests and medications for these chronic conditions, and have limited access to health care due to cost and coverage. Physicians are also more likely to perceive low SES patients as less intelligent, less independent, less responsible, less adherent to medical advice, and less likely to return for follow-up visits [16]. Undoubtedly, this can serve as a barrier to care.

The prevalence of overweight and obese individuals is increasing. According to the Centers for Disease Control and Prevention, between 2017 and 2018, approximately 75% of adults aged 20 and over were overweight or obese [17]. Being overweight and obese can be stigmatizing for patients and present a challenge when receiving care. These patients are often viewed as less likely to adhere to self-care or treatment, lazy, undisciplined, and weak-willed [18]. Physicians may over-attribute patient symptoms and problems to obesity. Furthermore, they may fail to refer patients for diagnostic testing or consider other treatment options beyond weight loss advisement [18].

23.3 Impact of Unconscious Bias on Patient Care and Outcomes

Healthcare disparities are well known. Race and ethnicity were previously the main factors thought to contribute to healthcare disparities. It is now recognized that social determinants of health, which are conditions in which individuals are born, live, learn, work, play, and pray, influence health and health outcomes much more than the previously prescribed constructs [19]. Studies have demonstrated that unconscious bias can impact physician decision-making on patient care. For example, Green et al. found physicians were more likely to diagnose a black patient presenting with chest pain as having coronary artery disease than a white patient. However, physicians with anti-black bias were less likely to offer black patients thrombolytic therapy over white patients [20]. Similarly, in a study conducted by Sabin et al., pediatricians with higher pro-white bias were more likely to agree to prescribe white patients narcotics for postsurgical pain than black patients [21].

Unconscious bias has the potential to impact diagnosis and treatment for patients, which can have devastating consequences and ultimately affect outcomes. Young patients presenting with stroke are often misdiagnosed in comparison to older patients. This is due to a multitude of factors, such as atypical stroke presentation, stroke mimics such as seizures, and the need for a broader differential diagnosis in this population. Physician bias also plays a role due to the failure to recognize the importance of traditional stroke risk factors in young patients, such as smoking, hypertension, diabetes, and atherosclerotic disease [22]. Misdiagnosis and treatment have also been documented in the field of psychiatry, where it has been shown that black patients with affective disorders are more likely to be diagnosed with schizophrenia than white patients. Reasons for this include physicians not performing a thorough interview for affective symptoms, noting psychotic symptoms with periods of recovery or occurring in the absence of affective symptoms, attributing more negative symptoms such as a blunted affect to black patients, and underemphasizing affective symptoms [23].

Patient outcomes are subject to the influence of provider implicit bias. Hausman and colleagues found spinal cord injury patients had a greater likelihood of disability in social integration, higher levels of depression, and lower life satisfaction when cared for by a physician with implicit racial bias [24]. The impact of bias can be felt by patients directly in the clinical setting. Cooper et al. found that black patients experienced longer office visits, more clinician verbal dominance during the clinic visit, less patient-centered dialogue, less perceived involvement in their care and respect by the clinician, lower trust and confidence in the physician, and were less likely to recommend the physician to others when seen by a physician with more implicit bias in comparison to white patients [25]. Unconscious bias has many effects on patients, which conveys the need to address it early in medical education.

23.4 How to Recognize Unconscious Bias

The Implicit Association Test (IAT) is commonly used in research and medical education to measure bias. The IAT involves participants sorting words into groups as quickly and accurately as possible [2]. It measures the strength of associations between concepts, stereotypes, or evaluations, relying on the notion that choosing a response is easier when closely associated items share the same response key [26]. When participating in an IAT, the user is asked to quickly sort words into categories on the left and right side of the computer screen corresponding to the "e" key and "i" key, respectively. The IAT is divided into five parts [26]. During the first part of the test, the user sorts words relating to the concepts into categories. In an example where the concept is "obese people" or "thin people," if the category of "obese people" is on the right side of the screen and a photo of an obese person appears, the user presses the "i" key to designate the photo to the right under its appropriate category. In the second part, the user sorts words relating to evaluation, such as "good" or "bad." If the category "good" is on the left side of the screen and a pleasant word such as "happiness" appears on the screen, the user should press the "e" key. The third part combines the categories, requiring the user to sort both concept and evaluation words. Using the prior examples, "obese people/good" are on the left side of the screen while "thin people/bad" are on the right side. The user would then have to sort the words and photos appropriately. In the fourth part, the concepts switch places so that in this example, "obese people" would now be on the right side of the screen while "thin people" would be on the left. The evaluations ("good" and "bad") would remain in their original positions. In the fifth part, the categories are combined in the opposite way that was previously [26].

The IAT score comprises how long it takes the user, on average, to sort words in the third part of the test versus the fifth part of the test. In the prior example, an implicit preference is noted if the user is faster to categorize words when "thin people" and "good" share a response key and "obese people" and "bad" share a response key relative to the reverse associations [26]. The IAT has different categories, such as age, race, weight, and gender. The IAT is not a perfect tool, and many opponents note deficiencies of the test, such as the lack of clarity for what the test measures and difficulty in identifying associations. Others suggest that the results of the IAT may stem from other associations such as victimization, maltreatment, and oppression rather than reflecting authentic negative attitudes. It is designed to be used as a self-reflection tool to understand better one's preferences and biases [27, 28].

23.5 Strategies for Mitigating Unconscious Bias

Recognition of unconscious bias can be complex and requires intentional action by the individual and organization to identify and reduce it. Deliberate reflection can be a valuable tool to mitigate bias individually. It requires the user to assess how their experiences and identity shape their interactions with those around them. This method has been shown to reduce stereotype activation [29]. Engaging in this method allows the individual to have an open discussion with others to discuss and ameliorate behaviors should they unknowingly behave in a discriminatory manner. Along with deliberate reflection, perspective-taking is another strategy that can be utilized to reduce unconscious bias. It involves a conscious effort to understand another individual's point of view and has been shown to reduce unconscious bias in social interactions [30].

Healthcare professionals should practice cultural humility, also known as cultural sensitivity, which implies that the individual focuses on the willingness to care for others from various backgrounds. It requires that the individual be aware that they cannot be experts in all cultures they encounter but are willing to learn [31]. By practicing cultural humility, individuals acknowledge that the lens through which they view the world is not exhaustive, and others are likely to have a different perspective [31]. Cultural humility can be further augmented by integrating its discussion into training, allowing participants to practice interacting with individuals from diverse backgrounds to provide and receive feedback in a non-threatening environment [32]. In addition to cultural humility, individuation has been shown to reduce bias. It involves evaluating a person based on personal attributes rather than associating them with group attributes [33].

Intentional efforts can be made for individuals to connect with others from different backgrounds to diversify their circle. Examples include reading a book or article from a new author, meeting new people at a conference, and trying new cuisine with a friend [34]. In doing so, we can become more comfortable with individuals we view as unfamiliar and form a mutual understanding and respect, which can positively alter our interactions with others. Individuals must also acquire the tools to counteract bias should they experience it or witness it from others. The Kirwan Institute at the Ohio State University has developed strategies to empower others to respond to bias as active bystanders. This includes tactics such as refusing to rely on the assumption, asking questions to invite discussion, acknowledging that the statement made you uncomfortable, and using "I statements" to directly communicate your feelings [35]. Although not exhaustive, these strategies can allow individuals to confront bias by starting a dialogue and advocating for themselves and others.

23.6 Summary

Bias is inherent to human nature and is a form of automatic thinking that allows for rapid decision-making. It can have positive and negative effects on individuals and groups alike. Unconscious bias can result in the differential care of patients based on characteristics such as race, ethnicity, religion, and gender. It differs from explicit bias in that it is formed outside of the individual's awareness. As healthcare providers, we must be aware of our biases and their associated implications on decision-making. Deliberate intention is needed to identify and mitigate unconscious bias in everyday interactions. In doing so, we can work towards providing more equitable care for patients.

References

1. Chapman EN, Kaatz A, Carnes M. Physicians and implicit bias: how doctors may unwittingly perpetuate health care disparities. J Gen Intern Med. 2013;28(11):1504–10. https://doi.org/10.1007/s11606-013-2441-1.
2. Gopal DP, Chetty U, O'Donnell P, Gajria C, Blackadder-Weinstein J. Implicit bias in healthcare: clinical practice, research and decision making. Future Healthc J. 2021;8(1):40–8. https://doi.org/10.7861/fhj.2020-0233.
3. Croskerry P, Singhal G, Mamede S. Cognitive debiasing 1: origins of bias and theory of debiasing. BMJ Qual Saf. 2013;22 Suppl 2(Suppl 2):ii58–64. https://doi.org/10.1136/bmjqs-2012-001712.
4. Ogunleye TA. Unconscious Bias. Dermatol Clin. 2023;41(2):285–90. https://doi.org/10.1016/j.det.2022.08.003.
5. Greenwald AG, Banaji MR. Implicit social cognition: attitudes, self-esteem, and stereotypes. Psychol Rev. 1995;102(1):4–27. https://doi.org/10.1037/0033-295x.102.1.4.
6. Blair IV, Steiner JF, Havranek EP. Unconscious (implicit) bias and health disparities: where do we go from here? Perm J. 2011;15(2):71–8. https://doi.org/10.7812/TPP/11.979.
7. Varkey B. Principles of clinical ethics and their application to practice. Med Princ Pract. 2021;30(1):17–28. https://doi.org/10.1159/000509119.
8. Smedley BD, Stith AY, Nelson AR. Unequal treatment: confronting racial and ethnic disparities in health care. Washington, DC: National Academy Press; 2003.
9. Rogers SE, Thrasher AD, Miao Y, Boscardin WJ, Smith AK. Discrimination in healthcare settings is associated with disability in older adults: health and retirement study, 2008-2012. J Gen Intern Med. 2015;30(10):1413–20. https://doi.org/10.1007/s11606-015-3233-6.
10. Allen JO, Solway E, Kirch M, Singer D, Kullgren JT, Moise V, Malani PN. Experiences of everyday ageism and the health of older US adults. JAMA Netw Open. 2022;5(6):e2217240. https://doi.org/10.1001/jamanetworkopen.2022.17240.
11. Adelman RD, Greene MG, Ory MG. Communication between older patients and their physicians. Clin Geriatr Med. 2000;16(1):1–24, vii. https://doi.org/10.1016/s0749-0690(05)70004-5.
12. Peake MD, Thompson S, Lowe D, Pearson MG, Participating C. Ageism in the management of lung cancer. Age Ageing. 2003;32(2):171–7. https://doi.org/10.1093/ageing/32.2.171.
13. Samulowitz A, Gremyr I, Eriksson E, Hensing G. "Brave men" and "emotional women": a theory-guided literature review on gender bias in health care and gendered norms towards patients with chronic pain. Pain Res Manag. 2018;2018:6358624. https://doi.org/10.1155/2018/6358624.

14. Casey LS, Reisner SL, Findling MG, Blendon RJ, Benson JM, Sayde JM, Miller C. Discrimination in the United States: experiences of lesbian, gay, bisexual, transgender, and queer Americans. Health Serv Res. 2019;54 Suppl 2(Suppl 2):1454–66. https://doi.org/10.1111/1475-6773.13229.
15. Zajacova A, Lawrence EM. The relationship between education and health: reducing disparities through a contextual approach. Annu Rev Public Health. 2018;39:273–89. https://doi.org/10.1146/annurev-publhealth-031816-044628.
16. Arpey NC, Gaglioti AH, Rosenbaum ME. How socioeconomic status affects patient perceptions of health care: a qualitative study. J Prim Care Community Health. 2017;8(3):169–75. https://doi.org/10.1177/2150131917697439.
17. Prevention CfDCa: Prevalence of overweight, obesity, and severe obesity among adults aged 20 and over: United States, 1960–1962 through 2017–2018. 2020. https://www.cdc.gov/nchs/data/hestat/obesity-adult-17-18/obesity-adult.htm. Accessed 14 Dec 2023.
18. Phelan SM, Burgess DJ, Yeazel MW, Hellerstedt WL, Griffin JM, van Ryn M. Impact of weight bias and stigma on quality of care and outcomes for patients with obesity. Obes Rev. 2015;16(4):319–26. https://doi.org/10.1111/obr.12266.
19. Braveman P, Egerter S, Williams DR. The social determinants of health: coming of age. Annu Rev Public Health. 2011;32:381–98. https://doi.org/10.1146/annurev-publhealth-031210-101218.
20. Green AR, Carney DR, Pallin DJ, Ngo LH, Raymond KL, Iezzoni LI, Banaji MR. Implicit bias among physicians and its prediction of thrombolysis decisions for black and white patients. J Gen Intern Med. 2007;22(9):1231–8. https://doi.org/10.1007/s11606-007-0258-5.
21. Sabin JA, Greenwald AG. The influence of implicit bias on treatment recommendations for 4 common pediatric conditions: pain, urinary tract infection, attention deficit hyperactivity disorder, and asthma. Am J Public Health. 2012;102(5):988–95. https://doi.org/10.2105/AJPH.2011.300621.
22. Bhat A, Mahajan V, Wolfe N. Implicit bias in stroke care: a recurring old problem in the rising incidence of young stroke. J Clin Neurosci. 2021;85:27–35. https://doi.org/10.1016/j.jocn.2020.12.017.
23. Hairston DR, Gibbs TA, Wong SS, Jordan A. Clinician bias in diagnosis and treatment. In: Medlock MM, Shtasel D, Trinh N-HT, Williams DR, editors. Racism and psychiatry: contemporary issues and interventions. Cham: Springer International Publishing; 2019. p. 105–37.
24. Hausmann LR, Myaskovsky L, Niyonkuru C, Oyster ML, Switzer GE, Burkitt KH, et al. Examining implicit bias of physicians who care for individuals with spinal cord injury: a pilot study and future directions. J Spinal Cord Med. 2015;38(1):102–10. https://doi.org/10.1179/2045772313Y.0000000184.
25. Cooper LA, Roter DL, Carson KA, Beach MC, Sabin JA, Greenwald AG, Inui TS. The associations of clinicians' implicit attitudes about race with medical visit communication and patient ratings of interpersonal care. Am J Public Health. 2012;102(5):979–87. https://doi.org/10.2105/AJPH.2011.300558.
26. Implicit P: Project implicit. 2011. https://implicit.harvard.edu/implicit/iatdetails.html. Accessed 21 Nov 2023.
27. Sukhera J, Wodzinski M, Milne A, Teunissen PW, Lingard L, Watling C. Implicit bias and the feedback paradox: exploring how health professionals engage with feedback while questioning its credibility. Acad Med. 2019;94(8):1204–10. https://doi.org/10.1097/ACM.0000000000002782.
28. Sukhera J, Wodzinski M, Rehman M, Gonzalez CM. The Implicit association test in health professions education: a meta-narrative review. Perspect Med Educ. 2019;8(5):267–75. https://doi.org/10.1007/s40037-019-00533-8.
29. Devine PG, Forscher PS, Austin AJ, Cox WT. Long-term reduction in implicit race bias: a prejudice habit-breaking intervention. J Exp Soc Psychol. 2012;48(6):1267–78. https://doi.org/10.1016/j.jesp.2012.06.003.

30. Galinsky AD, Moskowitz GB. Perspective-taking: decreasing stereotype expression, stereotype accessibility, and in-group favoritism. J Pers Soc Psychol. 2000;78(4):708–24. https://doi.org/10.1037/0022-3514.78.4.708.
31. Juarez JA, Marvel K, Brezinski KL, Glazner C, Towbin MM, Lawton S. Bridging the gap: a curriculum to teach residents cultural humility. Fam Med. 2006;38(2):97–102.
32. Teal CR, Gill AC, Green AR, Crandall S. Helping medical learners recognise and manage unconscious bias toward certain patient groups. Med Educ. 2012;46(1):80–8. https://doi.org/10.1111/j.1365-2923.2011.04101.x.
33. Vela MB, Erondu AI, Smith NA, Peek ME, Woodruff JN, Chin MH. Eliminating explicit and Implicit biases in health care: evidence and research needs. Annu Rev Public Health. 2022;43:477–501. https://doi.org/10.1146/annurev-publhealth-052620-103528.
34. Marcelin JR, Siraj DS, Victor R, Kotadia S, Maldonado YA. The impact of unconscious bias in healthcare: how to recognize and mitigate it. J Infect Dis. 2019;220(220 Suppl 2):S62–73. https://doi.org/10.1093/infdis/jiz214.
35. Ethnicity LT-KIftSoR: Being an active bystander: strategies for challenging the emergence of bias. 2017. https://u.osu.edu/activebystander/. Accessed 22 Nov 2023.

Chapter 24
Strategies for Promoting Diversity and Inclusion in Surgical Specialties

Ariel Nehemiah

Abstract Representation in the field of surgery is historically homogeneous and does not reflect the increasingly diverse patient population in the United States. Diversity in surgery is important for delivering culturally competent and empathetic surgical care, which can have implications for patient outcomes. Representation in surgery that mirrors the general population also reduces biases among care team members and improves interpersonal communication and working environments. Successful strategies for promoting diversity and inclusion in surgery exist and are discussed. From residency recruitment to retention efforts, mentorship to sponsorship, this chapter provides medical students with a framework for effectively navigating a journey to academic surgery and seeking the best opportunities to advance in the field.

24.1 The Importance of Diversity and Inclusion in Surgery

Surgery has a centuries-long history of exclusion, creating a field of medicine in the United States with a workforce that often does not reflect the patient populations it serves [1–4]. Though efforts are ongoing to eliminate this representation gap, it still exists, particularly for people from racial and ethnic populations underrepresented in medicine (UIM) and people who do not identify as cisgender male [1–4]. Systemic barriers to access to medical education, including but not limited to the financial burden of higher education and biases in medical school selection criteria, are some notable contributors to this disparity [4, 5]. As a field of medicine that provides care to a diverse population of people, surgery needs providers to have the cultural competency required to effectively treat them. Surgical providers who are cognizant of and sensitive to their patients' perceptions of health, whether informed

A. Nehemiah (✉)
Department of Surgery, Perelman School of Medicine, University of Pennsylvania, Philadelphia, PA, USA
e-mail: ariel.nehemiah@pennmedicine.upenn.edu

A. Gillis, C. B. Aarons (eds.), *A How To Guide For Medical Students*, Success in Academic Surgery, https://doi.org/10.1007/978-3-031-66011-5_24

by culture, experience, religion, etc., can better meet their patients where they are and provide patient-centered care [6].

Studies show that racial and/or ethnic concordance between patients and their physicians leads to high levels of trust and better care experiences [6–9]. Similarly, gender concordance between patients and surgeons can lead to lower rates of post-operative complications and more optimal post-operative courses in the eyes of patients [10–12]. In fact, research suggests that female surgeons are more likely to provide guideline-concordant care to their patients regardless of their gender identity [11, 12]. People seem to be more at ease and better able to navigate their care when they share an identity with their physician or when they feel understood by them.

While the systemic barriers to medical education are slowly dismantled, how do we strive for high-quality and equitable surgical care experiences for patients? The answer: diversity and inclusion. A surgical workforce with people of diverse races, ethnicities, gender identities, with diverse world views, backgrounds, and skillsets, provides a greater opportunity for patients to identify in some way with their providers [13]. Furthermore, interactions among individuals of a diverse care team can foster a culture of understanding and drive innovation. This can help providers eliminate their own biases and become more empathetic and culturally competent [13–15]. This empathy and cultural competency not only enhance interactions between patients and providers, but also strengthen relationships among care team members, building community and empowerment in the workplace.

An empathetic and culturally competent surgical provider is better equipped to deliver trustworthy and understandable care to a much broader patient population than a provider who lacks exposure to diversity [14]. Patients are also more likely to maintain relationships with an understanding provider and continue seeking care when needed, which has numerous implications for patient outcomes [9]. In surgery, that could quite literally mean the difference between life and death.

24.2 Recruiting a Diverse Surgical Workforce

As the calls for social justice in the United States rose to deafening levels in 2020, medical organizations like the Association of American Medical Colleges (AAMC) devised plans to "transform rhetoric into action [16]." Included in these plans were nationwide efforts to promote diverse representation in surgery, some of which will be discussed in this chapter.

One method to promote diversity and inclusion in surgery is the visiting clerkship. Visiting clerkship programs directed to students who identify as UIM are employed by some medical institutions to enhance the diversity of the surgical workforce. These programs typically supplement existing visiting clerkship opportunities offered by medical institutions. Targeted outreach to UIM students aims to provide equitable access to sub-internship experiences and broader mentorship networks.

Visiting clerkships are excellent opportunities for students from all backgrounds to demonstrate their capabilities as future trainees and boost their chances of successful matriculation into residency [17–20]. Furthermore, they can give students exposure to subspecialties they may not otherwise get exposure to at their home institutions. Unfortunately, they can be cost-prohibitive for many students who identify as UIM, giving them a competitive disadvantage in the residency application process. Some programs offer stipends or scholarships to offset this burden and level the playing field [18, 19]. The result is a more diverse group of students with an interest in surgery who will be much more likely to apply to the field and successfully matriculate [18–20].

Along with the visiting clerkship, holistic review is a successful method to increase diversity in surgery. According to the AAMC, the holistic review "allows admissions committees to consider the 'whole' applicant, rather than disproportionately focusing on any one factor [21]." This method implores reviewers to consider characteristics and experiences of applicants that equip them for a career in medicine, rather than limit their evaluations strictly to grades and test scores. Holistic review of medical school and residency applications also reduces opportunities for bias to influence applicant selection.

Increasing numbers of surgical residency programs utilize holistic review for residency selection, leading to enhanced diversity in their trainee cohorts [22, 23]. Programs have published data on their holistic review processes, showing that high academic achievement and board exam performance (i.e., United States Medical Licensing Exam or USMLE) can be maintained with these methods [24, 25]. These data challenge concerns that the caliber of surgical residency matriculants is somehow compromised by holistic review. With many medical schools using pass/fail grading systems and the transition of USMLE Step 1 to pass/fail scoring, holistic review methods are now almost necessary to distinguish between candidates.

Efforts to recruit diverse surgical residents are very important components of increasing representation in surgery, but alone are not enough. Diverse representation must also be reflected in the faculty members of a surgical department. The Accreditation Council for Graduate Medical Education (ACGME) requires its programs to have diverse workforces [26]. Some institutions employ holistic review of faculty applications that mirrors the process for residency interview selection [27]. Others implement initiatives that lead to equitable representation in search committees which aids in the recruitment of diverse faculty members [28]. The presence of a faculty cohort that reflects the diversity of its residency and patient population allows for higher quality of patient care and reduced biases in trainee evaluations and promotion metrics for faculty [29].

24.3 Retention and the Role of Mentorship

Recruitment is an important first step toward building a surgical workforce that reflects the population it serves. This representation cannot happen without recruiting people to medical institutions who represent the diversity of their patients. That *brings* people to surgical departments, but what makes them *stay*? The answer: retention efforts.

For many professions, retention refers to the ability of an employer to keep its employees and minimize their turnover [30]. In surgery, retention may look like maintaining residency trainees from matriculation to graduation without transfer or attrition. With attrition rates as high as 20–26%, surgery *needs* retention efforts [31, 32]. Moreover, the people who leave the field are often those who identify as UIM and/or women [31, 32]. These statistics suggest that recruiting diverse candidates into a field with a history of exclusion without the proper retention strategies will not yield success.

Surgery is an inherently hierarchical field that expects medical students, residents, fellows, and attendings alike to respect their seniors and "work their way up" to the next rung of the milestone achievement ladder. In what can seem like a very rigid structure, mentorship is an important retention strategy for building a culture of inclusivity in surgery that fosters success [33, 34]. Mentorship is a relationship between a more experienced and knowledgeable mentor who provides guidance and assistance to a mentee who wants to learn and gain the necessary skills to accomplish their goals. This relationship can help demystify academic surgery and provide needed support through residency training and beyond.

For mentorship to be an effective retention strategy, buy-in from surgical department stakeholders at every level is essential [34]. This means that chairs, vice chairs, senior faculty, junior faculty, and trainees must understand the benefits of mentorship and invest in its implementation in their departments. Chairs and vice chairs can incorporate mentorship into promotion criteria and allocate administrative time to faculty to carry out mentorship work [35]. Faculty can advocate for and use administrative time to participate in mentorship activities with their mentees [35]. Trainees can commit to consistently meeting with their mentors. The documented benefits of mentorship in surgery are convincing and include increased matriculation of mentored students into surgical residency, greater likelihoods of matriculating UIM and women trainees, increased retention of UIM and women trainees as surgical faculty, increased research productivity, improved rates of promotion, and greater career satisfaction [23, 34, 36–38].

24.4 Securing Mentors and Cultivating a Strong Relationship

The first challenge often encountered by medical students interested in academic surgery is identifying potential mentors. Who should hold this role and what characteristics should they have? It is important to understand that people in many positions in medicine can serve as mentors in some capacity, be they fellow medical students, residents, or attendings. In fact, having multiple mentors (a mentorship network) is encouraged, as a diverse mentorship team provides medical students with a more comprehensive education, a larger set of skills, and broader support system [39]. Additionally, the earlier students can obtain mentors, the better they can navigate their journey to academic surgery [40].

Medical students in their preclinical years of medical school do not have the same access to clinical surgical faculty as medical students in their clerkships, which can add an additional layer of difficulty to seeking out potential mentors. Talking with preclinical faculty or fellow medical students about recommendations for mentors can be a great first step. Attending medical conferences sponsored by organizations like the American College of Surgeons (ACS), the Society of Black Academic Surgeons (SBAS), the Latino Surgical Society (LSS), the Association of Women Surgeons (AWS), the Society of Asian Academic Surgeons (SAAS), and the Association of Out Surgeons and Allies (AOSA) can provide excellent opportunities to network with potential mentors and cultivate relationships [40].

It helps to understand one's learning style preferences and personality, as these can influence the types of teaching styles and personalities one seeks in a mentor. Mentees may seek mentors who share an identity with them such as race, ethnicity, or gender, but that is not always essential or feasible. Cross-cultural mentorship also has significant benefits, as it provides mentees diverse perspectives that can inform their academic careers [41–43].

To create an optimal list of potential mentors, there are some best practices to consider. Dedicated time should be set aside for deliberate reflection on the goals one wants to achieve and the skills one wants to master. Writing these down can help organize and clarify one's thoughts. With these goals and skills in mind, one should identify domains in which mentorship is needed. Examples of such domains are personal development, professional development, and research. One should think broadly about the network available and who in that network could provide the best mentorship in the necessary domains. This can require one to look outside of surgery to other specialties and even other institutions. Faculty at one's institution and connections made from conference participation can help identify these individuals.

Once a preliminary list of mentors is created, the next step is to reach out, preferably electronically via email versus phone call, to set up a meeting. During this meeting, goals and needs should be clearly stated to the mentor so they can decide if and how they can provide appropriate guidance [39]. Not every person will have the bandwidth to become a mentor, but they can refer students to other potential mentors and offer informal support in other spaces such as research, surgical education, and surgical residency application.

After establishing a mentorship team, mentees should schedule regular check-ins with their mentors [39, 44]. These check-ins help keep mentees on track to accomplish the goals they previously outlined with their mentors. This allows for better communication, stronger relationships, and quicker resolution of any issues faced by the mentees [39].

Surgical mentors are the front-facing representatives of the surgical field for medical students. The quality of their mentorship can show students the endless possibilities of the field, or conversely steer them clear of it. Proper guidance from surgical mentors allows medical students to feel empowered to explore their curiosities about the field and gain exposure to the different facets of it that will inform their decision to pursue a career in academic surgery. Strong mentors use their capital in their institutions to advance their mentees toward their goals while providing oversight and instilling insight along the way.

A medical student interested in a career in academic surgery is much more likely to maintain interest in the field if they have abundant support from mentors [36, 40]. They are more likely to continue to a surgical residency, potentially a surgical fellowship, and then successful surgical practice. Maintaining and growing their mentorship team through all these phases of their surgical career will preserve their support systems and help them advance in their respective institutions. They can then try their hands at being mentors for the next generation of mentees.

24.5 From Mentorship to Sponsorship

Some mentors can, should, and will become sponsors of their mentees. In fact, many mentoring relationships naturally progress to sponsorship. Sponsorship involves advocacy and active support by the sponsor to help their mentees obtain promotions, awards, or other indicators of achievement within their institution [40, 45]. Sponsors often work behind closed doors, leveraging their position to help their mentees advance in their careers, while mentors work face-to-face with their mentees to aid in their growth. Both relationships are essential for the success of mentees [45].

Establishing good mentorship behaviors like open lines of communication and frequent, regular meetings strengthens the relationship between mentor and mentee [39, 44]. As the mentee progresses through training or faculty appointments, their strong relationship with their mentor can create a path to sponsorship. The groundwork laid down by both parties enables the mentor to transition to sponsor and comfortably advocate for the advancement of their mentee's career to department leadership.

Sponsorship is not unidirectional but in fact bidirectional, with both the sponsor and mentee having opportunities to achieve success. For the mentee, the gain is obvious: academic promotion, committee appointments, funding, etc. [40] For the sponsor, the gain is less conspicuous and comes with risk. When a sponsor advocates for a mentee, they "stick their neck out" for them, using their own position and achievements as collateral of sorts [40]. If their risk is rewarded and their mentee advances, their mentee's successes reflect their success as a sponsor. Similarly, if their mentee does not achieve, that may be seen as failure or miscalculation.

Sponsorship is a powerful tool for young surgeons to create optimal working conditions for them as they ascend the surgery ranks [39, 46, 47]. Strong mentoring relationships with the characteristics discussed allow mentors to have a solid understanding of what their mentees want and need. The mentor can then transition to a sponsor and appropriately advocate for the needs and wants of their mentee. If these conditions are met, the mentees will have much less risk of burnout and dissatisfaction with their department [42].

If the recruitment efforts described matriculate a more diverse surgical workforce, and that workforce works in surgical departments that emphasize and invest in early and frequent mentorship, the opportunities for sponsorship will likely increase exponentially. This exponential increase in sponsorship opportunities allows for the retention and advancement of a much more diverse population of surgeons at every level of the academic surgery continuum. This diverse surgery cohort can then continue to foster an inclusive environment from within its departments and provide culturally competent and high-quality surgical care to its patients in the community.

24.6 Becoming Agents of Change

With the challenges associated with transitioning from medical school to surgical residency and beyond, it can be difficult to be an active contributor to progress within an institution. The important thing to know is that creating and maintaining positive change in surgical programs does not require overextension nor a position of seniority. Small but intentional efforts can help develop a lasting culture of inclusion and support. The following are examples of such efforts:

- Create a mentorship network.

- Everyone does not start at the same place in surgical residency, therefore varying levels of support are needed. Like in medical school, mentors should be secured early and often. Be intentional in self-reflection and creating a plan for development with mentors. Engage with them often. They can make the transition into and journey through residency much smoother.
- Understand that "impostor syndrome" is normal.
- "Impostor syndrome" is a colloquialism that refers to impostor phenomenon, or when high-achieving people fear they will be viewed as incompetent and undeserving of their successes [48]. This fear can lead to self-doubt and burnout. Impostor phenomenon happens to many people at different levels in academic surgery. It is important to share these feelings with peers, mentors, and other

trusted colleagues [48]. This can build a surgical community that is supportive and that validates and celebrates its members [48].

- Lean into passions inside and outside of medicine.
- Surgical training is challenging, but it is not a time to sacrifice one's passions, particularly those that promote diversity and inclusion in the field. Create affinity groups to strengthen support and provide safe spaces for discussion of pertinent issues. Join and participate in national organizations like those listed earlier in this chapter. These groups can provide resources and support to foster change and inclusion in surgery. Engage in community outreach, particularly with populations that are underserved and marginalized. Conduct research that addresses health equity and aims to eliminate healthcare disparities. Maintain hobbies and interests outside of the hospital to stay grounded and avoid burnout. Remember, time outside of training is limited and everything cannot be done at once. However, with intention and scheduling, one can continue pursuing one's passions within and aside from medicine.
- Lift as you climb.
- Trainees can be agents of change in the representation and mentorship pipeline. Intentional peer mentorship within and outside of one's institution is extremely important for network and community building. Peer mentorship can look like many things, including wellness check-ins, knowledge-sharing, or advocating to program leadership. Peer mentorship can empower junior residents and medical students to be more engaged in team dynamics, improve camaraderie among trainees, secure research experiences, and even create job opportunities down the road.
- Do not accept the status quo.

- The learning environment in residency is dynamic. Questioning existing practices, policies, and norms of an institution is an important part of meaningful change. Do not be afraid to ask questions when they arise. Mentors and peer mentors can give advice on how to best approach certain issues and can also be sources of support and advocacy. There is strength in numbers. An inclusive community of residents can move the needle in the direction they need.

If the above efforts are performed by even a fraction of the members of a surgical program, positive change can happen. Medical students and residents are key stakeholders in academic surgery programs at teaching hospitals. As such, they hold a tremendous amount of capital, and their opinions carry weight in the system. Together, they can use this capital to mold surgery into a diverse and inclusive field that also mirrors the patient populations they care for.

References

1. Abelson JS, Symer MM, Yeo HL, Butler PD, Dolan PT, Moo TA, Watkins AC. Surgical time out: our counts are still short on racial diversity in academic surgery. Am J Surg. 2018;215(4):542–8. https://doi.org/10.1016/j.amjsurg.2017.06.028.
2. Cortés-Guiral D, Mayol J, Wexner SD. Diversity in surgery: a historical, international, and contemporary perspective. Curr Surg Rep. 2021;9(5):14.
3. Green RL, Kling SM, Dunham P, Erkmen CP, Kuo LE. Gender diversity in surgery: a review. Curr Surg Rep. 2022;10(6):71–82.
4. Strong BL. Diversity, equity and inclusion in acute care surgery: a multifaceted approach. Trauma Surg Acute Care Open. 2021;6(Suppl 1):e000647. https://doi.org/10.1136/tsaco-2020-000647.
5. Weir K. Inequality at school: What's behind the racial disparity in our education system. Monit Psychol. 2016;47(10):44–7.
6. Butler PD, Longaker MT, Britt LD. Major deficit in the number of underrepresented minority academic surgeons persists. Ann Surg. 2008;248(5):704–11. https://doi.org/10.1097/SLA.0b013e31817f2c30.
7. Takeshita J, Wang S, Loren AW, et al. Association of racial/ethnic and gender concordance between patients and physicians with patient experience ratings. JAMA Netw Open. 2020;3(11):e2024583. https://doi.org/10.1001/jamanetworkopen.2020.24583.
8. Shen MJ, Peterson EB, Costas-Muñiz R, Hernandez MH, Jewell ST, Matsoukas K, Bylund CL. The effects of race and racial concordance on patient-physician communication: a systematic review of the literature. J Racial Ethn Health Disparities. 2018;5(1):117–40. https://doi.org/10.1007/s40615-017-0350-4.
9. Ma A, Sanchez A, Ma M. The impact of patient-provider race/ethnicity concordance on provider visits: updated evidence from the medical expenditure panel survey. J Racial Ethnic Health Disparities. 2019;6:1011–20. https://doi.org/10.1007/s40615-019-00602-y.
10. Khan MMM, Munir MM, Woldesenbet S, Endo Y, Rawicz-Pruszyński K, Katayama E, Ejaz A, Cloyd J, Dilhoff M, Pawlik TM. Association of surgeon-patient sex concordance with postoperative outcomes following complex cancer surgery. J Surg Oncol. 2023;129:489–98. https://doi.org/10.1002/jso.27527.
11. Wallis CJD, Jerath A, Coburn N, Klaassen Z, Luckenbaugh AN, Magee DE, Hird AE, Armstrong K, Ravi B, Esnaola NF, Guzman JCA, Bass B, Detsky AS, Satkunasivam R. Association of Surgeon-Patient sex Concordance with Postoperative Outcomes. JAMA Surg. 2022;157(2):146–56. https://doi.org/10.1001/jamasurg.2021.6339.
12. Wallis CJ, Jerath A, Ikesu R, Satkunasivam R, Dimick JB, Orav EJ, Maggard-Gibbons M, Li R, Salles A, Klaassen Z, Coburn N, Bass BL, Detsky AS, Tsugawa Y. Association between patient-surgeon gender concordance and mortality after surgery in the United States: retrospective observational study. BMJ (Clinical Research ed). 2023;383:e075484. https://doi.org/10.1136/bmj-2023-075484.
13. Cohen JJ, Gabriel BA, Terrell C. The case for diversity in the health care workforce. Health Aff (Project Hope). 2002;21(5):90–102. https://doi.org/10.1377/hlthaff.21.5.90.
14. Saha S, Guiton G, Wimmers PF, Wilkerson L. Student body racial and ethnic composition and diversity-related outcomes in US medical schools. JAMA. 2008;300(10):1135–45. https://doi.org/10.1001/jama.300.10.1135.
15. Marrast LM, Zallman L, Woolhandler S, Bor DH, McCormick D. Minority physicians' role in the care of underserved patients: diversifying the physician workforce may be key in addressing health disparities. JAMA Intern Med. 2014;174(2):289–91. https://doi.org/10.1001/jamainternmed.2013.12756.
16. "Addressing and Eliminating Racism at the AAMC and Beyond." AAMC. www.aamc.org/addressing-and-eliminating-racism-aamc-and-beyond. Accessed 10 Jan 2024.

17. Mueller PS, McConahey LL, Orvidas LJ, Jenkins SM, Kasten MJ. The visiting medical student clerkship program at mayo clinic. Mayo Clin Proc. 2010;85(8):723–7. https://doi.org/10.4065/mcp.2009.0511.
18. Butler PD, Aarons CB, Ahn J, Wein AJ, Ruckenstein MJ, Lett E, DeMatteo RP, Serletti JM. Leading from the front: an approach to increasing racial and ethnic diversity in surgical training programs. Ann Surg. 2019;269(6):1012–5. https://doi.org/10.1097/SLA.0000000000003197.
19. Nellis JC, Eisele DW, Francis HW, Hillel AT, Lin SY. Impact of a mentored student clerkship on underrepresented minority diversity in otolaryngology-head and neck surgery. Laryngoscope. 2016;126(12):2684–8. https://doi.org/10.1002/lary.25992.
20. Mason BS, Ross W, Ortega G, Chambers MC, Parks ML. Can a strategic pipeline initiative increase the number of women and underrepresented minorities in orthopaedic surgery? Clin Orthop Relat Res. 2016;474(9):1979–85. https://doi.org/10.1007/s11999-016-4846-8.
21. "Holistic Review." AAMC. www.aamc.org/services/member-capacity-building/holistic-review. Accessed 10 Jan 2024.
22. Burks CA, Russell TI, Goss D, Ortega G, Randolph GW, Varvares MA, Brown DJ, Gray ST, Bergmark RW. Strategies to increase racial and ethnic diversity in the surgical workforce: a state of the art review. Otolaryngol Head Neck Surg. 2022;166(6):1182–91. https://doi.org/10.1177/01945998221094461.
23. Mabeza RM, Christophers B, Ederaine SA, Glenn EJ, Benton-Slocum ZP, Marcelin JR. Interventions associated with racial and ethnic diversity in US graduate medical education: a scoping review. JAMA Netw Open. 2023;6(1):e2249335. https://doi.org/10.1001/jamanetworkopen.2022.49335.
24. Nehemiah A, Roberts SE, Song Y, Kelz RR, Butler PD, Morris JB, Aarons CB. Looking beyond the numbers: increasing diversity and inclusion through holistic review in general surgery recruitment. J Surg Educ. 2021;78(3):763–9. https://doi.org/10.1016/j.jsurg.2020.08.048.
25. Steward L, Nehler M, Zweck-Bronner S, Christian N. Implementation of a holistic review process of US allopathic medical students eliminates non-comparable metrics and bias in general surgery residency interview invitations. J Surg Educ. 2023;80(11):1536–43. https://doi.org/10.1016/j.jsurg.2023.07.008.
26. Common Program Requirements—Residency—ACGME. www.acgme.org/globalassets/pfassets/programrequirements/cprresidency_2023.pdf. Accessed 15 Jan 2024.
27. Harris TB, Jacobs NN, Fuqua CF, Lyness JM, Smith PO, Poll-Hunter NI, Piggott C, Monroe AD. Advancing equity in academic medicine through holistic review for faculty recruitment and retention. Acad Med. 2022;97(5):631–4. https://doi.org/10.1097/ACM.0000000000004568.
28. Arjani S, Tasnim S, Sumra H, Zope M, Riner AN, Reyna C, Henry M, Anand T. It begins with the search committee: promoting faculty diversity at the source. Am J Surg. 2022;223(2):432–5. https://doi.org/10.1016/j.amjsurg.2021.08.027.
29. Ajayi AA, Rodriguez F, de Jesus Perez V. Prioritizing equity and diversity in academic medicine faculty recruitment and retention. JAMA Health Forum. 2021;2(9):e212426. https://doi.org/10.1001/jamahealthforum.2021.2426.
30. Retention | English Meaning. Cambridge Dictionary, dictionary.cambridge.org/dictionary/english/retention. https://dictionary.cambridge.org/dictionary/english/retention. Accessed 10 Jan2024.
31. Hope C, Reilly JJ, Griffiths G, Lund J, Humes D. Factors associated with attrition and performance throughout surgical training: a systematic review and meta-analysis. World J Surg. 2021;45(2):429–42. https://doi.org/10.1007/s00268-020-05844-0.
32. Yeo HL, Abelson JS, Symer MM, Mao J, Michelassi F, Bell R, Sedrakyan A, Sosa JA. Association of time to attrition in surgical residency with individual resident and programmatic factors. JAMA Surg. 2018;153(6):511–7. https://doi.org/10.1001/jamasurg.2017.6202.
33. Bernstein DN, Mesfin A. What's important: cross-cultural mentorship in orthopaedic surgery: reflections from a black Mentor and white mentee. J Bone Joint Surg Am. 2022;104(3):293–5. https://doi.org/10.2106/JBJS.21.00328.

34. Choi AMK, Moon JE, Steinecke A, Prescott JE. Developing a culture of mentorship to strengthen academic medical centers. Acad Med. 2019;94(5):630–3. https://doi.org/10.1097/ACM.0000000000002498.
35. Maisel NC, Halvorson MA, Finney JW, Bi X, Hayashi KP, Blonigen DM, Weitlauf JC, Timko C, Cronkite RC. Institutional incentives for mentoring at the U.S. department of veterans affairs and universities: associations with Mentors' perceptions and time spent mentoring. Acad Med. 2017;92(4):521–7. https://doi.org/10.1097/ACM.0000000000001507.
36. Ulloa JG, Viramontes O, Ryan G, Wells K, Maggard-Gibbons M, Moreno G. Perceptual and structural facilitators and barriers to becoming a surgeon: a qualitative study of African American and Latino Surgeons. Acad Med. 2018;93(9):1326–34. https://doi.org/10.1097/ACM.0000000000002282.
37. Boatright D, London M, Soriano AJ, Westervelt M, Sanchez S, Gonzalo JD, McDade W, Fancher TL. Strategies and best practices to improve diversity, equity, and inclusion among US graduate medical education programs. JAMA Netw Open. 2023;6(2):e2255110. https://doi.org/10.1001/jamanetworkopen.2022.55110.
38. DeCastro R, Griffith KA, Ubel PA, Stewart A, Jagsi R. Mentoring and the career satisfaction of male and female academic medical faculty. Acad Med. 2014;89(2):301–11. https://doi.org/10.1097/ACM.0000000000000109.
39. Villano Anthony. Surgical mentorship and the mentee to mentor transition. Association for Academic Surgery (AAS), 5 Dec. 2022. www.aasurg.org/blog/surgical-mentorship-and-the-mentee-to-mentor-transition/.
40. Williams-Karnesky RL, Kashyap M, Courtney C, Park C, Ritter KA, Hanke R. Shoring up the pipeline: increasing diversity in surgery by enhancing equity and inclusion in the surgical learning environment. Bulletin of the American College of Surgeons; 2021.
41. Campbell KM, Rodríguez JE. Mentoring underrepresented minority in medicine (URMM) students across racial, ethnic and institutional differences. J Natl Med Assoc. 2018;110(5):421–3.
42. Johnson-Bailey J, Cervero RM. Mentoring in black and white: the intricacies of cross-cultural mentoring. Mentor Tutor. 2004;12(1):7–21.
43. Campbell KM, Rodríguez JE. Addressing the minority tax: perspectives from two diversity leaders on building minority faculty success in academic medicine. Acad Med. 2019;94(12):1854–7. https://doi.org/10.1097/ACM.0000000000002839.
44. Nassour I, Balentine C, Boland GM, Chu D, Habermann E, Holscher C, Idrees K, In H, Kimbrough MK, Mitchem J, Warner SG, Karakousis G, Committee on Academic Advancement of the Association for Academic Surgery. Successful mentor-mentee relationship. J Surg Res. 2020;247:332–4. https://doi.org/10.1016/j.jss.2019.09.066.
45. Patton EW, Griffith KA, Jones RD, Stewart A, Ubel PA, Jagsi R. Differences in mentor-mentee sponsorship in male vs female recipients of national institutes of health grants. JAMA Intern Med. 2017;177(4):580–2. https://doi.org/10.1001/jamainternmed.2016.9391.
46. Bickel J, Brown AJ. Generation X: implications for faculty recruitment and development in academic health centers. Acad Med. 2005;80(3):205–10. https://doi.org/10.1097/00001888-200503000-00003.
47. Shanafelt TD, West CP, Sloan JA, Novotny PJ, Poland GA, Menaker R, Rummans TA, Dyrbye LN. Career fit and burnout among academic faculty. Arch Intern Med. 2009;169(10):990–5. https://doi.org/10.1001/archinternmed.2009.70.
48. "How to Overcome Impostor Phenomenon." Monitor on Psychology, American Psychological Association, 1 June 2021. www.apa.org/monitor/2021/06/cover-impostor-phenomenon.

Chapter 25
Understanding the Importance of Self-Care and Mental Health

Simryn Covarrubias, Steven Molina, Emon K. Javadi, and Carter C. Lebares

Abstract Purpose: In this review, we use available literature and data to describe the current understanding of self-care in medical training and practice, discuss its relationship to academic performance, and review the landscape of existing self-care programs within academic surgery. Practical suggestions on how to best maintain mental health and resilience throughout surgical residency and a surgical career will be provided.

Summary: Given the rigorous nature of academic surgery, it is crucial to anticipate stress and its overwhelming effects. Simultaneously, within medicine, burnout is becoming increasingly recognized as a growing workplace hazard that has negative impacts on physicians, patients, and the healthcare economy. While workplace systems and culture play a role in both stress and burnout, emerging evidence shows that individual actions and interventions are also important factors. Recent literature

---

S. Covarrubias
Center for Mindfulness in Surgery, University of California San Francisco, San Francisco, CA, USA
e-mail: scovarrubias@dons.usfca.edu

S. Molina
Center for Mindfulness in Surgery, University of California San Francisco, San Francisco, CA, USA

UCR School of Medicine, University of California Riverside, Riverside, CA, USA
e-mail: Steven.Molina@medsch.ucr.edu

E. K. Javadi
Center for Mindfulness in Surgery, University of California San Francisco, San Francisco, CA, USA

St. George's University School of Medicine, Saint George, Grenada
e-mail: ejavadi@sgu.edu

C. C. Lebares (✉)
Center for Mindfulness in Surgery, University of California San Francisco, San Francisco, CA, USA

Department of Surgery, University of California San Francisco, San Francisco, CA, USA
e-mail: Carter.Lebares@ucsf.edu

A. Gillis, C. B. Aarons (eds.), *A How To Guide For Medical Students*, Success in Academic Surgery, https://doi.org/10.1007/978-3-031-66011-5_25

reveals that adopting self-care practices extends beyond stress reduction, impacting overall quality of life, career trajectory, and resilience. Therefore, learning to prioritize one's well-being, both in theory and in individual practice, is essential for success in academic surgery.

Self-care in medical training and practice is now recognized as a necessary and essential skill. Research involving current medical students, residents and practicing physicians has demonstrated that self-care is an integral part of healthy work-life balance, mitigating the repercussions of burnout which include reduced career longevity, clinical performance, and work satisfaction. Many institutions have made efforts to address these issues with initiatives that focus primarily on physical health (free gym access or increased access to healthy food) and social well-being (happy hours or outings). However, current offerings have been minimally effective to date, and few evidence-based self-care programs exist for residents or attendings. Some interventions, such as facilitated mentorship and peer support, are institutionally supported with growing evidence of benefit and increasing uptake. Nevertheless, individuals preparing for success in today's academic landscape are wise to have a personal plan of self-care that includes (1) consistent basics like exercise, sleep, and healthy food; (2) periodic boosters like social contact outside of work if possible; and (3) prophylactic steps such as cognitive skills training, outside mental health support, and trusted confidantes.

Practical suggestions are explored throughout this chapter. In summary, self-care practices are critical and require individual commitment and preparation, ideally against a back-drop of academic program support and healthy organizational culture.

25.1 Introduction

Academic Surgery is known for being a demanding and challenging field with substantial responsibilities related to research, teaching, and clinical care. By its very nature, academic surgery can cause significant strain on a surgeon's well-being. In recent years, maintaining a healthy work-life balance has gained substantial traction as rates of physician burnout continue to grow, and the associated human and economic costs are recognized. As our understanding of work-life balance continues to evolve, we are observing a shift in culture. Mental health and self-care are now recognized as integral parts of sustaining a healthy work-life balance for all healthcare professionals, especially those who practice within academia.

"Burnout," a clinical syndrome characterized by emotional exhaustion, depersonalization, and a decreased sense of accomplishment, is rooted in workplace systems and culture. Consensus holds that when workplace demands outweigh resources, burnout ensues [1, 2]. The consequences of burnout include a myriad of poor personal health outcomes, notably suicidal ideation, and alcohol/substance abuse. Recent studies have shown that medical students and surgical residents are more likely to experience burnout and mental health disorders such as depression when compared to age-matched peers [3]. While the precise systemic and cultural factors that drive burnout in medicine and surgery are coming to light, there is also growing empirical evidence that individual-level interventions are an important part of the solution.

In this chapter, we explore the link between self-care and mental health and the impact they can have on maintaining the attitudes and behaviors required to achieve academic and professional goals in academic surgery. We will also discuss the current landscape of self-care programs in academic surgery and provide suggestions on how to best maintain mental health throughout surgical residency and a surgical career.

25.2 The Surgeon's Journey: Challenges and Demands

The role of a surgeon necessitates maintaining composure in high-pressure situations, requiring the ability to navigate dynamic situations and make critical decisions swiftly. The stress faced by surgeons can easily become overwhelming, leading to burnout and associated increases in attrition rates, job dissatisfaction, and their associated costs [4]. As mentioned, workplace systems and culture can contribute to stress load (and burnout) and require their own unique solutions and interventions. However, factors such as split-second decision making, high-stakes outcomes, immense responsibility, and inevitable complications are intrinsic to surgical work. This means that, no matter how much we humanize the healthcare/workplace environment, some stress will always remain. Individualized self care practices are particularly important and useful in this area. Optimizing the management of inherent stressors through purposeful training and practices is crucial for surgeons to thrive in their demanding profession. The only resource available to you in every setting and scenario is your own mind, a malleable and trainable resource perpetually at your disposal.

In the next section, we will begin to outline the modern definition of self-care and mental health. This will lay down the foundation required to devise a personalized approach to combat feelings of burnout that you may encounter throughout your career.

25.3 Mental Health + Self-Care

The General Adaptation Syndrome, a model framed by Hans Selye, describes our response to stress in three phases: alarm, resistance, and exhaustion. In the context of medical education, particularly for surgical trainees, the application of the General Adaptation Syndrome model underscores the significant chronic stress experienced during training, contributing to high levels of burnout within surgical specialties [5]. Burnout affects physicians but also undermines the physician-patient relationship and patient outcomes [5]. No group is spared the negative implications of this condition.

It is noteworthy that burnout has been reported at every level of medical training, emphasizing the need to directly address this pervasive issue using a multifaceted approach. Here, we will explore two crucial components: mental health and self-care.

Mental health encompasses a person's emotional, psychological, and social well-being, making it an integral part of one's overall well-being and health. Emotional well-being involves our ability to balance and process our emotions while psychological well-being revolves around aspects of self-acceptance, personal growth, and satisfaction. Lastly, social well-being refers to our interactions with others and our ability to contribute positively to society.

Being in a state of good mental health means that a person is capable of navigating through and coping with various stressful situations and environments, while maintaining a high level of productivity. A common misconception is that the absence of good mental health is synonymous with having a mental health disorder. However, it is important to understand that a person who does not have a mental health disorder may still have poor mental health. Conversely, a person who has been diagnosed with a mental health disorder may still exhibit signs of good mental health.

Our mental health is dynamic and can change over time. It exists on a spectrum and can be influenced by a variety of external factors such as transitions in our work, relationships, or environments. By recognizing that our mental health is susceptible to change and improvement, we can learn how to adapt and maintain our mental well-being through different self-care practices.

Mental health and self-care are undeniably interconnected. Self-care practices vary from individual to individual, but uniformly involve regularly engaging in activities aimed at alleviating our stress and improving our mental health. Practicing self-care is the key to establishing and maintaining a healthy and sustainable relationship with our bodies and minds. This holistic approach to well-being is shaped by family, physical health, socioeconomic well being, and professional culture, among other factors. Self-care practices for medical students encompass a spectrum of activities including nutrition, stress management, physical activity, health responsibility, interpersonal relationships, and spiritual growth.

A comprehensive study identified ten clusters of self-care activities for medical students, encompassing nourishment, hygiene, intellectual and creative health, physical activity, and spiritual care [6, 7] greatly from prioritizing self-care. It is imperative to foster a culture that values self-care and provides support for students to develop these essential skills, particularly during critical transition periods, ensuring their well-being and paving the way for academic success.

In the context of academic surgery, self-care can involve a proactive and personalized approach that prioritizes the health and well-being of surgical providers inside and outside the hospital. While a variety of activities can contribute to self-care, the most effective strategies are mental approaches, such as maintaining a positive outlook, learning to manage stress, and finding meaning in work [8, 9]. There are several ways that individuals may develop these attitudes and skills, but an underlying attribute to each is the ability to identify and manage one's emotional state. In a later section, we will be discussing suggestions in regards to wellness and self care in medical students specifically.

In summary, mental health plays a crucial role as it encompasses emotional, psychological, and social well-being. Emphasizing the dynamic spectrum of mental well-being, we debunked the misconception that its absence is synonymous with mental health disorders. Shifting focus to self-care, we underscored a range of universally essential practices for stress alleviation and mental health enhancement. Within the realm of academic surgery, the importance of fostering a culture that values mental health and self-care becomes evident, stressing the need for a personalized, proactive approach for building resilience and sustainability in surgical practice [9].

25.4 The Link Between Self-Care and Academic Success

As mentioned, self-care is undeniably paramount for medical students and physicians, especially given the rigorous nature of medical education and practice. Decades of research unequivocally demonstrate that overwhelming stress negatively impacts cognition, individual physiology, and long-term performance [10]. Stress can be influenced by family, physical health, and professional culture, among other factors. Notably, research on human social genomics carried out by Slavich and Cole highlights how changes to our environment and external social conditions can influence gene expression [11]. Recognizing that social or environmental changes can impact an individual's level of stress is crucial to our understanding of stress management. Furthermore, stress can also have direct implications on career longevity and clinical performance. Specifically, work-related burnout in surgeons is associated with decreased work satisfaction and is the greatest predictor of intent to leave practice. Studies indicate that adopting multiple self-care strategies can bolster resilience and mitigate distress levels [12].

Johnson et al. examined the impact of mindfulness training on resilience mechanisms among active-duty marines preparing for deployment. This study focused on active marines because of the observed effects that military deployment can have on one's physical and mental health. It is important to note that the authors highlight a current knowledge gap regarding stress recovery and our ability to adapt our behaviors prior to facing stressful situations. In order to gain more insight, they used a specific mindfulness-based intervention aimed at understanding this mechanism related to stress recovery. This study found beneficial effects across three different categories (heart and breathing rate, biomarkers, neuroimaging results) [13]. These findings suggest a crucial role for mindfulness interventions in enhancing stress recovery. While the study centered on military deployments, its implications reach beyond, as evidenced by the similar positive outcomes in a non-clinical sample.

This emphasizes the potential for mindfulness-based interventions to extend their benefits beyond the military context.

These insights carry particular relevance to the growing burnout rates experienced by healthcare professionals. As mentioned previously, burnout is deeply embedded in our workplace systems.

Al-Ghunaim et al. conducted a systematic review to investigate the association between surgeon burnout and patient safety and surgical professionalism. This review found that surgeon burnout was "significantly associated with a higher incidence of medical errors" and "poorer patient safety" [14]. Thus, there is a growing need for interventions that can help mitigate this burnout and improve overall well-being for surgeons.

Luton et al. studied the impact of enrolling new surgical trainees into a five-week Enhanced Stress Resilience Training (ESRT) course as well as the feasibility of delivering an ESRT course to surgical trainees [15]. This course was designed to teach surgical trainees and provide them with tools to manage their work stress and burnout. The study's findings indicate not only the feasibility of implementing an ESRT course but also reveals "themes alluding to trainees wanting formalized methods to manage stress, to care for their mental health and engage in mindfulness."

It is evident that self-care practices are a necessary aspect of medical education and career development. It involves proactively mitigating unnecessary stressors and maintaining grounded and realistic expectations. By defining self-care on an individual level, medical students can enhance their well-being and approach their careers with confidence. Integrating self-care into the academic environment can be achieved through various techniques. For instance, establishing structured study hours has been found to be beneficial for reducing stress among medical students. By implementing a study schedule, students can create a clear boundary between study time and personal time, allowing them to prioritize self-care activities and feel recharged for the following day. Additionally, rewarding small achievements, such as successful exam completion, with leisure activities can serve as a positive reinforcement for the hard work and dedication required in medical training [12].

In conclusion, the integration of self-care practices with medical training is not just about promoting well-being; it is a strategic investment for the success and resilience of future physicians. Further, by fostering a culture that values self-care and providing support for its development, academic institutions can significantly contribute to the overall success of medical trainees as they develop into attending physicians, ultimately benefiting the healthcare system as a whole.

25.5 Current Status of Self-Care Programs in Academic Surgery

As stated above, the landscape of academic surgery has undergone a transformative shift, with an increased focus on the holistic well-being of surgical residents. This shift responds to the alarming statistic that physician burnout now affects 44% of practicing physicians in the United States, marking it not just as an individual concern but as a systemic issue requiring comprehensive intervention [16]. Individual-level interventions, such as purposeful self-care practices, have growing evidence of value and impact in this area. Specifically, a strong body of research in medicine and other high-stakes professions have demonstrated the direct impact of overwhelming stress and burnout on performance, longevity and success. This section delves into the current state of self-care programs in academic surgery, exploring precipitating factors, two case studies exemplifying innovative approaches (UPMC Neurosurgery Wellness Initiative and Stanford's "Balance in Life" program), challenges faced, and the promising path forward.

25.6 Historical Context

Burnout is pervasive through surgical training, with recent studies showing a prevalence as high as 69%, linked to high stress, depression, and suicidal ideation [3]. In the early 2000's, the Accreditation Council for Graduate Medical Education (ACGME) implemented the 80-h work week to combat burnout, yet the effects of this policy have been mixed. However, a recent study found that resident mistreatment contributes more to burnout than frequent duty hour violations [17].

Recognizing the importance of trainee well-being, the ACGME has included well-being as a common program requirement and required that schools include "policies and programs that encourage optimal resident and faculty member well-being." Broadly, the ACGME policies call for the creation of formalized systems to identify burnout and depression, fostering a culture that values wellness. In addition, the 2021 Clinical Learning Environment Review (CLER) reported an overarching theme that programs are focused on individual resilience and responsibility, and a need for "identifying and addressing systems-based factors adversely affecting the well-being of all members of the care team." This is underpinned by literature supporting the notion that burnout is a systemic issue rather than an individual one, with organizational interventions showing more or the same efficacy as individual-level interventions.

In response to the current landscape and ACGME policies, academic institutions have also implemented various self-care programs. Two case studies illustrate the complexities of these initiatives.

25.7 UPMC Neurosurgery Wellness Initiative

Published literature from the University of Pittsburgh Medical Center Neurosurgery Wellness Initiative highlights challenges in implementation and evaluation of programs, as the group did not find significant changes to resident self-care, burnout, or perceived social support after a series of initiatives that were designed to combat burnout were implemented.

The studied program consisted of a bimonthly wellness lecture series, free access to the hospital gym for residents, group gym visits, and faculty mentorship. At the end of the program, 36% of residents agreed with the statement that they had focused more on their health during the first year of the program, and free gym access was a major contributor to helping residents focus on their physical health. Though most (60%) of participants felt that the lectures were very or mildly helpful, lectures on mental health, mindfulness, and meditation were not well received, mainly because of the esoteric nature of the topics. Importantly, residents anecdotally reported concerns about a lack of perceived faculty and departmental support, the perception that they would be shamed by their peers if they took time to focus on wellness rather than work, and feelings of guilt for making their own wellness a priority over that of their patients.

The program has sought to accept and implement responses to resident feedback. One striking example was in response to trainee reports that revealed difficulty in making medical and dental appointments given the limited hours of community healthcare providers. As a result, collaborations with the School of Dentistry and department of internal medicine have provided residents with off-hours dental cleanings and special office hours for primary care checkups between cases or in the evenings.

25.8 Stanford's "Balance in Life" for General Surgery Residents

Stanford's "Balance in Life" program adopts a multifaceted approach to surgical residency wellness. In 2017, Salles et al. described in a paper the program's focus around 6 main components within 4 broad categories of well-being (physical, psychological, professional, and social). The following bullet points will demonstrate how each category of well-being is respectively supported:

- Physical Well-being: Access to a 24-h stocked refrigerator with healthy snacks and drinks, and an "After Hours" guide showcasing local restaurants, gyms, and local healthcare providers with weekend and late evening hours.
- Psychological Well-being: Regular scheduled confidential group meetings with an experienced psychologist, allowing a space for discussing concerns and coping strategies.

- Professional Well-being: Mentorship and leadership training with peer mentorship and a Class Representation System that meets regularly with the Residency Program Director.
- Social Well-being: Organized events such as sporting events and outdoor activities.

Residents found the fully stocked refrigerator to be extremely valuable, with psychological counseling services and organized social events reported as moderately valuable. However, the Resident Mentorship Program was considered somewhat valuable, while the Class Representation System and After Hours guide were rarely taken advantage of, possibly due to residents' unawareness of these resources.

Salles et al. expanded on these findings, reporting no change to burnout or psychological well-being among residents [18]. Nevertheless, residents exhibited significantly more grit and reported improved sleep and exercise habits. The lack of measured benefit in burnout and psychological well-being can be attributed to continued exposure to the demanding hospital environment and the sacrifice of personal well-being for patient care. Intense and stressful daily interactions further contribute to challenges, including resistance from both faculty and residents regarding perceived inefficiencies and financial expenses. Despite challenges, the path forward involves a commitment to fundamental changes in training programs, with both organizational and individual interventions.

25.9 Individual Strategies for Self-Care in Academic Surgery

Here, we will focus on how one can implement self-care on an individual level. Personalized interventions can target both emotional self-care as well as psychosocial self-care.

25.10 Emotional Self-Care in Academic Surgery

Emotional self-care stands as a cornerstone of overall well-being, especially in the demanding and high-stakes environment of academic surgery. Developing emotional intelligence and establishing robust support systems are integral strategies for medical students and surgeons to navigate the challenges, pressures, and emotional demands intrinsic to their profession.

In surgery, the significance of technical expertise is undisputable. However, the evolving landscape of healthcare has underscored an equally crucial facet of surgical ability—emotional intelligence (EI). Composed of the ability to recognize, understand, manage, and leverage one's own emotions and those of others, EI has emerged as a vital aspect in surgical practice. As the academic surgical community grapples with burnout rates, high-stakes decision fatigue, and the complex dynamics of patient interactions, the cultivation of EI emerges as an indispensable tool for enhancing overall well-being, resilience, and ultimately, the quality of patient care.

Here we offer several evidence-based methods to increase your emotional intelligence, based on 2 important EI traits: self-awareness and self-regulation.

Self-awareness serves as the foundational step in emotional intelligence, involving an understanding of one's emotions, strengths, limitations, biases, beliefs, and motivation. Only after gaining a clear understanding of yourself can you effectively make values-based decisions, communicate, and empathize with others.

One way to cultivate enhanced self-awareness is through meditation, which focuses on improving our moment-to-moment awareness. While many programs and institutions offer meditation-based classes or services, meditation does not need to be a formalized or structured process. Simple, everyday activities such as doing laundry, washing dishes, exercising, or walking can serve as opportunities to notice and enhance awareness of the five senses, emotions, and one's overall state of mind.

Here are some other ways to practice mindful meditation:

- Body scans: While taking deep breaths, bring attention to your body from head to toe, noticing and letting go of any discomforts.
- The Raisin Exercise: Hold a raisin. What do you taste, feel, smell, see, hear?
- Progressive Muscle Relaxation: Go from one muscle to the next, from head to toe, squeezing and relaxing.

If you recognize that you are feeling intense emotions, it can become vital to take a step back, objectively re-evaluate those emotions, and move forward in a way that aligns with your values and goals. We want to mention self-compassion here as well, as practicing kindness with ourselves allows us to maintain well-being and move forward from troubling thoughts.

By investing in building emotional intelligence you can cultivate resilience, enhance your ability to navigate emotional challenges, and contribute to a healthier and more sustainable academic surgical environment.

25.11 Cognitive Skills Training (Mindfulness)

Psychological self-care focuses on both our mental and emotional well-being. A widely embraced practice of psychological self-care is mindfulness, which emphasizes being aware in the present moment. Mindfulness involves being able to recognize the interconnected nature of emotions and thus consciously respond to them rather than reacting on impulses. In recent years, mindfulness has emerged as a potential intervention to reduce and protect against burnout among physicians, reduce medical errors, and increase professionalism.

A pilot clinical trial followed first-year surgical residents at University of California, San Francisco who were randomly assigned to an 8-week "Mindfulness-Based Stress Reduction (MBSR) course [19]." The trial assessed the surgical residents in six different categories—demand, implementation, practicality, acceptability, adaptation, and integration. The study found that implementing mindfulness-based training is both "feasible and acceptable for surgical interns at a tertiary academic medical center." However, it is important to note that while change on an institutional level is necessary, we also recognize that implementation of such an intervention into an academic setting can be a time-consuming process. Mindfulness-based training on an individual level can serve as a valuable intervention in the interim.

Engaging in regular mindfulness practices can help to improve focus, regulate emotions, control impulses and executive functioning. Mindfulness practice can significantly benefit and improve the lives and well-being of both medical students and academic surgeons.

Mindfulness meditation involves four main components:

1. Regular and Intentional Practice
2. Gratitude
3. Mini Meditations Throughout the Day
4. Learning to Reframe Negative Thoughts

Incorporating these four elements into mindfulness-based practices can allow individuals to improve their well-being both in the present and over the long-term. It is important to note that there are also other ways to learn and practice mindfulness through mindfulness-based courses, guest speakers and mindfulness apps. These alternatives can serve as foundational tools to guide medical trainees as they navigate this demanding profession and learn how to establish sustainable self-care and well-being practices. Mindfulness courses such as Enhanced Stress Resilience Training (ESRT) have been shown to have "potential benefits to well being and executive function in the time-compressed and high-stake surgical training environment [20]."

25.12 Implementing Self-Care Strategies in Medical School

In the demanding field of academic surgery, where the rigors of research, teaching, and clinical care converge, self-care is indispensable. As medical students navigate this challenging journey, prioritizing personal well-being becomes crucial. This section briefly revisits the significance of self-care among medical students, emphasizing its crucial role in maintaining optimal mental health, integral to the overall success and resilience on their path to becoming surgery residents, while specifically focusing on a detailed exploration of tailored strategies and coping methods designed to enhance well-being and academic achievement.

25.13 Significance of Self-Care in Medical School

Medical school introduces a myriad of stressors that significantly impact the well-being of students. The rigorous academic demands, coupled with the weight of intense workloads, create an environment where individuals are constantly challenged. In addition to academic pressures, medical trainees struggle with the psychological toll of their responsibilities, often facing personal life events that add to the complexity of their experiences.

Studies show that the primary source of stress for medical students revolves around the medical curriculum [21]. Among the stressors identified, the top three perceived as highly stressful include examinations, coping with a substantial amount of content, and the perceived lack of time for review. Medical students deal with an overwhelming volume of information to be mastered within a constrained time frame for examinations. The resulting information overload gives rise to sentiments of academic dismay, with numerous medical students experiencing a sense of incapacity to adequately review all subjects to achieve their individual examination performance objectives.

Recent research underscores the prevalence of burnout and mental health challenges among medical students, with alarming statistics revealing that 49% met criteria for burnout, 17% experienced moderate to severe depression, and 23% attributed the development of depression to their coping challenges [22]. These findings emphasize the necessity for self-care strategies and coping behaviors which influence the mental health and academic performance of medical students, ultimately shaping the quality of patient care they provide.

Recognizing and understanding these stressors are pivotal for effective implementation of self-care strategies tailored to the unique challenges faced during medical training. Once the stressors are acknowledged, the next necessary step involves identifying personalized self-care approaches that resonate with individual preferences and situations [23]. While not all strategies are universally applicable, our findings are scientifically validated through analysis of common stressors in medical students.

25.14 Self-Care Strategies Tailored to Medical Students

Earlier, we explored strategies tailored for medical students, such as structured study hours, positive reinforcement for small achievements, cultivating emotional intelligence through practices like meditation, and prioritizing psychological well-being with mindfulness. However, here we will discuss additional and distinct strategies to further enhance the well-being of medical students throughout their academic journey.

What remains indisputable is the essential role of adopting healthy lifestyle behaviors including nutritious eating, adequate rest, relaxation techniques, exercise, and humor. This assertion is reinforced by a study conducted at the University of Pittsburgh School of Medicine, where results revealed substantial correlation between decreased exercise frequency and lower professional efficacy, as well as a connection between pathological sleepiness and a higher prevalence of burnout [24]. Furthermore, inadequate sleep was linked to lower professional efficacy and higher exhaustion scores. In light of these findings, it becomes evident that maintaining healthy lifestyle behaviors is not just a matter of personal well-being but also plays a pivotal role in mitigating burnout risks among medical residents.

In this context, fostering resilience emerges as a key element of academic success, tightly connected to the adoption of healthy lifestyle behaviors. Resilience is nurtured through mindful awareness, adhering to safety precautions, managing fatigue, and recognizing when wellness strategies are necessary. Various elements such as nutrition, exercise, sleep hygiene, gratitude, spirituality, cognitive restructuring, setting boundaries, and incorporating humor contribute to building resilience. The narrative one crafts, language choices, and the cultivation of creativity also play pivotal roles in fostering resilience and mitigating distress for a successful academic and professional trajectory [25].

To reinforce this perspective, medical students are encouraged to cultivate a positive and health-oriented perspective regarding academic pursuits. An effective approach documented for enhancing this mindset is the utilization of the DEAL-based practice [25]. This psychoeducational tool provides a systematic and effective method for medical students to manage stress sources, thereby contributing to the reduction of psychological pressures [26].

The DEAL model comprises four key components: **D**etection of stressors, **E**valuation of stressors, **A**ction towards stressors, and **L**earning from stressors through self-reflection. Several guiding principles have been established through the DEAL model. These principles involve instructing students in early problem detection and promoting a positive outlook toward challenges. Additionally, they guide students in positively and appropriately appraising problems, teach effective coping strategies for problems, and foster an environment that encourages students to extract valuable lessons from challenges for continuous self-improvement. Through engaging in DEAL-based intervention, individuals gain deeper insights into their personal stress management abilities, facilitated by heightened self-awareness, experiential learning, and conscious effort [27]. The intervention effectively alleviated perceived academic stressors, a significant concern for medical students, as those who perceived high academic stress were 16 times more likely to develop psychological distress [28]. The DEAL model's ability to reduce such stressors supports its potential as a valuable self-care strategy tailored to the unique challenges faced by medical students.

Our exploration here sets the stage for the next section, where we discuss the broader landscape of surgical careers. This involves acknowledging ongoing challenges and advocating for a pervasive culture of well-being at every stage of a medical professional's journey.

25.15 The Ongoing Journey

Research underscores the importance of integrating self-care strategies into medical education. Despite this, medical schools and residency programs struggle with implementation due to the lack of established guidelines for effective integration. Effective strategies to address these challenges include conducting targeted needs assessments, implementing mental and physical health improvements, identifying and addressing barriers to self-care, and continuously evaluating interventions.

Kern's six-step curriculum development model highlights the importance of starting with a targeted needs assessment and focusing on identifying a specific population's specific needs and problems (e.g., residents in a particular training program). Key metrics to consider when selecting appropriate assessment tools include cost, frequency, ease of completion, and whether it has been studied in target populations.

A recent study revealed that only a fraction of medical schools have a structured and defined well-being competency, with effectiveness being primarily measured through participation and satisfaction rates. Recommended tools by the ACGME for institutional and individual assessment include: The Maslach Burnout Inventory for healthcare professionals (MBI-HSS) and Mayo Clinic Well-Being Index.

On an institutional level, recommendations include creating schedules with designated time off for health and well-being appointments and fostering a culture that prioritizes self-care. Initiatives such as team-based care models and facilitated-group interventions showcase the potential impact of organizational changes, ultimately aiming to create an environment where residents not only survive but thrive, recognizing the symbiotic relationship between physician well-being and the quality of patient care.

To successfully integrate a self-care curriculum into medical education, well-being must become an institutional priority. The establishment of a wellness committee, composed of both residents and faculty, can aid developing effective wellness learning and interventions. Promoting a culture of well-being in any organization requires a collective effort towards the prioritization of mental health and self-care practices.

Program directors (PDs) and faculty play a critical role in fostering student wellness. They can actively help students recognize signs of distress and connect them to the appropriate resources and care. Residents are more inclined to both seek and accept wellness assistance when recommended by their PDs or faculty, highlighting the critical role of faculty mentorship, especially for women and underrepresented minorities.

25.16 Conclusion: Thriving in Academic Surgery Through Self-Care and Mental Health

To summarize, we dived into the intricate interplay between self-care, mental health, and the challenging landscape of academic surgery. Recognizing the unique stresses faced by surgeons, we have emphasized the critical need for tailored strategies in optimizing stress management. The concept of self-care has emerged as a pivotal element, with implications extending beyond individual well-being to impact the broader surgical community.

Linking self-care to academic success, we examined the multifaceted nature of this concept, acknowledging its profound influence on medical students and physicians. Our work revealed that adopting self-care practices not only to reduce stress but also to enhance overall quality of life and resilience. Analysis of current self-care programs in academic surgery, such as the UPMC Neurosurgery Wellness Initiative and Stanford's "Balance in Life" program, offered insights into the potential benefits and challenges of integrating well-being programs into surgical residency.

Moreover, we also described individual strategies for self-care, focusing on emotional and psychological well-being. Recognizing the significance of emotional intelligence in surgery, we explored evidence-based methods that can be used to enhance self-awareness and self-regulation. Mindfulness, highlighted as a powerful tool, showcased feasibility and acceptability among surgical interns. Our discussion of the ongoing journey of maintaining mental health throughout a surgical career, emphasized the importance of integrating self-care strategies into both medical education and residency programs.

In conclusion, this chapter underscores the pivotal role of self-care in the holistic well-being of surgeons and the potential impact on the quality of patient care. The recommendations provided, including fostering a culture prioritizing mental health, offer a roadmap for creating environments where surgical professionals not only navigate challenges but thrive in their careers. As we contemplate the future, we are compelled to embrace innovative approaches and expand our thinking to foster a culture where well-being is not just encouraged but embedded in the fabric of academic surgery.

References

1. Maslach C, Leiter MP. Understanding the burnout experience: recent research and its implications for psychiatry. World Psychiatry. 2016;15(2):103–11. https://doi.org/10.1002/wps.20311. PMID: 27265691; PMCID: PMC4911781
2. Van Doorn JR. Marylène Gagné (Ed.), the oxford handbook of work engagement, motivation, and self-determination theory. Psychol Learn Teach. 2015;14(2):205–9. https://doi.org/10.1177/1475725715584700.

3. Golisch KB, Sanders JM, Rzhetsky A, Tatebe LC. Addressing surgeon burnout through a multi-level approach: a national call to action. Curr Trauma Rep. 2023;9(2):28–39. https://doi.org/10.1007/s40719-022-00249-x. Epub 2023 Jan 17. PMID: 36688090; PMCID: PMC9843106
4. Patel RS, Bachu R, Adikey A, Malik M, Shah M. Factors related to physician burnout and its consequences: a review. Behav Sci (Basel). 2018;8(11):98. https://doi.org/10.3390/bs8110098. PMID: 30366419; PMCID: PMC6262585
5. Scheepers RA, Boerebach BC, Arah OA, Heineman MJ, Lombarts KM. A systematic review of the impact of physicians' occupational well-being on the quality of patient care. Int J Behav Med. 2015;22(6):683–98. https://doi.org/10.1007/s12529-015-9473-3. PMID: 25733349; PMCID: PMC4642595
6. Ayala EE, Omorodion AM, Nmecha D, Winseman JS, Mason HRC. What do medical students do for self-care? A student-centered approach to well-being. Teach Learn Med. 2017;29(3):237–46. https://doi.org/10.1080/10401334.2016.1271334. Epub 2017 Feb 16
7. Schuster M. The case for self-care among physicians. Med Econ. 2023;100(2):28. Gale Academic OneFile. link.gale.com/apps/doc/A737640435/AONE?u=anon~9d9cf069&sid=googleScholar&xid=4269d a43. Accessed 6 Jan 2024
8. Shanafelt TD, Balch CM, Dyrbye L, et al. Special report: suicidal ideation among American surgeons. Arch Surg. 2011;146(1):54–62. https://doi.org/10.1001/archsurg.2010.292.
9. Ball S, Bax A. Self-care in medical education: effectiveness of health-habits interventions for first-year medical students. Acad Med. 2002;77(9):911–7.
10. McEwen BS, Sapolsky RM. Stress and cognitive function. Curr Opin Neurobiol. 1995;5(2):205–16. https://doi.org/10.1016/0959-4388(95)80028-x.
11. Slavich GM, Cole SW. The emerging field of human social genomics. Clin Psychol Sci. 2013;1(3):331–48. https://doi.org/10.1177/2167702613478594.
12. Ayala EE, Winseman JS, Johnsen RD, et al. U.S. medical students who engage in self-care report less stress and higher quality of life. BMC Med Educ. 2018;18:189. https://doi.org/10.1186/s12909-018-1296-x.
13. Johnson DC, Thom NJ, Stanley EA, Haase L, Simmons AN, Shih PA, Thompson WK, Potterat EG, Minor TR, Paulus MP. Modifying resilience mechanisms in at-risk individuals: a controlled study of mindfulness training in marines preparing for deployment. Am J Psychiatry. 2014;171(8):844–53. https://doi.org/10.1176/appi.ajp.2014.13040502.
14. Al-Ghunaim TA, Johnson J, Biyani CS, Alshahrani KM, Dunning A, O'Connor DB. Surgeon burnout, impact on patient safety and professionalism: a systematic review and meta-analysis. Am J Surg. 2022;224(1):228–38.
15. Luton OW, James OP, Mellor K, Eley C, Hopkins L, Robinson DBT, et al. Enhanced stress-resilience training for surgical trainees. BJS Open. 2021;5(4):zrab054.
16. Berg S. Physician burnout: new AMA effort to close solutions research gap. American Medical Association; 2019. https://www.ama-assn.org/practice-management/sustainability/physician-burnout-new-ama-effort-close-solutions-research-gap
17. Hu YY, Ellis RJ, Hewitt DB, Yang AD, Cheung EO, Moskowitz JT, et al. Discrimination, abuse, harassment, and burnout in surgical residency training. N Engl J Med. 2019;381(18):1741–52.
18. Salles A, Cohen GL, Mueller CM. The relationship between grit and resident Well-being. Am J Surg. 2014;207(2):251–4. https://doi.org/10.1016/j.amjsurg.2013.09.006.
19. Lebares CC, Hershberger AO, Guvva EV, Desai A, Mitchell J, Shen W, et al. Feasibility of formal mindfulness-based stress-resilience training among surgery interns: a randomized clinical trial. JAMA Surg. 2018;153(10):–e182734.
20. Dave U, Taylor-Robinson SD. Maintaining resilience in today's medical environment: personal perspectives on self-care. Int J Gen Med. 2022;15:2475–8.
21. Yusoff MSB, Rahim AFA, Baba AA, Ismail SB, Pa MNM. Prevalence and associated factors of stress, anxiety and depression among prospective medical students. Asian J Psychiatr. 2013;6(2):128–33.

22. Rahimi B, Baetz M, Bowen R, Balbuena L. Resilience, stress, and coping among Canadian medical students. Can Med Educ J. 2014;5(1):e5–e12.
23. Brissie JS, Hoover-Demprey KV, Bassler OC. Individual, situational contributors to teacher burnout. J Educ Res. 1988;82(2):106–12.
24. Wolf MR, Rosenstock JB. Inadequate sleep and exercise associated with burnout and depression among medical students. Acad Psychiatry. 2017;41:174–9.
25. Yusoff MSB. Promoting resilience and minimizing burnout. Wellbeing in Higher Education; 2018. p. 70–93.
26. Yusoff MSB. Interventions on medical students' psychological health: a meta-analysis. J Taibah Univ Med Sci. 2014;9(1):1–13.
27. Yusoff MSB, Yaacob MJ, Naing NN. The effectiveness of a DEAL-based intervention to reduce stress and depression symptoms. Educ Med J. 2015;7(1)
28. Yusoff MSB, Yee LY, Wei LH, Siong TC, Meng LH, Bin LX, Rahim AFA. A study on stress, stressors and coping strategies among Malaysian medical students. Int J Stud Res. 2011;1(2):45–50.

Index

A. Gillis, C. B. Aarons (eds.), *A How To Guide For Medical Students*, Success in Academic Surgery, https://doi.org/10.1007/978-3-031-66011-5

MIX
Papier aus verantwortungsvollen Quellen
Paper from responsible sources
FSC® C105338

If you have any concerns about our products,
you can contact us on
ProductSafety@springernature.com

In case Publisher is established outside the EU,
the EU authorized representative is:
Springer Nature Customer Service Center GmbH
Europaplatz 3, 69115 Heidelberg, Germany

Printed by Libri Plureos GmbH
in Hamburg, Germany